Practical Psychiatric
Epidemiology

Oxford Medical Publications

Practical Psychiatric Epidemiology

Edited by

Martin Prince
Institute of Psychiatry, King's College London, UK

Robert Stewart
Institute of Psychiatry, King's College London, UK

Tamsin Ford
Institute of Psychiatry, King's College London, UK

Matthew Hotopf
Guy's King's and St Thomas' School of Medicine
King's College London, UK

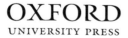

OXFORD
UNIVERSITY PRESS

OXFORD

UNIVERSITY PRESS

Great Clarendon Street, Oxford OX2 6DP

Oxford University Press is a department of the University of Oxford.
It furthers the University's objective of excellence in research, scholarship,
and education by publishing worldwide in

Oxford New York

Auckland Cape Town Dar es Salaam Hong Kong Karachi
Kuala Lumpur Madrid Melbourne Mexico City Nairobi
New Delhi Shanghai Taipei Toronto

With offices in

Argentina Austria Brazil Chile Czech Republic France Greece
Guatemala Hungary Italy Japan South Korea Poland Portugal
Singapore Switzerland Thailand Turkey Ukraine Vietnam

Oxford is a registered trade mark of Oxford University Press
in the UK and in certain other countries

Published in the United States
by Oxford University Press Inc., New York

© Oxford University Press 2003

The moral rights of the author have been asserted

Database right Oxford University Press (maker)

First published 2003

Reprinted 2004 (with corrections), 2006 (twice), 2007, 2008

A catalogue record for this title is available from the British Library

ISBN 978–0–19–851551–7 (Pbk)

10 9 8 7 6

Typeset by Newgen Imaging Systems (P) Ltd., Chennai, India

Printed in Great Britain
on acid-free paper by Biddles Ltd., King's Lynn, Norfolk

Preface

Epidemiology and statistics are two of the cornerstones of biomedical research, and as such are relevant to almost all fields of psychiatric research. Epidemiology has been defined as

> the study of the distribution and determinants of disease or other health related states or events in specified populations, and the application of these findings to the control of health problems.
>
> (Last 1995)

Epidemiologists first *describe* the extent and pattern of a public health problem; *who* becomes ill, and *when* and *where* do they do so? Next they try to *explain* these observations; *why* do people become ill? The description of disease patterns provides clues about possible risk factors, leading to hypotheses that can be tested in carefully designed analytical studies. Trials of interventions aimed at specific risk factors can occasionally provide further persuasive evidence of causality. Thus epidemiology is, above all, a *practical* discipline involving the systematic study of health, disease, and human behaviour in the natural world. As such, it is the basic science of public health medicine. Description identifies priorities for health policy and delivery of services. Explanation should lead to effective, feasible primary and secondary preventive interventions. Epidemiology and public health are thus complimentary, even co-dependent disciplines.

The four editors of this book work at the Institute of Psychiatry in London. They have each previously studied epidemiology at the London School of Hygiene and Tropical Medicine, where MP and MH have also held appointments in the Epidemiology Unit. Most of the chapter authors have similar backgrounds in psychiatry and epidemiology. Our aim has been to adapt the tried and tested methods used to teach generic epidemiology at LSHTM to the special circumstances of psychiatric epidemiology. Epidemiology is like a cocktail blended from equal parts of science, art, and craft, laced with liberal applications of intellectual rigour and scepticism. Students should be taught to suspect easy certainties, challenge orthodoxies and embrace and explore controversy; they should be encouraged to defend, debate, and dispute. These essential skills are best passed on by teachers who can communicate to their students some of the enthusiasm they feel for the subject, in the practical context of real studies addressing real research questions. We have sought, where possible to illustrate our points with relevant examples taken from psychiatric epidemiology, drawing attention to the particular methodological issues arising from the study of mental health outcomes. We have thus sought to provide a comprehensive introduction, of interest to clinicians as well as to those embarking upon a career in mental health research. It is, however, intended more as a study guide than as a definitive textbook of psychiatric epidemiology, for which interested students already have a choice of texts available.

Martin Prince   March 2003
Robert Stewart
Tamsin Ford
Matthew Hotopf

Acknowledgements

The editors and many of the authors have benefited from the support and encouragement of colleagues at the Institute of Psychiatry. We are especially grateful to Professor Anthony Mann, whose Section of Epidemiology and General Practice provided a haven where many of us developed. Robin Murray, Simon Wessely, Glyn Lewis, and Robert Goodman have also all variously supported, challenged, cajoled, and encouraged the editorial team. We are especially grateful to Marie Eagle for her unstinting and patient secretarial support.

Contents

Contributors

Professor Sube Banerjee
Health Services Research Department
Institute of Psychiatry
De Crespigny Park
Denmark Hill
London SE5 8AF, UK

Dr Daniel Chisholm
EQC Team
Department of Evidence for Health
Policy (GPE)
World Health Organisation
CH-1211 Geneva 27
Switzerland

Ms Rachel Churchill
Health Services Research Department
Institute of Psychiatry
De Crespigny Park
Denmark Hill
London SE5 8AF, UK

Dr David Collier
Division of Psychological
Medicine
Institute of Psychiatry
De Crespigny Park
Denmark Hill
London SE5 8AF, UK

Dr Michael E. Dewey
Trent Institute for Health Services
Research
Medical School
Queen's Medical Centre
Nottingham NG7 2UH, UK

Dr Tamsin Ford
Department of Child Psychiatry
Institute of Psychiatry
De Crespigny Park
Denmark Hill
London SE5 8AF, UK

Dr Matthew Hotopf
Department of Psychological
Medicine
GKT School of Medicine
103 Denmark Hill
London SE5 8AZ, UK

Dr Anthony S. Kessel
Health Promotion Research Unit
London School of Hygiene and
Tropical Medicine
Keppel Street
London WC1E 7HT, UK

Dr Tao Li
Division of Psychological
Medicine
Institute of Psychiatry
De Crespigny Park
Denmark Hill
London SE5 8AF, UK

Dr Paul McCrone
Health Services Research
Department
Institute of Psychiatry
De Crespigny Park
Denmark Hill
London SE5 8AF, UK

Dr Joanna Moncrieff
Department of Psychiatry and
Behavioural Sciences
University College London
48 Riding House Street
London W1N 8AA, UK

Ms Joanna Murray
Health Services Research
Department
Institute of Psychiatry
De Crespigny Park
Denmark Hill
London SE5 8AF, UK

Dr Jan Neeleman
Department of Social Psychiatry
University of Groningen
P O Box 30.001
9700 RB Groningen
The Netherlands

Dr Vikram Patel
London School of Hygiene
and Tropical Medicine
Sangath Centre 841/1 Porvorim
Goa 403521
India

Professor Martin Prince
Section of Epidemiology
Institute of Psychiatry
De Crespigny Park
Denmark Hill
London SE5 8AF, UK

Dr Frühling Rijsdijk
Social, Genetic and Developmental
Psychiatry Research Centre

Institute of Psychiatry
De Crespigny Park
Denmark Hill
London SE5 8AF, UK

Professor Pak Sham
Social, Genetic and Developmental
Psychiatry Research Centre
Institute of Psychiatry
De Crespigny Park
Denmark Hill
London SE5 8AF, UK

Ms Francesca Silverton
London School of Hygiene and
Tropical Medicine
Keppel Street
London WC1E 7HT, UK

Dr Robert Stewart
Section of Epidemiology
Institute of Psychiatry
De Crespigny Park
Denmark Hill
London SE5 8AF, UK

Dr Scott Weich
Department of Psychiatry and
Behavioural Sciences
Royal Free and University College
Medical School
Royal Free Campus
Rowland Hill Street
London NW3 2PF, UK

Section 1

Basic principles

Chapter 1

The development of psychiatric epidemiology

The Editors

Probably for as long as mankind has considered its condition it was intuitively evident that vulnerability to disease might relate to external (environmental) as well as internal (innate) factors. Certainly Hippocrates expressed this view as early as the fifth century BC. However, systematic, quantitative attempts to describe patterns of disease in populations and to study their relationship to environmental factors had to await the development of civil society. In 1662, John Graunt published 'the nature and political observations made upon the Bills of mortality', in which he documented the patterns of births and deaths in London by various demographic characteristics. Progress was particularly rapid in the Victorian age. The London Epidemiological Society was established in 1850, and the Oxford English Dictionary first records a definition for 'epidemiology' in 1873. Geoffrey Rose has pointed to the confluence of three key influences: the impetus from clinicians who found they could not cure the common infectious diseases and sought instead to prevent them; the development and increasing application of the new science of statistics; and the concern of social reformers and environmentalists that created the political climate for preventive interventions. The 'statistical movement' of this period saw the introduction of the decennial census (1801), the civil registration of births marriages and deaths (William Farr and the General Registry Office (GRO) 1837) and the work of Edwin Chadwick on the Poor Law Commission. Farr's GRO data on the number and causes of deaths in England and Wales were used by John Snow to develop and test his hypothesis that the cholera epidemics in London in the 1850s were caused by drinking Thames water contaminated by effluent. In the 1854 cholera epidemic in Soho, Snow showed that the cases tended to cluster in residences close to the Broad Street public well. He famously caused the pump-handle of the well to be removed, an act described as the first effective public health intervention and commemorated to this day in the public house on Broad Street that bears his name. Inconveniently for the annals of public health medicine, the incidence of cholera had been declining for several days before Snow's dramatic intervention, presumably as herd immunity was established.

Since the time of John Snow, epidemiological research has successfully guided public health interventions in the battle to control infectious disease. Indeed, it has been argued that health improvements arose more from social changes and public health interventions than from the development of new treatments. For example, the decline in the incidence of tuberculosis preceded the development of effective chemotherapy. With the control of infectious disease and the resulting increase in life expectancy, in developed countries mid-life chronic diseases have emerged as the leading cause of death and disability (1996). Epidemiology has shifted its focus accordingly. With these new epidemics came the need to develop new study designs such as the case–control study, and the prospective and historical cohort study to examine the effect of exposures that may have occurred years or even decades before the onset of illness. 'Exposures' came to be defined increasingly in terms of social status (income, social class, housing status) and lifestyles and behaviours (smoking, drinking, diet, exercise). The yield of knowledge, particularly since the Second World War, has been impressive. Doll and Hill identified smoking as the major and preventable cause of lung cancer in their Brompton Hospital case–control study (Doll and Hill 1950) and the later British Doctor's Survey (Doll et al. 1994); a series of publications from the Framingham study delineated the role of smoking, hypertension, and hyperlipidaemia in the aetiology of heart disease and stroke (D'Agostino et al. 1994, 2000). Cervical carcinoma has been clearly linked to exposure to the human papillomavirus and the epidemic of this condition to secular changes in sexual behaviour (Schlecht et al. 2001). Some have detected a slowing in the pace of discoveries over recent years and have attributed this to the identification of most of the major determinants of cancer and vascular disease, leaving only difficult to detect small effects to be discovered (Taubes 1995). However, imaginative hypothesis formulation combined with innovative hypothesis testing continues to push the boundaries of knowledge. Barker's life course epidemiological research is a good example. Through the elegant use of historical cohort designs, he demonstrated the role of intra-uterine growth and nutrition in the foetus' propensity to develop hypertension, heart disease, and type II diabetes in mid-life (Barker et al. 1990; Hales et al. 1991).

It has been argued that epidemiological research into psychiatric disorders has been slow to develop compared with research into other non-communicable disorders (Kessler 2000). Kessler attributes this partly to a lack of understanding of the basis of psychiatric disorders and to a lack of any notably effective interventions until the latter half of the twentieth century. In this he echoes Eaton (1986)

> Epidemiology is a branch of medicine, and thus the assumptions of the medical model of disease are implicit. The most important assumption is that the disease under study actually exists . . . In psychiatry this assumption is assuredly more tenuous than in other areas of medicine, because psychiatric diseases tend to be defined by failure to locate a physical cause . . . .

Arguably however, the history of development of methods in psychiatric epidemiology, and the acquisition of knowledge through their application at least matches that of its companion disciplines.

In Victorian England there was already a lively debate regarding the existence or otherwise of 'an epidemic of insanity' based upon a detailed study and analysis of steady upward trends in numbers of asylum residents. The sophistication of this debate is illustrated particularly by the work of Daniel Hack Tuke. He distinguished between *existing* (prevalent) and *occurring* (incident) insanity, and described how better care and reduced case mortality might lead to an increase in the former while the latter had barely changed. He also commented on the need for comparable case ascertainment procedures to make meaningful comparisons between populations and across different time periods. Above all, he understood that treated incidence was not at all the same thing as population incidence, and that the former might be influenced by a range of factors that had nothing to do with the latter. He noted particularly 'a large exodus of patients from workhouses and the care of relatives to country asylums' and that 'the value and comfort of asylums was increasingly appreciated' (Tuke 1894).

1897 saw the first publication (in France) of Durkheim's 'Suicide', in which he had studied regional, national, and temporal variations of European suicide rates (see also Chapter 6). Durkheim's work was remarkable for its scope, for its ecological perspective, and for its synthesis of empirical and theoretical approaches. A quantitative analysis of ecological variation in suicide rates is accompanied by an attempt to explain this variation with a unifying socio-anthropological theory. For Durkheim, suicide needed to be understood not merely as an individual act, determined by that person's character, but also as a 'social' phenomenon, a property of the population in aggregate; specifically its anomie, characterized by a relative lack of moral goals, social cohesion and social connectedness. Over a century later Durkheim continues to exert a strong influence on mainstream epidemiology, with a renewed interest in the role of supraindividual characteristics, for example, social capital in explaining between-population differences in health experience.

We tend to forget that in the early part of the twentieth century two of the earliest successes for epidemiology were in the field of mental health. At that time both pellagra and general paresis of the insane (GPI) were clinical syndromes, matching in most respects Eaton's description for the current status qua diagnosis of mental disorders. The aetiology of pellagra was unknown, while that of GPI was suspected to be syphilis (on the grounds of clinical observations). There was no effective treatment for either condition and they collectively accounted for many admissions to asylums. Mattauschek and Pilcz followed up 4000 Austrian army officers who had contracted syphilis in the 1880s and 1890s. The incidence of GPI was 5%. Those who had escaped GPI had had more severe fevers in the early years after first exposure. This informed the 'fever therapy' intervention that was, until the development of penicillin the standard and partly effective treatment for GPI. Goldberger *et al.* (1920) studied the incidence of pellagra in South Carolina and found a strong association with socio-economic status, an association that he argued was mediated by dietary deficiency. In a landmark experimental trial (Goldberger and Tanner 1923) he subsequently demonstrated that the incidence of pellagra in institutions was eliminated by a change in institutional dietary regime, concluding that 'fresh meat and milk supplied some factor or factors which operate to prevent the development of pellagra . . . pellagra may be completely prevented by diet'. Goldberger's work neatly illustrates a feature of epidemiological research. It is an empirical discipline, and identification of risk factors and indeed of effective interventions can precede in many cases by decades the identification of the precise causal mechanism. Only in 1937 did Conrad Elvehjem establish that nicotinic acid, or niacin, prevented and cured pellagra in dogs.

Dohrenwend and Dohrenwend (1982) described three overlapping stages in the development of methodology for psychiatric epidemiology (with particular reference to surveys, although their classification applies to some extent to other designs). In the first phase dating approximately from the 1930s to the 1960s most studies used unstructured, non-standardized clinical diagnoses. Many studies limited their enquiry to treated cases, and used diagnoses applied by clinicians in the course of their routine work (Shepherd 1957). The underlying assumption, possibly valid to some extent for serious mental illnesses such as schizophrenia, was that most incident cases would come to the attention of secondary care services in short order. The few truly population-based studies also involved clinicians as investigators using their clinical skills to interview all participants and apply diagnoses according to their usual practice (Sjogren 1948). The assumption here (evidently much less tenable) was that the common clinical training for psychiatrists would in some way ensure reliability and validity for their diagnostic assessments.

In the second phase of methodological development, dating from the late 1950s and early 1960s, growing understanding of the weaknesses of phase one studies led to attempts to standardize assessments. However, rather than clinical diagnoses these were, as in the US Stirling County Study (Leighton *et al.* 1963), based upon self-reports providing a standard coverage of a list of possible symptoms. Psychopathology was scaled using symptom counts as a continuum from health to disease. This was certainly no blind alley in the history of psychiatric epidemiology; from this approach can be traced directly the contemporary interest in, for example, studies of 'well-being' as a counterpoint to clinical diagnosis. Latterly the use of continuous traits has been advocated as an efficient approach for identification of polygenes, the multiple genes of small to moderate effect that are likely account for much of the genetic aetiology of mental disorders from anxiety and depression (Sham *et al.* 2000) to schizophrenia (Cardno *et al.* 2001).

The third phase of development in psychiatric epidemiology can be traced, first, to the concerns raised by the US–UK joint diagnostic project. Gross differences in the clinical diagnostic practices of English and American psychiatrists led to a disturbing level of disagreement particularly in relation to schizophrenia and depression (Cooper *et al.* 1972). This material was grist to the mill for those who had argued that psychiatric diagnoses were no more than stigmatizing labels for behaviours perceived as deviant from societal norms (Szasz 1961). A critical review of psychiatric classification ensued on both sides of the Atlantic (Klerman 1990; Weissman 1995). Rapid developments in psychopharmacology in the 1950s and 1960s may to some extent have stimulated the re-emergence of the medical model of psychiatry. It became necessary systematically to assess psychopathology to identify indications for and assess the efficacy of the new psychotropic drugs (Weissman 1995). Researchers in both the United States and Europe began to develop consensus diagnostic criteria, which were eventually incorporated into Diagnostic and Statistical Manual III (DSM III) and International Classification of Disease 8 (ICD 8) (Klerman 1990). Fully structured interviews were developed to map on to the new criteria, standardizing the process of enquiring after symptoms, rating symptoms and codifying symptom profiles into diagnoses using standard algorithms (see Chapters 2 and 7 for further details). While the reliability of such methods is likely to be high, their validity, all too often remains adequately to be established. There have been particular concerns regarding the unconsidered application of criteria and methods that reflect western psychiatric orthodoxy to people from other cultures (Kleinman 1987). Parallel to the development of epidemiological methods in psychiatric research has been a development in the agenda for that research. Early studies were mainly cross-sectional in design and descriptive in intent. Prospective studies were preoccupied either with clinical course and outcome or with the identification of secular trends in disease frequency. Analytical epidemiology has been slower to develop. The ECA study, for example, gathered relatively little data on potential risk factors for mental disorders, and limited itself to descriptions of prevalence stratified by socio-demographic factors (e.g. age and gender) (Weissman *et al.* 1988). Ten years later the US National Comorbidity Survey and the UK National Psychiatric Morbidity Survey were much more focused upon theory- and hypothesis-driven aetiologic research, considering, for example, the association between common mental disorder and economic deprivation (Lewis *et al.* 1998) and depression and child sexual abuse (Molnar *et al.* 2001). The real development, however, has been in the use, and increasing sophistication of analytical designs, both case–control and cohort studies for the elegant and efficient testing of specific research hypotheses, for example, (a) historical cohort designs to study long latency associations relevant to the neurodevelopmental theory of schizophrenia (Susser and Lin 1992; Jones *et al.* 1994), and the association between midlife exposures and risk for dementia in late-life (Seshadri *et al.* 2002); (b) twin cohorts studies of the interplay over the life course of genetic and environmental factors in the aetiology of child and adult mental disorders (Kendler *et al.* 1993; Caspi *et al.* 2000); (c) the increasing use of analytical study designs in the developing world promoting the salience of mental health to the acknowledged public health priorities for those regions; infectious disease, reproductive health, and child development (Patel *et al.* 2002).

Most psychiatric outcomes have a clearly multi-factorial aetiology with strong familial tendencies and a presumed underlying genetic basis. However, environmental factors are evidently also important, and researchers are becoming increasingly interested in the potential interactions between genetic and environmental factors in disease causation. The discovery in 1992 of the association between the APOE gene and risk for both the dementia syndrome and Alzheimer's disease (Saunders *et al.* 1993) has ushered in a new phase in epidemiological research that will undoubtedly serve as a model for research into other chronic conditions. The finding of the association with the APOE gene is now among the most replicated findings in biomedicine, with over 1000 positive reports in the literature. Research has now moved on to second order considerations, in particular the identification of gene–environment interactions, thus the following observations were made.

(1) The association appears to be modified by age (decreasing effect size with increasing age) and by race (lower effect sizes in Africans and Asians, compared with Caucasians; Farrer *et al.* 1997). The age effect may be explained by differential mortality; those who survive to a great age despite the APOE e4 allele may have other genetic or constitutional characteristics that protect against neurodegeneration. Alternatively AD may be a heterogenous disorder and later onset variants may have a different aetiology.

(2) Observational epidemiology has already suggested that APOE may interact with a variety of environmental exposures that have the capacity to insult the brain at different stages over the life course. Thus ApoE seems to modify mortality after stroke (Corder *et al.* 2000), the association between atherosclerosis and both cognitive decline (Slooter *et al.* 1998) and dementia (Hofman *et al.* 1997), the association between white matter lesions and dementia (Skoog *et al.* 1998), and the associations between both head injury (Mayeux *et al.* 1995) and Alzheimer's Disease and boxing trauma and chronic brain injury (Jordan *et al.* 1997). These findings suggest a mechanism for the operation of APOE as a neuroprotective factor influencing the growth and regeneration of peripheral and central nervous system tissues in normal development and in response to injury (Prince 1998).

Rapid advances in biotechnology, including the recent mapping of the human genome are certain soon to yield similar discoveries with respect to other mental health outcomes. This is an exciting time for psychiatric epidemiologists.

References

1996, *The Global Burden of Disease. A comprehensive assessment of mortality and disability from diseases, injuries and risk factors in 1990 and projected to 2020.* The Harvard School of Public Health, Harvard University Press.

Barker, D.J., Bull, A.R., Osmond, C., and Simmonds, S.J. (1990) Fetal and placental size and risk of hypertension in adult life [see comments]. *British Medical Journal,* **301** (6746), 259–62.

Cardno, A.G., Sham, P.C., Murray, R.M., and McGuffin, P. (2001) Twin study of symptom dimensions in psychoses. *British Journal of Psychiatry,* **179**, 39–45.

Caspi, A., Taylor, A., Moffitt, T.E., and Plomin, R. (2000) Neighborhood deprivation affects children's mental health: environmental risks identified in a genetic design. *Psychological Science,* **11** (4), 338–42.

Cooper, J.E., Kendell, R.E., Gurland, B.J., Sharpe, L., Copeland, J.R.M., and Simon, R. (1972) *Psychiatric diagnosis in New York and London.* Oxford University Press, London.

Corder, E.H., Basun, H., Fratiglioni, L., Guo, Z., Lannfelt, L., Viitanen, M., Corder, L.S., Manton, K.G., and Winblad, B. (2000) Inherited frailty. ApoE alleles determine survival after a diagnosis of heart disease or stroke at ages 85$^+$. *Annals of the New York Academy of Sciences,* **908**, 295–8.

D'Agostino, R.B., Russell, M.W., Huse, D.M., Ellison, R.C., Silbershatz, H., Wilson, P.W., and Hartz, S.C. (2000) Primary and subsequent coronary risk appraisal: new results from the Framingham study. *American Heart Journal,* **139** (2 Pt 1), 272–81.

D'Agostino, R.B., Wolf, P.A., Belanger, A.J., and Kannel, W.B. (1994) Stroke risk profile: adjustment for antihypertensive medication. The Framingham Study. *Stroke,* **25** (1), 40–3.

Dohrenwend, B.P. and Dohrenwend, B.S. (1982) Perspectives on the past and future of psychiatric epidemiology. The 1981 Rema Lapouse Lecture. *American Journal of Public Health,* **72** (11), 1271–9.

Doll, R. and Bradford Hill, A. (1950) Smoking and carcinoma of the lung. *British Medical Journal*, ii, 739–48.

Doll, R., Peto, R., Wheatley, K., Gray, R., and Sutherland, I. (1994) Mortality in relation to smoking: 40 years' observations on male British doctors [see comments]. *British Medical Journal*, **309** (6959), 901–11.

Eaton, W. (1986) *The Sociology of Mental Disorders*. Praeger, New York.

Farrer, L.A., Cupples, L.A., Haines, J.L., Hyman, B., Kukull, W.A., Mayeux, R., Myers, R.H., Pericak-Vance, M.A., Risch, N., and van Duijn, C.M. (1997) Effects of age, sex, and ethnicity on the association between apolipoprotein E genotype and Alzheimer disease. A meta-analysis. APOE and Alzheimer Disease Meta Analysis Consortium. [see comments.]. *Journal of the American Medical Association*, **278** (16), 1349–56.

Goldberger, J., Wheeler, G.A., and Sydenstricker, E. (1920) A study of the relation of family income and other economic factors to pellagra incidence in seven cotton mill villages of South Carolina in 1916. *Public Health Reports*, **35** (46), 2673–714.

Goldberger, J.W.C.H. and Tanner, W.F. (1923) Pellagra prevention by diet among institutional inmates. *Public Health Reports*, **38** (41), 2361–8.

Hales, C.N., Barker, D.J., Clark, P.M., Cox, L.J., Fall, C., Osmond, C., and Winter, P.D. (1991) Fetal and infant growth and impaired glucose tolerance at age 64 [see comments]. *British Medical Journal*, **303** (6809), 1019–22.

Hofman, A., Ott, A., Breteler, M.M.B., Bots, M.L., Slooter, A.J.C., van Harskamp, F., van Duijn, C.N., Van Broeckhoven, C., and Grobbee, D.E. (1997) Atherosclerosis, apolipoprotein E, and prevalence of dementia and Alzheimer's disease in the Rotterdam Study. *Lancet*, **349**, 151–4.

Jones, P., Rodgers, B., Murray, R., and Marmot, M. (1994) Child development risk factors for adult schizophrenia in the British 1946 birth cohort. *Lancet*, **344** (8934), 1398–402.

Jordan, B.D., Relkin, N.R., Ravdin, L.D., Jacobs, A.R., Bennett, A., and Gandy, S. (1997) Apolipoprotein E epsilon4 associated with chronic traumatic brain injury in boxing [see comments.]. *Journal of the American Medical Association*, **278** (2), 136–40.

Kendler, K.S., Kessler, R.C., Neale, M.C., Heath, A.C., and Eaves, L.J. (1993) The prediction of major depression in women: toward an integrated etiologic model. *American Journal of Psychiatry*, **150**, 1139–48.

Kleinman, A. (1987) Anthropology and psychiatry. The role of culture in cross-cultural research on illness. *British Journal of Psychiatry*, **151**, 447–54.

Klerman, G.L. (1990) Paradigm shifts in USA psychiatric epidemiology since World War II [Review] [28 refs]. *Social Psychiatry and Psychiatric Epidemiology*, **25** (1), 27–32.

Leighton, D.C., Harding, J.S., Macklin, D.B., MacMillan, A.M., and Leighton, A.H. (1963) *The character of danger* Basic Books, New York.

Lewis, G., Bebbington, P., Brugha, T., Farrell, M., Gill, B., Jenkins, R., and Meltzer, H. (1998) Socioeconomic status, standard of living, and neurotic disorder. *Lancet*, **352** (9128), 605–9.

Mayeux, R., Ottman, R., Maestre, G., Ngai, C., Tang, M.X., Ginsberg, H., Chun, M., Tycko, B., and Shelanski, M. (1995) Synergistic effects of traumatic head injury and apolipoprotein-epsilon 4 in patients with Alzheimer's disease [see comments]. *Neurology*, **45** (3 Pt 1), 555–7.

Molnar, B.E., Buka, S.L., and Kessler, R.C. (2001) Child sexual abuse and subsequent psychopathology: results from the National Comorbidity Survey. *American Journal of Public Health*, **91** (5), 753–60.

Patel, V., Rodrigues, M., and DeSouza, N. (2002) Gender, poverty, and postnatal depression: a study of mothers in Goa, India. *American Journal of Psychiatry*, 159 (1), 43–7.

Prince, M.J. (1998) Is chronic low-level lead exposure in early life an aetiological factor in Alzheimers disease? *Epidemiology*, 9, 618–21.

Saunders, A.M., Strittmatter, W.J., Schmechel, D., St.George-Hyslop, P.H., Pericak-Vance, M.A., Joo, S.H., Rosi, B.L., Gusella, J.F., Crapper-Maclachlan, D.R., Alberts, M.J., Hulette, C., Crain, B., Goldgaber, D., and Roses, A.D. (1993) Association of apolipoprotein E allele e4 with late-onset familial and sporadic Alzheimer's disease. *Neurology*, 43, 1467–72.

Schlecht, N.F., Kulaga, S., Robitaille, J., Ferreira, S., Santos, M., Miyamura, R.A., Duarte-Franco, E., Rohan, T.E., Ferenczy, A., Villa, L.L., and Franco, E.L. (2001) Persistent human papillomavirus infection as a predictor of cervical intraepithelial neoplasia. *Journal of the American Medical Association*, 286 (24), 3106–14.

Seshadri, S., Beiser, A., Selhub, J., Jacques, P.F., Rosenberg, I.H., D'Agostino, R.B., Wilson, P.W., and Wolf, P.A. (2002) Plasma homocysteine as a risk factor for dementia and Alzheimer's disease [see comments.]. *New England Journal of Medicine*, 346 (7), 476–83.

Sham, P.C., Sterne, A., Purcell, S., Cherny, S., Webster, M., Rijsdijk, F., Asherson, P., Ball, D., Craig, I., Eley, T., Goldberg, D., Gray, J., Mann, A., Owen, M., and Plomin, R. (2000) GENESiS: creating a composite index of the vulnerability to anxiety and depression in a community-based sample of siblings. *Twin Research*, 3 (4), 316–22.

Shepherd, M. (1957) *A Study of the Major Psychoses in an English County*. Chapman and Hall, London.

Sjogren, T. (1948) Genetic-statistical and psychiatric investigations of a west Swedish population. *Acta Psychiatrica et Neurologica*, (Suppl. 52), 239–307.

Skoog, I., Hesse, C., Aevarsson, O., Landahl, S., Wahlstrom, J., Fredman, P., and Blennow, K. (1998) A population study of apoE genotype at the age of 85: relation to dementia, cerebrovascular disease, and mortality. *Journal of Neurology, Neurosurgery and Psychiatry*, 64 (1), 37–43.

Slooter, A.J., van Duijn, C.M., Bots, M.L., Ott, A., Breteler, M.B., De Voecht, J., Wehnert, A., de Knijff, P., Havekes, L.M., Grobbee, D.E., Van Broeckhoven, C., and Hofman, A. (1998) Apolipoprotein E genotype, atherosclerosis, and cognitive decline: the Rotterdam Study. *Journal of Neural Transmission*, (Suppl. 53), 17–29.

Susser, E.S. and Lin, S.P. (1992) Schizophrenia after prenatal exposure to the Dutch Hunger Winter of 1944–1945 [see comments]. *Archives of General Psychiatry*, 49 (12), 983–8.

Szasz, T. (1961) *The myth of mental illness*. Free Press, New York.

Taubes, G. (1995) Epidemiology faces its limits [see comments]. *Science*, 269 (5221), 164–9.

Tuke, D.H. (1894) Alleged increase of insanity. *Journal of Mental Science*, 40, 219–31.

Weissman, M.M. (1995) The epidemiology of psychiatric disorders: past, present, and future generations. *International Journal of Methods in Psychiatric Research*, 5, 69–78.

Weissman, M.M., Leaf, P.J., Tischler, G.L., Blazer, D.G., Karno, M., Bruce, M.L., and Florio, L.P. (1988) Affective disorders in five United States communities [published erratum appears in Psychol Med 1988 Aug;18(3): following 792]. *Psychological Medicine*, 18, 141–53.

Chapter 2

Measurement in psychiatry

Martin Prince

Introduction

The science of the measurement of mental phenomena (psychometrics) is central to quantitative research in psychiatry. Without appropriate, accurate, stable, and unbiased measures, our research is doomed from the outset. Much effort has been expended over the last 40 years in the development of a bewildering array of assessments. Most of our measurement strategies are based on eliciting symptoms, either by asking the participant to complete a self-report questionnaire, or by using an interviewer to question the participant. Some are long, detailed, and comprehensive clinical diagnostic assessments. Others are much briefer, designed either to screen for probable cases, or as scalable measures in their own right, of a trait or dimension such as depression, neuroticism or cognitive function or as measures of an exposure to a possible risk factor for a disease.

Researchers in other medical disciplines sometimes criticise psychiatric measures for being vague or woolly, because they are not based on biological markers of pathology. For this very reason, psychiatry was among the first medical disciplines to develop internationally recognized operationalized diagnostic criteria. At the same time the research interview has become progressively refined, such that the processes of eliciting, recording, and distilling symptoms into diagnoses or scalable traits are now also highly standardized. These criticisms are therefore largely misplaced. Thanks to the careful construction and extensive validation of the better established measures in psychiatric research we can now afford to be slightly more confident of their appropriateness, accuracy, and stability than would be the case even for some biological measurements. This confidence is based on our understanding of the *validity* and *reliability* of our measures.

Levels of measurement

One way of classifying measures is according to the level of organization of the data that they generate. This data is coded in *variables*. In general, measures may be categorical or continuous.

Categorical variables

These may have two or more levels but they describe categories to which no meaningful numerical value can be ascribed. Examples would include gender, ethnicity, and marital status (married, never married, widowed, separated, and divorced). These measures describe types rather than quantities.

(1) *Binary or dichotomous variables* are the simplest categorical variables having only two levels, for example, exposed or unexposed, case or non-case. Examples would include gender, victim of child sexual abuse—yes/no, current DSM major depression—yes/no. Some more complex variables are reduced to binary form to simplify an analysis. For example, data on lifetime smoking habit could be reduced to a binary variable, ever smoked—yes/no.

(2) *Polychotomous variables* may be *simple* or *ordered*. *Ordered categorical variables* still describe discrete categories, but with some meaningful trend in the quantity of what is being described in each level of the variable. Examples would include current smoking status (classified as non-smoker, 1–10 cigarettes daily, 10–20 cigarettes daily and >20 cigarettes daily) and number of life events (classified as none, one and two or more).

Simple categorical variables display no such trend or progression from level to level of the variable. Examples would include eye colour, country of birth or ICD diagnostic group.

Continuous variables

These are, strictly speaking, measures of attributes or *traits* that can be indexed at any point along a scale. Thus weight can be measured as 70 or 70.1 kg or even more precisely as 70.09 kg. Age and temperature are other examples of true continuous variables. Number of children is not a continuous variable, as only integer values are possible. Such measures generate *discrete quantitative variables*. True continuous variables should also ideally conform to the properties of an arithmetic scale. Thus an adult who is 1.80 m tall is twice as tall as a child of 90 cm. Also they are 90 cm taller. However, somebody scoring 20 points on the CES-D depression symptoms scale is probably not twice as depressed as somebody scoring 10 points. Likewise the difference in levels of depression between persons scoring 10 and 14, and 14 and 18 may not be the same. It should be apparent from the above that many 'scales' in common use in psychiatric and psychological research are neither continuous nor arithmetical, and should in fact properly be considered to be closer in character to ordered categorical variables. Sometimes these are referred to as ordinal scales.

Domains of measurement

Measures in common use in psychiatric epidemiology can be thought of as covering six principal domains

1 Demographic status—Age, gender, marital status, household circumstances, and occupation.

2 Socio-economic status—Social class, income, wealth, and debt.

3 Social circumstances—Social network and social support.

4 Activities, lifestyles, and behaviours—A very broad area, its contents are dictated by the focus of the research—examples would include tobacco and alcohol consumption, substance use, diet, and exercise. Some measures such as recent exposure to positive and negative life events may be particularly relevant to psychiatric research.

5 Opinions and attitudes—An area of measurement initially restricted to market research organisations, but increasingly being adopted by social science and biomedical researchers.

6 Health status—Measures can be further grouped into:

   (a) specific measures of dichotomous diagnoses (schizophrenia or psoriasis), or continuously distributed traits (blood pressure level, serum cholesterol, mood, anxiety, neuroticism, and cognitive status);

   (b) global measures, for example, subjective or objective global health assessment, disablement (impairment, activity, and participation), and health-related quality of life;

   (c) measures reflecting the need for, or use of health services.

Selecting a measure

Selection of an appropriate measure for a research project is an essential element of the study design. In general it is neither necessary nor desirable to develop a measure of your own. It is highly likely that someone, somewhere will have already developed an applicable measure for that you could use, perhaps after some appropriate adaptations have been made. The amount of work involved in developing and validating a new measure should not be underestimated. This is certainly true for diagnostic assessments and scale-based measures. However, even apparently simple or trivial single questions eliciting information about, for example, household composition or smoking behaviour may be very sensitive to phrasing or presentation. Developing your own questions without adequate piloting and validation may lead to unforeseen error or bias.

The following is a simple checklist:

1 Do you have a clear concept and definition of what it is that you want to measure?

2 Are you clear about why you want to measure it?

3 Is there already a suitable measure around? that is, one that is:

   (a) Feasible? Existing measures may be too long and complex. You will not want to spend 1 h eliciting recent life events if this is simply one of several potential confounders and not directly relevant to the testing of the main hypothesis. Equally, existing measures may be too brief, and lack appropriate precision for assessment of a key exposure or outcome.

   (b) Ecologically appropriate? Instruments should be validated *for the population in which they are being used*. Some instruments have been validated for clinical populations, but not for community samples. Existing measures have commonly been developed and validated in an English speaking country in the developed world. What if your study is to be conducted in Tanzania? Will the measure have good construct and content validity (see below) in that setting. Is the phrasing of the questions appropriate, even after translation. An example would be the assessment of instrumental activities of daily living in older persons. An instrument developed in the west, which focussed upon activities such as using the telephone, handling money, and going shopping may fail to reflect the typical roles and responsibilities of older adults in Tanzania. Establishing validity for an instrument in a different culture will necessitate pilot work, including

   ◆ translation and back translation;

   ◆ checking conceptual validity using ethnographic procedures, for example, focus group discussions involving local clinicians, community leaders, and potential survey participants.

      Field trialling for feasibility, and for criterion validity against a local gold standard (emic) diagnosis, and internationally recognised (etic) diagnosis. The local gold standard might, for instance, be that of a local clinician, a traditional healer, or a community leader.

   (c) Psychometrically robust? This refers to the validity and reliability of a measure, and in the special case of a scale measure to its internal consistency (see below).

Developing a new measure

If existing measures fail adequately to meet each of the three criteria listed above, then *may be* you will need to develop your own. The caution is there, because a good deal of diligent work is required if your new measure is to be superior to those that already exist.

An example of instrument development

The procedure for the development of scale-based measures is perhaps most clearly established. One of many good examples is that of a maternal self-report scale intended to assess the extent of parent–child joint activity in toddlers (with a view to assessing its potential as a protective factor against behavioural disorder in pre-schoolers (Kumari *et al.* 2000).

The stages in instrument development

(1) *Definition of the construct.* What is the trait that is to be measured. What does it include? What does it exclude?

(2) *Review of the construct definition.* This is usually carried out both by experts in the field, and by lay persons similar to those to whom the measure will be administered. Is it clear? Does it make sense? Is it culturally appropriate?

(3) *Item drafting.* Drawing up a long list of potential items felt to address the construct.

(4) *Item review.* Expert and lay review of these items for content validity (do all the items address the construct? Have some aspects of the construct not been covered by the items?) and comprehensibility. Poorly drafted items are discarded.

(5) *Alpha testing.* Remaining items are tested for test–retest reliability, ceiling and floor effects, and internal scale consistency. Fifty to 100 participants usually suffice. Unreliable items, those endorsed by nearly everyone (ceiling effects) or no one (floor effects), and items that reduce internal scale consistency as evidenced by poor correlations between the item score and the total scale score are discarded.

(6) *Beta testing.* In a separate sample, the surviving items, and the scale as a whole, are tested for criterion or more usually concurrent validity (see below). The internal consistency of the scale is retested, and often a factor analysis (principal components analysis) is carried out to see whether the scale is a unidimensional scale in which all items are measuring the same single underlying trait, or if two or more factors are extracted, whether the scale may effectively consist of subscales measuring related yet to some extent distinct underlying traits.

> ## Box 2.1 **Stages in the development of a scale**
>
> (1) Definition of the construct
> (2) Review of the construct definition
> (3) Item drafting
> (4) Item review
> (5) Alpha testing (test–retest reliability, ceiling and floor effects, and internal scale consistency)
> (6) Beta testing (criterion or more usually concurrent validity)
> (7) Post-development testing

(7) *Post-development testing*. Validation of a measure is never completed by its developers. Widespread use by other investigators in different settings will, over time, establish the extent and limitations of its validity (Box 2.1).

Psychometric properties

Validity refers to the extent to which a measure really does measure what it sets out to measure. Reliability refers to the consistency of a measure when applied repeatedly under similar circumstances. Put simply, a measure is reliable if you use it twice to measure the same thing and arrive at the same answer. A measure is valid if you measure the same thing twice using two different measures, one known to be valid, and come to the same answer. The reliability and validity of all measures need to be cited in research grant proposals and research publications. If they have not been adequately established, particularly if the measure is new, then the investigators need to do this themselves in a pilot investigation.

Validity

Construct validity

This refers to the extent to which the construct that the measure seeks to address is a real and coherent entity, and then also to the salience of the measure to that construct. Construct validity cannot be demonstrated empirically, but evidence can be sought to support it. The scope and content of the construct can be identified in open-ended interviews and focus group discussions with key informants. These same informants can review the proposed measure and comment on the appropriateness of the items (face or content validity). An exploratory factor analysis may suggest whether the construct is homogenous or multi-dimensional.

Concurrent validity

This is tested by the extent to which the new measure relates, as hypothesized, to other measures taken at the same time (hence concurrent). There are four main variants: criterion, convergent, divergent, and known group validity.

Criterion validity is tested by comparing measures obtained with the new instrument to those obtained with an existing criterion measure. The criterion is the current 'gold standard' measure and is usually more complex, lengthier or more expensive to administer, otherwise there would be little point in developing the new measure! In psychiatry there are generally no biologically based criterion measures as, for example, bronchoscopy and biopsy for carcinoma of the bronchus. The first measures developed for psychiatric research were compared with the criterion or 'gold standard' of a competent psychiatrist's clinical diagnosis. More recently, detailed standardized clinical interviews such as SCAN have taken the place of the psychiatrist's opinion. (*Note*: For convenience, details of this, and all other instruments referred to in this chapter are given in the Appendix.)

Convergent and divergent validity should be tested in relation to each other. A measure will be more closely related to an alternative measure of the same construct than it will be to measures of different constructs. Thus, the general health questionnaire should correlate more strongly with the CES-D and the CIS-R than to a physical functioning scale, or to a measure of income.

Known group validity can be assessed where no established gold standard external criterion exists. Thus a new questionnaire measuring the amount of time parents spend in positive joint activities with their children could be applied to two groups of parents, identified by their health visitors or teachers as having contrasting levels of involvement with their children (Box 2.2).

Box 2.2 **Assessment of validity**

(1) *Construct validity*: The extent to which the thing being measured is a real, coherent, and meaningful entity, addressed appropriately by the scale or measure.

(2) *Concurrent validity*:

+ Criterion validity: Agreement with what is being measured.

+ Convergent and divergent validity: Correlation as predicted with something associated with what is being measured.

+ Known group validity: Differences as predicted between groups with evidently high and low levels of the trait being measured.

(3) *Predictive validity*: An association as predicted with a likely outcome stemming from what is being measured.

Predictive validity

Predictive validity assesses the extent to which a new measure can predict future occurrences. Thus depression may predict time off work, or use of health services; alcohol dependency may predict alcoholic liver disease; cognitive impairment may predict dementia.

Measuring validity

Concurrent validity of a continuous measure against another continuous measure as criterion is measured with a Pearson's (parametric) or Spearman's (non-parametric) correlation coefficient.

Concurrent validity against a dichotomous criterion is usually expressed in terms of the validity coefficients, sensitivity, specificity, and positive and negative predictive value. When the same participants have been assessed using the new measure and the 'gold standard' criterion measure, the results can be summarized in a 2 $\times$ 2 table as:

The sensitivity of the new measure is the proportion of true cases correctly identified:

New measure	Gold standard	
	Case	Non-case
Case	a	b
Non-case	c	d

$$\text{Sensitivity} = a/a + c$$

The specificity of the new measure is the proportion of non-cases correctly identified:

$$\text{Specificity} = d/b + d$$

Note that for screening tests based upon scale scores with validated cutpoints (e.g. the Centre for Epidemiological Studies Depression Scale, used to screen for the category of DSM major depression) there is evidently a trade-off between sensitivity and specificity. As the cutpoint is raised there are fewer false positives and the specificity increases. However, at the same time, there are fewer true positives and the sensitivity of the test declines.

The positive predictive value (PPV) of the new measure is the proportion of participants it identifies as cases that actually are cases according to the gold standard:

$$\text{PPV} = a/a + b$$

The negative predictive value (NPV) of the new measure is the proportion of participants it identifies as non-cases that actually are non-cases according to the gold standard:

$$NPV = d/c + d$$

Note that sensitivity and specificity are independent of the prevalence of the condition in the population being studied. However, for a given sensitivity and specificity, the PPV necessarily falls with the prevalence of the condition. Even with high sensitivity and specificity, false positives (b) will tend to overwhelm true positives (a). For NPV, true negative (d) will tend to overwhelm false negatives (c), and thus the NPV rises with falling prevalence. The implication is that, for example, for a screening test for schizophrenia, the favourable and high PPV recorded in a high prevalence clinical population will fall sharply when the same screen is used in the low prevalence general population context

Likelihood ratios

The overall predictiveness of a given test result can be conveniently summarized as the likelihood ratio (LR). The likelihood ratio is easily calculated:

$$LR = \frac{\text{the probability of a given test result in diseased persons}}{\text{the probability of that test result in non-diseased persons}}$$

Using Bayes' theorem we can calculate the post-test probability of disease given knowledge of the pre-test probability (in this case disease prevalence) and the LR associated with different test results.

For example, The Apolipoprotein E e4 (ApoE e4) genotype is strongly associated with risk for Alzheimer's disease (AD). A typical finding for the association is given as:

	Controls (%)	AD cases (%)
Homozygous (two e4 alleles)	3	13
Heterozygous (one e4 allele)	19	50
No e4 alleles	78	37

Use of these prevalence rates, and the presence of any ApoE e4 allele as the test criterion, suggests a test with 78% specificity and 63% sensitivity for a diagnosis of AD.

The LRs derived from the ApoE e4 frequencies given above are

Homozygous (two e4 alleles)	0.13/ 0.03 = 4.3
Heterozygous (one e4 allele)	0.50/ 0.19 = 2.5
No e4 alleles	0.37/ 0.78 = 0.48

The likelihood ratio for a positive test result (e.g. one or two e4 alleles) is sometimes known as a likelihood ratio positive and that for a negative test result (e.g. no e4 alleles) as a likelihood ratio negative.

The LR for a given test result is related to the pre- and post-test probability of disease, for

$$\text{pre-test odds of disease} \times \text{LR} = \text{post-test odds of disease}$$

If the pre-test probability of Alzheimer's disease is 0.10 (a generous estimate for the eventual lifetime prevalence for those who have already survived into their sixties) then the pre-test odds are $0.1/(1 - 0.10) = 0.11$. If a subject is then found to be homozygous for ApoE e4 their post-test odds, given this additional information, become $0.11 \times 4.3 = 0.47$. This translates into a post-test probability of disease (PPV for the test) of: $0.47/ (1 + 0.47) = 0.32$. The post-test probabilities for heterozygosity and for no ApoE e4 allele are 0.22 and 0.05, respectively. The positive predictive values (0.32 and 0.22) therefore encompass too much uncertainty to be of use to screened subjects and their clinicians. One reason for this shortcoming is the low prevalence rate of AD. For a test with given predictive power the post-test probability of disease is crucially dependent on the pre-test probability. Rarely can a single test be used as an early indicator of a disease with as low a population prevalence as AD. This demonstrates in another way the impact of disease prevalence upon PPV mentioned above. It can be shown that a test with a given LR will provide a maximum 'gain' of post-test diagnostic probability when the pre-test probability is in the region of 0.4–0.6. One solution then might be to apply the test to a target population with a known high lifetime prevalence of the disease; in the case of ApoE e4 and AD for instance the test might work satisfactorily in subjects with a strong family history of AD. Alternatively Bayes' theorem can be used to combine a number of moderately predictive tests into a more effective package. Given the assumption of conditional independence (i.e. that the results of the second test do not depend on the results of the first) then:

$$\text{pre-test odds} \times \text{LR (test 1)} \times \text{LR (test 2)} = \text{post-test odds (tests 1 and 2)}$$

ROC curves

Given the trade off between sensitivity and specificity for a scaleable screening test as the cutpoint is shifted up or down, the sensitivity and specificity of a given cutpoint may fail to convey the *overall predictiveness* of the measure. This is best estimated as the area under the *receiver operating characteristic (ROC) curve* so called because of its derivation from transistor physics. An ROC curve plots sensitivity (on the *y*-axis) against 1-specificity (on the *x*-axis). A useless predictive screening test follows a diagonal line as below, with a perfect trade off between sensitivity and specificity.

A useless screening test:

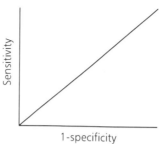

The area under the ROC curve is 0.5. A useful predictive test has the character-istic that for a given decline in specificity, there is a greater increase in sensitivity, and the ROC curve arches progressively up and to the left. The area under the ROC curve lies somewhere between 0.5 (a useless test) and 1.0 (a perfect test).

A useful screening test:

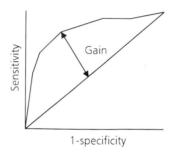

One way of identifying the optimal cutpoint is to drop an arc from the top left hand corner of the plot, with a radius just sufficient to meet the ROC curve. The cutpoint corresponding to the sensitivity and 1-specificity at this point should simultaneously maximize sensitivity and specificity.

ROC curves can be plotted and the areas under ROC curves estimated, using SPSS statistical software. Other packages offer the additional facility of comparing areas under ROC curves for two possible screening tests with p-values for the statistical significance of the observed difference. Thus, for example, one may test the hypothesis that a new screening test is superior to an existing standard screening test.

Reliability

Test re-test reliability (intra-measurement reliability)

Intra-measurement reliability tests the stability of a measure over time. The measure is administered to a participant, and then after an interval of time is administered again to the same participant, under the same conditions (e.g by the same interviewer). The selection of the time interval is a matter of judgement. Too short and the participant may simply recall and repeat their response from the first testing. Too long, and the trait that the measure was measuring may have changed, for example, they may have recovered from their depression.

Inter-observer reliability

Inter-observer reliability tests the stability of the measure when administered or rated by different investigators. Administering the measure to the same participant under the same conditions by several interviewers tests inter-interviewer reliability. These test conditions are for practical reasons evidently difficult to achieve. More usually therefore inter-rater reliability is tested; several raters view a video recording of one or more interviews and all rate the participants responses.

Measuring agreement

Intra-measurement and inter-observer reliability are assessed using measures of agreement. For a continuous scale measure the appropriate statistic would be the intra-class correlation. For a categorical measure the appropriate statistic is Cohen's kappa; this takes into account the agreement expected by chance:

$$\text{Cohen's Kappa} = \frac{P_0 - P_c}{1 - P_c}$$

where P_0 is the proportion of individuals tested upon whom there is agreement between the new test and the criterion, and P_c is the proportion of agreements expected by chance.

Values of kappa range from -1 (perfect disagreement) to $+1$ (perfect agreement) with a kappa of zero indicating a random relationship between test and criterion. Another measure sometimes used is the criterion of agreement. This is independent of the prevalence of the condition being assessed, and is given by the proportion of true positives among all those testing positive on either measure. Values range from 0 to 1.

Internal consistency

The internal consistency of a measure indicates the extent to which its component parts, in the case of a scale the individual items, address a common underlying construct. Each item will correlate to a greater or lesser extent with the total score (e.g. the association between responses on a single question about feelings of hopelessness with the total score for a depression screen). Alpha testing (see above) will have refined these items to those which correlate satisfactorily. For the whole scale these individual correlations (i.e. the internal consistency) can be summarized by a single statistic, the Cronbach's coefficient alpha, which varies between 0 and 1. Coefficient alpha scores of 0.6–0.8 are moderate but satisfactory, and scores above 0.8 indicate a highly internally consistent scale. Another measure of internal consistency is the split-half reliability, a measure of agreement between subscales derived from two randomly selected halves of the scale.

Measures of mental health status

Measures of 'caseness'

What is a case?

At first sight the concept of psychiatric caseness seems at best confusing and possibly even unhelpful. A recent comprehensive review of 40 community-based studies of the prevalence of late-life depression concluded that there was wide variation in reported prevalence, but that the most important source of variation was the diagnostic criteria that were used (Beekman *et al.* 1999). Fifteen studies measured DSM major depression; three quarters reported a prevalence of between 0% and 3%, with a weighted average of 2%. Twenty-five studies used other criteria; three-quarters of them reported a prevalence of between 9% and 18%, with a weighted average of 13%. Is the correct prevalence of late-life depression 2% or 13%? Surely both these contrasting estimates cannot be 'right'. In our confusion, we are led to ask the question 'What is a case of depression?'

Case criteria

Diagnostic criteria can be classified as broad or narrow, and as more or less operationalized. Broader criteria include diffuse and less severe forms of the disorder, narrow criteria exclude all but the most clear-cut and severe cases. Operationalized criteria make explicit a series of unambiguous rules according to which people either qualify or do not qualify as cases.

Major depression is defined according to DSM-IV (American Psychiatric Association 1994) criteria. ICD-10 (WHO 1990) has a very similar category of severe depressive episode. These are both narrow and strictly operationalized criteria. The DSM criteria require a depressed, disinterested or irritable mood (dysphoria) with associated loss of interest or pleasure in most activities (anhedonia) with at least four of eight 'criterion B' symptoms including, reduced capacity for enjoyment, reduced interest in surroundings, difficulty concentrating, lethargy, sleep disturbances, appetite disturbances, decreased self-esteem, and frequent ideas of guilt or worthlessness. In all the other studies described above depression is both more broadly and more loosely defined; operationalized criteria were not used. Depression in these studies incorporates both major and more minor degrees of depression, the threshold being defined here in terms of the concept of 'clinical significance'; a level of depression that a competent clinician would consider merited some kind of active therapeutic intervention. Thus the depression measures used in these studies define categories that do not quite correspond to DSM or ICD criteria.

A case for what?

The correct question is usually not so much 'What is a case?' as 'A case for what?'. One should not decide the optimal case criterion or measure without considering the purpose for which the measurement is being made.

The narrow criteria for major depression define a small proportion of persons with an unarguably severe form of depressive disorder, implying strong construct validity. Since the criteria are strictly operationalized they can also be applied reliably. This might be a good case definition for the first studies investigating the efficacy of a new treatment for depressive disorder; the criteria have indeed been widely used in randomized controlled trials. Major depression might also be a good 'pure' case definition for a genetic linkage study, aiming to identify gene loci predisposing to depression in a multiply affected family pedigree. However, these criteria will not suit all purposes. One cannot presume for instance that the findings from the drug efficacy studies will generalize to the broader group of depressed patients whom clinicians typically diagnose and treat, but who do not meet criteria for major depression. Also, major depression criteria arguably miss much of the impact of depressive disorder within a community population. Depressed persons are known to be heavy users of health and social services. However, the very small number of cases of major depression account for a tiny proportion of this excess, which is mainly made up of cases of 'common mental disorder'. Also, operationalized criteria can be capricious. Many persons might meet some but not all of the necessary case criteria, and nevertheless experience an equivalent, or lesser but still significant intensity of symptoms and loss of quality of life.

Measures of traits or dimensions

The idea of psychiatric disorder as a dimension can be difficult for psychiatrists to grasp. They are used to making a series of dichotomous judgements in their clinical practice. Is this patient depressed? Does he need treatment? Should he be admitted? Does he have insight? Is he a danger to himself? As Pickering commented (when arguing that hypertension was better understood as a dimensional rather than a dichotomous disorder) 'doctors can count to one but not beyond'. It is important to recognise that a dimensional concept need not contradict a categorical view of a disorder. As with the relativity of the concept of 'a case', it may be useful under some circumstances to think categorically and in others dimensionally. There is for instance a positive correlation between the number of symptoms of depression experienced by a person and

(a) the impairment of their quality of life,

(b) the frequency with which they use GP services,

(c) the number of days they take off work in a month.

Thus, the dimensional perspective can offer useful insights into the way in which the consequences of mental disorder are very widely distributed in the community. For example, Broadhead et al. (1990) showed in the USA that although major depression increased risk for 'disability days' nearly five-fold and lesser degrees of depression only one and a half-fold, because the lesser degrees of depression were much more prevalent they accounted for half as many disability days again as did major depression in the population as a whole. Therefore the impact of depression in the population would have been considerably underestimated if the narrowly-based clinical criterion had been used alone. While a public health perspective necessitates taking a broad view of a pathology, whether it be hypertension or common mental disorder, no one would argue that it would be helpful to medicalize this phenomenon by seeking to identify and treat all persons with any symptoms of depression at all. It might however be appropriate to identify population-based interventions that reduce the general level of depression symptoms in the community as a whole, rather than focussing interventions merely upon those at the extreme end of the distribution (Rose 2001).

From a technical point of view, continuous measures of dimensional traits such as depression, anxiety, neuroticism, and cognitive function offer some advantages over their dichotomous equivalents, major depression, generalized anxiety disorder, personality disorder, and dementia. These diagnoses tend to be rather rare; collapsing a continuous trait into a dichotomous diagnosis may mean that the investigators are in effect throwing away informative data; the net effect may be loss of statistical power to demonstrate an important association with a risk factor, or a real benefit of a treatment. In psychiatric genetics, for example, researchers are increasingly using as the phenotype for their linkage analyses the traits that at their extremes are postulated to underlie susceptibility for expression of the clinical condition thus hyperactivity for Attention Deficit Hyperactivity Disorder (Payton et al. 2001), or disorganised thinking for psychosis (Cardno et al. 2001). Trait based methods may offer considerable advantages in terms of statistical power for identification of genes of small to moderate effect.

Technical issues in measurement

The medium for the interview: face-to-face interview vs. postal interview vs. telephone interview

Face-to-face interviews offer the participant the convenience of being interviewed in their own home, by an interviewer who should

- be polite,
- be neatly and appropriately dressed,
- carry identification,
- be sensitive to their position as guests in the participant's home.

Some participants may prefer to be interviewed in a research centre rather than in their own homes, and provision should be made for this eventuality.

The postal method can obviously only be used for self-completion questionnaires. It may seem appealing at first sight because of the apparent savings in personnel time, cost, and efficiency. However, response rates can be very low, typically only 30–40% on first mailing. Non-responders tend to have lower socio-economic status and lower educational level (there is evidently a particular problem if literacy is limited) than responders, hence this is likely to lead to bias. Postal methods will thus only be acceptable if the questionnaire is exceptionally simple and clearly laid out, and if considerable resources can be allocated to pursuing non-responders by postal reminders, and if need be, with telephone calls or home visits (see below).

Telephone interviews may be an acceptable alternative that still offers economies in terms of time saved taken to travel to a participant's home. Repeated telephone calls can be made to gain access to subjects who are rarely at home. Response rates can therefore be quite high, and many instruments have been shown to be both feasible and valid when administered in this way. Evidently this method can only be used in settings where a substantial proportion of the population have a telephone in their home, effectively limiting its use to certain developed countries.

The source of information: participant vs. informant

It would seem self-evident that the participant should be the best source of information about mental phenomena that are in the realms of their personal experience. However, in clinical psychiatry a collateral history from a reliable informant plays an important part in the diagnostic process. In practice, such collateral information is rarely incorporated into research interviews. However informant-based measures have been widely used in the assessment of personality, and in screening for dementia (see Appendix for details).

Who administers the assessment?: self-report vs. interviewer administered

Simple scalable measures of traits such as the GHQ have been validated as self-report instruments. Recently more complex measures (e.g. CIS-R and CIDI) that were developed as semi-structured or structured clinical diagnostic assessments have been adapted and validated as self-administered instruments. This has been accomplished by computerizing the interview. The computer guides the participant through the interview skipping irrelevant sections and providing prompts on demand (hence mimicking in many ways the role of the clinical interviewer, but, through standardization, removing the risk of observer bias). Self-report assessments may be particularly useful for ascertainment of highly sensitive material, such as drug use, sexual experiences, or criminal behaviours, where the participant may be readier to make an accurate report on a self-report form or a computer than through the medium of an interviewer. Conversely, good rapport established in a research interview may assist full and accurate disclosure of mental phenomena. A major drawback of a self-report method is that if the participant does not understand the question they may give no response or an inaccurate response. Within limits (which apply particularly in a fully structured interview), the interviewer may be able to clarify or at least decline to code a meaningless response. It follows from the above that a self report questionnaire needs to be particularly clearly phrased and laid out.

The background and training of the interviewer/assessor: (a) lay interviewer vs. clinician administered and rated assessments; (b) unstructured vs. semi structured vs. fully structured assessments

Early epidemiological studies used unstructured clinician interviews to make diagnoses. In so doing, they placed an over-optimistic reliance on standardization in clinical training and practice. Nowadays interview schedules tend to be either semi-structured or fully structured. Semi-structured interviews (e.g. GMS, PSE, SCAN) are usually administered by a clinician and still allow some scope for clinical discretion to be exercised in the way in which questions are asked and responses coded. Fully structured interviews (e.g. CIDI) can be administered by clinical or by lay interviewers, who are trained to ask questions exactly as listed and to code the participant's answer accurately without interpretation. Structured assessments have standardized the way in which symptoms are elicited and recorded. Many diagnostic interviews have also standardized the way in which symptoms are used to generate diagnoses. Pre-defined diagnostic algorithms can be applied by an investigator, or even by a computer program hence removing the possibility of observer bias. Increasing standardization in assessment technology has led to more use of trained lay interviewers who are cheaper to employ, easier to recruit, and often more reliable (in terms of inter-interviewer reliability) than clinicians. The popularity of fully structured lay-administered assessments has been dented a little by the growing realization that their validity against the criterion of semi-structured clinical interviews is often relatively poor (Brugha *et al.* 1999*a,b*).

The style of measure: phenomenological vs. classificatory measures

The UK school of measurement in psychiatry tends to be phenomenologically based. Its instruments seek to mimic normal clinical interviewing style, and to combine elicited symptoms into realistic algorithms empirically devised to match normal diagnostic practice; the gold standard of the competent clinician. These instruments (the CIS-R, PSE/CATEGO, and GMS/AGECAT) therefore have their own criteria for caseness built into diagnostic algorithms that do not exactly correspond to DSM or ICD rubrics. However, the UK instruments have tended to fall into line and now include additional algorithms to generate ICD 10 and DSM IV diagnoses.

The classificatory approach, represented by DIS and CIDI, takes case criteria (usually DSM) as its starting point and tries to ask sufficiently precise questions to ensure that these can be matched. The resulting questions can be cumbersome, for example (from CIDI):

> For the next few questions, please think of the two week period during the past 12 months when you had the most complete loss of interest in things. During that two week period did the loss of interest usually last
>
> a) all day long
> b) most of the day
> c) about half of the day
> d) less than half of the day?

The equivalent question from the CIS-R is

> How is your interest in things?

Two phase (screening and diagnosis) vs. one phase assessment

The General Health Questionnaire (GHQ) identifies, using a validated cut-off score, individuals who have a high probability of having a psychiatric disorder (diagnosis unspecified). It is quick (5–10 min) and easy to use, and can even be administered as a self-report instrument. SCAN provides definitive diagnoses in a single assessment, but has to be administered by a specially trained clinician and takes up to an hour or more to complete. A two-phase survey technique might use GHQ as an initial brief screen; all participants scoring above the cut-off point (screen positives) would then be administered the SCAN, together with a randomly selected sub-group of the screen negatives. No screening instrument is perfect (otherwise there would be no point in the second stage assessment). The second stage will identify false positives. The selection of screen negatives is essential to identify false negatives; screening assessments are rarely perfectly sensitive; without this element the prevalence of a disorder is likely to be underestimated. The efficiency savings can be considerable, as shown in the following imaginary example of a two-phase survey of 1000 persons estimating the prevalence of ICD depressive episode or disorder. GHQ was used as a first phase screening assessment, and SCAN as the definitive second phase diagnostic assessment.

Phase 1 survey

GHQ$^-$	840
GHQ$^+$	160
Total	1000

Phase 1 duration = 1000 × 10 min = 166 h

Phase 2 survey (assuming all screen positives and 20% of screen negatives are selected)

	SCAN +ve	SCAN −ve	
GHQ$^-$	8	160	168
GHQ$^+$	110	50	160
Total	118	210	328

Phase 2 duration = 328 × 1 h = 328 h

The total interviewing time for the two phase design was therefore 166 + 328 = 494 h. Had no screening been carried out the interviewing time would have been 1000 h, a saving of over 50%.

The prevalence in the sample is now estimated by 'weighting back' by multiplying the numbers in the screen negative group by the inverse of the sampling fraction of 0.2, that is, five. The eight false negatives in the phase two assessment are therefore taken to represent 40 in the whole sample, the 160 true negatives 800 etc.

A weighted estimate of the prevalence of depressive episodes or disorders

	SCAN +ve	SCAN −ve	
GHQ⁻	8 (40)	160 (800)	168 (840)
GHQ⁺	110	50	160
Total	118 (150)	210 (850)	328 (1000)

The weighted prevalence is therefore 150/1000 or 15%. Note that if screen negatives had not been included in the phase two assessment (assuming wrongly that GHQ would be perfectly sensitive) then the prevalence would have been underestimated at only 110/1000 or 11%. A detailed discussion of the controversial question of the advantages and disadvantages of two phase against one phase survey methods is contained in chapter 7 on 'Cross-sectional surveys'.

Suggested classroom practical exercise

1. A new screening questionnaire has been developed for identifying cases of schizophrenia. The method was developed, and then validated in a 'first onset schizophrenia' service taking referrals of possible cases from primary care. The prediction provided by the questionnaire was validated against the gold standard of SCAN diagnosis in the clinic setting. Results of the validation in this sample were as follows.

Test/gold standard	SCAN −ve	SCAN +ve	
Test −ve	259	45	304
Test +ve	23	801	824
	282	846	1128

(a) What is the prevalence of schizophrenia in this sample?

(b) What are the psychometric properties of the test:
- ◆ the sensitivity
- ◆ the specificity
- ◆ the PPV
- ◆ the NPV.

2. The test is now tried out in the general population in the course of a national psychiatric morbidity survey. In this sample the prevalence of

schizophrenia is 0.5%. Assuming that the sensitivity and specificity of the test are the same as in the validation exercise, what is

(a) the PPV

(b) the NPV

of the test.

3. What is the relationship between PPV and prevalence (establish this for yourself empirically, if you like, by further varying prevalence in the above example, and keeping sensitivity and specificity constant)?

4. We assumed that sensitivity and specificity would not vary as prevalence of the disorder changed in moving from the high-risk clinic referral population to the low-risk general population sample. Is this a reasonable assumption? What if anything do you think would be the effect of changing prevalence on sensitivity and specificity?

What other factors might affect the sensitivity and specificity of a test from that reported in its initial validation study?

Answers

1. (a) What is the prevalence of Schizophrenia in this sample?

75%

(b) What are the psychometric properties of the test:

Sensitivity   94.7%

Specificity   91.8%

PPV   97.2%

NPV   85.2%

2. The test is now tried out in the general population in the course of a national psychiatric morbidity survey. In this sample the prevalence of schizophrenia is 0.5%. Assuming that the sensitivity and specificity of the test are the same as in the validation exercise, we would anticipate the following findings among (say) 10,000 participants.

Test/gold standard	SCAN −ve	SCAN +ve	
Test −ve	9134	3	9137
Test +ve	816	47	863
	9950	50	10,000

PPV   5.4%

NPV   99.97%

3. As the prevalence falls the PPV falls as well. For a very rare condition, even when the test has good specificity the number of false positives overwhelms the number of true positives. This is an important point to grasp, with major implications for clinical epidemiology. Most screening (and clinical) tests only work well when the *prior probability*, that is, the probability that someone is a case before any other information (i.e. test results) is known about them, is reasonably high. This is sometimes used as a justification for having primary care doctors as 'gatekeepers' responsible for referring people to specialist clinical services. Good primary care doctors quickly and efficiently screen out likely non-cases (e.g. 'innocent' headaches) before referring those at high risk (high prior probability) to a specialist (e.g. neurologist for MRI scans to exclude brain tumour).

4. This should be a reasonable assumption. Note that sensitivity and specificity are calculated within columns of the cross tab. PPV and NPV are calculated within rows, and hence are affected by prevalence.

What other factors might affect the sensitivity and specificity of a test from that reported in its initial validation study?

The validity coefficients of a test may vary from one setting to another, depending upon the nature of the test. Screening questionnaires may be affected by cultural or language factors, or by the characteristics of the interviewer administering the questionnaire. Tests requiring interpretation (e.g. MRI scans) may be affected by the skills of the clinician. In general, greater care is probably taken in research validation exercises, and the sensitivities and specificities from these studies may not be matched in realistic clinical practice.

Appendix

This is a selection of the more rigorously constructed, best validated, and most widely used measures. The choice reflects to some extent the author's bias towards briefer measures.

Note that some of these measures are copyrighted (e.g. GHQ and EPQ), and fees are charged for their use, although these are sometimes waived (e.g. for PhD students). For all copyrighted measures, it is essential that you seek permission to use the measure, and pay the copyright fee if required. In some cases a public domain alternative exists (e.g. you could use the SRQ-20 instead of the GHQ). For the public domain measures, you should still, as a matter of courtesy, contact the instrument developers for permission to use their measures. They will often be able to provide you with useful advice. All WHO measures are in the public domain and copyright free, however, again you should contact the

WHO Mental Health Division for the most up to date version of the measure (often available in a translated version suitable for use in your country).

Scalable measures with validated screening properties

Measuring psychiatric disorder

(1) *General adults (16–64)*

GHQ   General Health Questionnaire

A 12 (GHQ-12), 28 (GHQ-28) or 30 item (GHQ-30) self-administered (5–10 min) questionnaire with a validated cutpoint for identification of common mental disorder. The GHQ is copyrighted. Contact NFER Wilson for permission and information regarding copyright fees.

Goldberg, D.P., Gater, R., Sartorius, N., Ustun, T.B., *et al.* (1997) The validity of two versions of the GHQ in the WHO study of mental illness in general health care. Psychological Medicine **27**, 191–7.

Goldberg, G. and Williams, P. (1988) *A User's Guide to the General Health Questionnaire.* NFER Nelson, Windsor, Berkshire.

SRQ-20   Self Reporting Questionnaire—20

A 20 item self administered (5–10 min) questionnaire with a validated cutpoint for identification of common mental disorder. This is a WHO measure and therefore free of copyright charges. Very similar to the GHQ in its content, style and properties, but a useful alternative if you wish to avoid paying licence fees.

Araya, R., Wynn, R., and Lewis, G. (1992) Comparison of two self administered psychiatric questionnaires (GHQ-12 and SRQ-20) in primary care in Chile. *Social Psychiatry and Psychiatric Epidemiology,* **27**, 168–73.

CIS-R   Clinical Interview Schedule—Revised

Fully structured lay interviewer or self (computer) administered (20–30 min). The CIS-R can be used to screen for the presence of psychological morbidity with a scalable morbidity score, and a validated cutpoint of ≥12. More recently it has been adapted to generate ICD-10 diagnoses (neurosis only) using a computerised algorithm (PROQSY). Formal training is required. Contact Glyn Lewis (*Glyn.Lewis@bristol.ac.uk*) or Martin Prince (*m.prince@iop. kcl.ac.uk*) for details.

Lewis, G., Pelosi, A.J., Araya, R., and Dunn, G. (1992) Measuring psychiatric disorder in the community: a standardized assessment for use by lay interviewers. *Psychological Medicine,* **22**, 465–86.

(2) *Children*

SDQ   Strengths and difficulties questionnaire

25 item respondent-based questionnaire with identical parent, teacher, and self-report for common difficulties with emotional symptoms, behavioural difficulties, and hyperactivity.

Goodman, R. (2001) Psychometric properties of the Strengths and Difficulties Questionnaire (SDQ). *Journal of the American Academy of Child and Adolescent Psychiatry*, **40**, 1337–45, (Abstract) *www.sdqinfo.com*

CBCL   Child behaviour checklist

CBCL comprises 118 items and has different versions for parents (CBCL), teacher (TRF Teacher Report Form) and young person (Youth Self-Report).

Achenbach, T.M. (1994) Child Behavior Checklist and related instruments. In the use of psychological testing for treatment planning and outcome assessment (ed. Maruish, M.E.), pp. 517–49. Lawrence Erlbaum Associates, Inc., Hillsdale, NJ.

Measuring depression

CES-D   Centre for Epidemiological Studies—Depression
Self-administered (5–10 min)

Radloff, L.S. (1977) The CES-D scale: A self report depression scale for research in the general population. *Applied Psychological Measurements*, **1**, 385–401.

ZDS   Zung depression scale
Self-administered (5–10 min)

Zung, W.W.K. (1965) A self-rating depression scale. *Archives of General Psychiatry*, **12**, 62–70.

GDS   Geriatric Depression scale (over 65s)
Self-administered (5–10 min)

Yesavage, J., Rose, T., and Lum, O. (1983) Development and validation of a Geriatric Depression Screening Scale: a preliminary report. *Journal of Psychiatric Research*, **17**, 43–9.

Measuring fatigue

Self administered (5 min)

Chalder, T., Berelowitz, C., and Pawlikowska, T. (1993) Development of a fatigue scale. *Journal Psychosomatic Research*, **37**, 147–54.

An 11 item fatigue scale with mental and physical fatigue subscales.
Very similar to GHQ-12 in scoring with a cut off at 3/4 level for identification of clinically significant fatigue.

Measuring cognitive function (and screening for dementia)

MMSE   Mini-Mental State Examination
Interviewer administered (10–15 min)

Folstein, M.F., Folstein, S.E., and Mchugh, P.R. (1975) 'Mini-mental State': a practical method for grading the cognitive state of patients for the clinician. *Journal of Psychiatric Research*, **12**, 189–98.

TICS-m   The Telephone Interview for Cognitive Status
Interviewer administered (over the telephone: 10–15 min)

Brandt, J., Spencer, M., and Folstein, M. (1988) The telephone interview for cognitive status. *Neuropsychiatry, Neuropsychology and Behavioral Neurology* **1**, 111–7.

CSI-D   The Cognitive Screening Instrument for Dementia
Interviewer administered to participant (5–10 min) and informant (10 min)

Hall, K.S., Hendrie, H.H., Brittain, H.M., Norton, J.A., *et al.* (1993) The development of a
dementia screening interview in two distinct languages. *International Journal of
Methods in Psychiatric Research*, 3, 1–28.

IQ-CODE   The Informant Questionnaire on Cognitive Decline in the Elderly
Interviewer administered to informant (10 min)

Jorm, A.F. (1994) A short form of the Informant Questionnaire on Cognitive Decline in the
Elderly (IQCODE): development and cross-validation. *Psychological Medicine*, 24,
145–53.

Instruments generating diagnoses according to established algorithms

Assessing a comprehensive range of clinical diagnoses

(1)   *General adults (16–64 years)*
DIS   Diagnostic Interview Schedule
Interviewer administered (1.5–2 h)

A fully structured, lay interviewer administered comprehensive diagnostic
assessment. Used in the US ECA study, but probably of historical interest only,
superceded by the CIDI (see below).

Robins, L. and Helzer, J.E. (1994) The half-life of a structured interview: The NIMH
Diagnostic Interview Schedule (DIS). *International Journal of Methods in Psychiatric
Research*, 4, 95–102.

CIDI   Composite International Diagnostic Interview
A fully structured, lay interviewer administered comprehensive diagnostic
assessment. A computer algorithm generates DSM IV and/or ICD 10 diagnoses. (2 h in its full form, although shorter versions, CIDI-PC and UM-CIDI
have also been developed. The neurosis modules can be administered in
20–40 min only.) Formal training is essential. Contact the WHO for details of
local training centres.

World Health Organisation (1990) *Composite International Diagnostic
Interview (CIDI, Version 1.0)*, Geneva: World Health Organisation.

Wittchen, H.U. (1994) Reliability and validity studies of the WHO—Composite
International Diagnostic Interview (CIDI): A critical review. *Journal of Psychiatric
Research*, 28, 57–84.

SCAN and PSE
A semi-structured, clinician administered comprehensive diagnostic assessment. A computer algorithm generates DSM IV and/or ICD 10 diagnoses.
(1.5–2 h, but the neurosis modules can be administered in 20–40 min only).
Formal training is essential. Contact the WHO for details of local training
centres.

Wing (1996) SCAN and the PSE tradition. *Social Psychiatry and Psychiatric Epidemiology,* **31**, 50–4.

Wing (1983) Use and misuse of the PSE. *British Journal of Psychiatry,* **143**, 111–7.

(2)   *Older adults (65 and over)*

GMS   Geriatric Mental State

Lay or clinician interviewer administered (25–40 min). A semi-structured comprehensive diagnostic assessment for older (65 and over) participants, with a computerised algorithm to generate 'AGECAT' and ICD-10 or DSM IV diagnoses. Formal training is necessary. Contact Ken Wilson (K.C.M.Wilson@liverpool. ac.uk) or Martin Prince (*m.prince@iop.kcl.ac.uk*) for details of local centres.

Copeland, J.R.M., Dewey, M.E., and Griffith-Jones, H.M. (1986) A computerised psychiatric diagnostic system and case nomenclature for elderly participants: GMS and AGECAT. *Psychological Medicine,* 16, 89–99.

CAMDEX

Interviewer administered to participant and informant (1 h)

Roth, M., Tym, E., Mountjoy, C.Q., Huppert, F.A., *et al.* (1986) CAMDEX. A standardised instrument for the diagnosis of mental disorder in the elderly with special reference to the early detection of dementia. *British Journal of Psychiatry,* 149, 698–709.

(3)   *Childhood psychiatric disorder*

DAWBA

Development and well-being assessment for DSM IV or ICD 10 disorders in 5–17 year olds. Structured interview administered by computer or trained lay-interviewer, with versions for parents, teachers and young people.

Goodman, R., Ford, T., Richards, H., Gatward, R., and Meltzer, H. (2000) The Development and Well-Being Assessment: Description and initial validation of an integrated assessment of child and adolescent psychopathology. *Journal of Child Psychology and Psychiatry,* 41, 645–55 www.dawba.com

CAPA   Child and Adolescent Psychiatric Assessment

Semi-structured assessment administered by clinicians or lay people trained in the CAPA for 8–18 year olds.

Angold, A., Prendergast, M., Cox, A., and Harrington, R. (1995) The child and adolescent psychiatric assessment. *Psychological Medicine,* 25, 739–53.

DISC   Diagnostic Interview Schedule for Children

Highly structured interview for 6–17 year olds with parent, child and teacher versions.

Shaffer, D., *et al.* (1993). The Diagnostic Interview Schedule for Children—revised version (DISC_R) 1. Preparation, field testing, interrater reliability and acceptability. *Journal of the American Academy of Child and Adolescent Psychiatry,* 32, 643–50.

Assessing personality disorder

SAP   Standardized Assessment of Personality

Interviewer administered to informant (20–30 min). Formal training is required. Contact Martin Prince at *m.prince@iop.kcl.ac.uk* for details.

Pilgrim, J.A. and Mann, A.H. (1990) Use of the ICD-10 version of the Standardized Assessment of Personality to determine the prevalence of personality disorder in psychiatric in-patients. *Psychological Medicine*, **20**, 985–92.

Pilgrim, J.A., Mellers, B., and Mann (1993) Inter-rater and temporal reliability of the Standardized Assessment of Personality and the influence of informant characteristics. *Psychological Medicine*, **23**, 779–86.

Measures of other variables, relevant to mental disorder

Measuring stable traits

EPQ   Eysenck Personality Questionnaire (neuroticism, extroversion/introversion, psychoticism)

The EPQ is copyrighted. Contact Nfer Wilson for permission and information regarding copyright fees.

EYSENCK (1959) The differentiation between normal and various neurotic groups on the Maudsley Personality Inventory. *British Journal of Psychology*, **50**, 176–7.

PBI   Parental Bonding Inventory

Parker, G., Tupling, H., and Brown (1979) A parental bonding instrument. *British Journal of Medical Psychology*, **52**, 1–10.

Measuring life events

LTE   The List of Threatening Events
An 11-item self-report scale. Self or interviewer administered (5–10 min)

Brugha, T.S., Bebbington, P., Tennant, C., and Hurry, J. (1985) The list of threatening experiences: a subset of 12 life event categories with considerable long-term contextual threat. *Psychological Medicine*, **15**, 189–94.

Measuring social support

SPQ   The social problems questionnaire
Self or interviewer administered (10 min)

Corney, R.H., and Clare, A.W. (1985) The construction, development and testing of a self-report questionnaire to identify social problems. *Psychological Medicine*, **15**, 637–649.

CPQ   The Close Persons Questionnaire
Interviewer administered (10–20 min)

Stansfeld, S. and Marmot, M. (1992) Deriving a survey measure of social support: The reliability and validity of the Close Persons Questionnaire. *Social Science and Medicine*, **35**, 1027–35.

Describing social network

Social Network Assessment Instrument
Self or interviewer administered (5–10 min)

Wenger, G.C. (1989) Support networks in old age: Constructing a typology. In: Jeffreys, M. (ed.) *Growing Old in the Twentieth Century*. Routledge, London.

Quality of life

WHOQOL BREF

Self-report or interviewer administered (10–15 min). Contact the WHO for details.

World Health Organisation (1997) Measuring Quality of Life. The World Health Organization Quality of Life Instruments (The WHO-QOL – 100 and the WHOQOL-BREF. World Health Organization, Geneva. WHO/MNH/PSF/97.4. (*e-mail-whoqol@who.ch*)

Global health/disablement

LHS   The London Handicap Scale

Self or interviewer administered (5–10 min)

Harwood, R.H., Gompertz, P., and Ebrahim, S. (1994) Handicap one year after a stroke: validity of a new scale. *Journal of Neurology Neurosurgery and Psychiatry*, **57**, 825–29.

SF-36

A 36-item self-report or interviewer administered measure of health related quality of life (15–20 min). Perhaps the best validated and most widely used measure internationally. The SF-36 is copyrighted. Contact the instrument developers for permission to use.

McHorney C.A., Ware J.E., and Raczek, A.E. (1993) The MOS 36-Item Short-Form Health Survey (SF-36): II. Psychometric and clinical tests of validity in measuring physical and mental health constructs. *Medical Care*, **31**(3), 247–63.

McHorney, C.A., Ware, J.E., Lu, J.F., and Sherbourne, C.D. (1994) The MOS 36-item Short-Form Health Survey (SF-36): III. Tests of data quality, scaling assumptions, and reliability across diverse patient groups. *Medical Care* **32**(1), 40–66.

Ware, J.E. Jr. and Sherbourne, C.D. (1992). The MOS 36-item short-form health survey (SF-36). I. Conceptual framework and item selection. *Medical Care*, **30**(6), 473–83.

SF-12   Short Form—12 (Reduced version of MOS SF-36)

Self or interviewer administered (5–10 min). This shortened version generates simply a 'mental health component score' and a physical health component score' indicating respectively the consequences of heath impairments within these domains.

Jenkinson, C. and Layte, R. (1998) Development and testing of the UK SF-12. *Journal of Health Service Research Policy*, **2/1**, 14–18.

A fuller account of validated health measures, with particular reference to older participants, is contained in:

Prince, M.J., Harwood, R., Thomas, A., and Mann, A.H. (1997) Gospel Oak V. Impairment, disability and handicap as risk factors for depression in old age. *Psychological Medicine*, **27**, 311–21.

References

American Psychiatric Association. (1994) *Diagnostic and Statistical Manual of Mental Disorders*. AMA, Washington DC.

Beekman, A.T.F., Copeland, J.R.M., and Prince, M.J. (1999) Review of community prevalence of depression in later life. *British Journal of Psychiatry*, **174**, 307–11.

Broadhead, W.E., Blazer, D.G., George, L.K., and Tse, C.K. (1990) Depression, disability days, and days lost from work in a prospective epidemiologic survey. *Journal of the American Medical Association* **264**, 2524–8.

Brugha, T.S., Bebbington, P.E., Jenkins, R., Meltzer, H., Taub, N.A., Janas, M., *et al.* (1999*a*) Cross validation of a general population survey diagnostic interview: a comparison of CIS-R with SCAN ICD-10 diagnostic categories. *Psychological Medicine*, **29**, 1029–42.

Brugha, T.S., Bebbington, P.E., and Jenkins, R. (1999*b*) A difference that matters: comparisons of structured and semi-structured psychiatric diagnostic interviews in the general population. *Psychological Medicine*, **29**, 1013–20.

Cardno, A.G., Sham, P.C., Murray, R.M., and McGuffin, P. (2001) Twin study of symptom dimensions in psychoses. *British Journal of Psychiatry*, **179**, 39–45.

Kumari, G.L., Prince, M., and Scott, S. (2000) The development and validation of the Parent-Child Joint Activity Scale (PJAS). *International Journal of Methods in Psychiatric Research*, **8**, 219–27.

Payton, A., Holmes, J., Barrett, J.H., Sham, P., Harrington, R., McGuffin, P., *et al.* (2001) Susceptibility genes for a trait measure of attention deficit hyperactivity disorder: a pilot study in a non-clinical sample of twins. *Psychiatry Research*, **105**, 273–8.

Rose G. (2001) Sick individuals and sick populations. 1985. *Bulletin of the World Health Organization*, **79**, 990–6.

World Health Organisation. (1990) Mental and Behavioural Disorders (including disorders of psychological development). *Diagnostic Criteria for Research*, Geneva: MNH/ MEP/ 89.2 Rev. 1.

Chapter 3

Cultural issues in measurement and research

Vikram Patel

Introduction

We begin this chapter by considering the relevance of cultural issues in psychiatric research. Cultural issues are important because of the following reasons.

1 Cross-cultural studies can provide valuable insights into the social, environmental, economic and cultural variables which influence the aetiology and outcome of mental illness.

2 There is substantial evidence from 'multi-cultural' Western countries that the prevalence and outcome of mental illnesses, and in particular the way they are perceived and appropriate health services accessed, varies considerably between ethnic groups. There is also evidence that some types of mental illnesses are more or less common in some ethnic groups as compared to the 'host' population.

3 There is a growing recognition that psychiatric concepts (which form the core of any measurement process inherent in epidemiology) are strongly influenced by cultural factors. There are many examples of this, perhaps the most vivid one being that until recently homosexuality was considered a mental illness, but the liberal progressive influences on Western societies led to pressure on psychiatry to reconsider this status. Thus, epidemiological studies in non-Western settings will need to incorporate locally relevant concepts and idioms in their methods.

4 For research to be relevant to the needs of local communities and health services, it must be sensitive to the unique aspects of those communities, for example, the extent of mental health services, the provision of traditional and alternative medical systems, the availability and cost of psychotropics, and so on.

If we accept that culture plays a key role in influencing the epidemiology of psychiatric disorders, then by definition, cultural issues in measurement and research are relevant in every epidemiological investigation. The reality, however, is that the study of cultural influences on psychiatry has to a large extent been conducted from the platform of a biomedical diagnostic paradigm developed almost entirely in Europe and North America. The interest in the academic pursuit of cultural issues has most often been to describe how people from cultures different from Western cultures experience mental illnesses. There is an assumption that syndromes described in the cultures of Western Europe and USA around the middle of the twentieth century formed the basis of a universal categorization of mental illness. The need to establish psychiatry as a legitimate medical discipline was acute in the absence of any 'hard' biological definitions for disease states. This need was partly met by the acceptance of the dominant psychiatric nosologies, those originating from the West, as being globally valid. However, psychiatric disorders remained, at best, illnesses whose diagnoses relied on symptom reports from individual patients. Even today, all major diagnostic categories reified in various classification systems consist essentially of symptom constellations (Patel and Winston 1994), and there are few psychiatric diagnoses which are associated with the same demonstrable pathology globally. Despite these fundamental limitations, the overwhelming bulk of research on cultural influences on psychiatric disorder begins with an assumption of Western cultures as being the 'standard' against which other populations are compared. It is in this, somewhat warped context that this chapter is written.

Definitions

Culture

A problem with 'Cross-Cultural Psychiatry' has been a lack of consensus on what exactly 'culture' means. One definition of culture is that it is 'the customs, civilization and achievements of a particular time or people' (Concise Oxford Dictionary, 9th edn). As might be evident without the need for a definition, culture is a dynamic construct, particularly so in a shrinking world with increasing cultural admixture, assimilation, and mutual influence. With increasing mass migration between nations the cultures of both host and migrant communities are undergoing rapid and irrevocable change. Consider, for example, the recent acceptance of Asian food as part of British culture, or the adoption of European dress style by Asian migrants to the UK.

Race and ethnicity

In the face of the increasing ambiguity of 'culture', alternative terms such as race and ethnicity have been used to define national and international sub-populations. Race is, essentially, a descriptive term wherein people are grouped according to how they look to the observer based on pre-defined physical characteristics of presumed genetic or biological origin. However, great caution is needed in interpreting studies based on racial distribution of diseases since genetic or biological factors may be irrelevant in the face of social and cultural differences between groups defined in this way. For example, if rates of alcohol abuse are more commonly reported in black people in North America, these findings need to be carefully interpreted to take into account socio-economic differences between blacks and whites. The concept of ethnicity is seen as more acceptable. This term is used to describe a group of people who share a common identity (i.e. how they describe their origins), a common ancestry (historically and geographically) and, to some extent, shared beliefs and history. However, this term is also fraught with difficulties. Whereas people from the Indian sub-continent living in the UK may be defined as 'ethnic Asians', this does not capture the fact that this apparently related ethnic grouping is at least as internally diverse as an ethnic grouping of 'European'. Still, in what can turn out to be tautological nightmare, ethnicity is arguably the most useful term to describe sub-groups of people in the study of the epidemiology of diseases.

Comparative psychiatry

Comparative psychiatry is 'the study of the relations between mental disorder and the psychological characteristics which differentiate people, nations, or cultures. Its main goals are to identify, verify, and explain the links between mental disorder and these broad psychosocial characteristics' (Murphy 1982). This concept has, to an extent, gradually fallen into disuse. However it has advantages over 'cross-cultural psychiatry', because it does not seek to define the comparative groups only along the lines of preset criteria such as culture. In this sense, this term comes closest to the concept of an international psychiatry described later.

From cross-cultural to international psychiatry

The universalist 'etic' approach

A particular problem for cross-cultural studies in psychiatric epidemiology has been the variation of case identification techniques between settings and the lack of equivalence in symptom quantification. These inconsistencies led to a movement to standardize the process of psychiatric measurement and diagnosis, principally driven by psychiatric classification systems originating in Euro-American societies. Standardized interviews derived from the clinical psychiatric evaluation were developed to determine 'caseness' in epidemiological investigations (Williams *et al.* 1980). After validation in Euro-American cultures, the interview schedules were subsequently used in other cultures. This 'etic' or universalist approach, became the most popular method for epidemiological investigations of mental illness across cultures. The etic approach assumes that mental illness is broadly similar throughout the world, and that psychiatric taxonomies and measurements, and models of health care are also globally applicable. There are two dominant systems of psychiatric classification, the International Classification of Diseases developed by the World Health Organization and the Diagnostic and Statistical Manual developed by the American Psychiatric Association. Diagnostic criteria of syndromes can and do change over time as is well demonstrated by the regular revisions of international psychiatric classifications; these revisions are considerably influenced by political factors.

Deficiencies in etic frameworks

Etic investigations involve implicit, and often untested assumptions, as highlighted in Box 3.1. Although many researchers in non-Western cultures have argued for the effectiveness and universal applicability of current classification systems (e.g. Sen and Mari 1986), some have raised concerns over this process. A particular caution has been the risk of confounding culturally distinctive behaviour with psychopathology on the basis of other superficial similarities of behaviour patterns or phenomena in different cultures (Kleinman 1987). In particular, it has been contested that classification of psychiatric disorders largely reflects American and European concepts of psychopathology based on implicit cultural concepts of normality and deviance. Some authors have

Box 3.1 **Implicit assumptions in universalist, 'etic' research**

- ◆ Universality of mental illnesses: The assumption that 'disorders' described in Euro-American classifications occur everywhere.

- ◆ Syndrome invariance: The assumption that the core features of psychiatric syndromes do not vary between cultures.

- ◆ Inherent validity: The assumption that, although refinement is possible, the diagnostic categories of current classifications are universally valid clinical constructs (Beiser *et al.* 1994).

proposed that cross-cultural psychiatry should examine the influence of culture on mental illness in Euro-American societies itself, rather than assume that these illnesses are 'natural' and free of any cultural bias in these contexts. Critics have accused the etic approach of contributing to a worldview which 'privileges biology over culture' (Eisenbruch 1991) and ignores the cultural and social contexts of psychiatric disorders.

The emic approach

The field of medical anthropology has exerted a growing influence on health research, particularly in low-income countries. This influence has seen a paradigm shift within Public Health and Epidemiology from unifocal and positivist 'scientific' viewpoints towards a recognition that illness is the result of a 'web of causation' which includes an individual's socio-cultural environment (Heggenhougen and Draper 1990). Medical anthropology has been one of the key influences which fuelled the development of the 'emic' approach in cross-cultural psychiatry. At a general level it is argued that the culture-bound aspects of biomedicine (such as its emphasis on medical disease entities) limits its universal applicability. More specifically, culture plays such an influential role in the presentation of psychiatric disorders that Euro-American psychiatric categories cannot be assumed to be universally appropriate (Littlewood 1990). Part of this argument lies in the lack of specific pathophysiological changes associated with psychiatric disorders, so that diagnostic categories can only represent 'illnesses' rather than 'diseases'. The emic approach involves an evaluation of phenomena from within a culture and its context, aiming to understand their significance and relationship with other intra-cultural elements.

Drawbacks with the emic approach

'Pure' emic studies have also drawn their share of criticism. An important problem is that they are unable to provide data which can be compared across cultures. Emic studies are usually small in scale and are usually of insufficient size to address questions concerning the long-term course and treatment outcome (Kirmayer 1989). The reliability of emic studies may be limited by the lack of standardization of research methods. The emic approach has also been criticized for not suggesting plausible alternatives, such as a set of principles which would help ensure cultural sensitivity, or models upon which to fashion culturally sensitive nosologies (Beiser et al. 1994). It is argued that culture is not a static concept. All cultures are constantly evolving and changing and with the increasing influence of Euro-American values and urbanization in many low-income societies, 'traditional' beliefs may not be as rigidly held as is supposed. Furthermore, any individual may hold a multiplicity of ideas regarding his illness and any or all of these ideas may change with time (Eisenbruch 1990).

Integrating emic and etic approaches

Despite major strides in the international classification of mental disorders and in the ethnographic approach to studying mental illness, a truly international psychiatry does not exist. There are strengths and weaknesses of both the etic and emic approaches in cross-cultural psychiatry. It is widely accepted that the integration of their methodological strengths is essential for the development of the 'new cross-cultural psychiatry' or a culturally sensitive psychiatry (Kleinman 1987; Littlewood 1990). Value must be given to folk beliefs about mental illness as well as to the biomedical system of psychiatry. It is important to investigate patients' 'explanatory models' (i.e. how a patient understands a particular problem, its nature, origins, consequences, and likely remedies) since these can radically assist patient–doctor negotiations over appropriate treatment (Kleinman 1980). Similarly, researchers should investigate the psychiatric symptoms of individuals who are considered to be mentally ill by their local population and to determine the relationship of the diagnoses used by local health care providers with 'international' classification systems. In essence, the central aim of the 'new' cross-cultural psychiatry is to describe mental illness in different cultures using methods which are sensitive and valid for the local culture but which still result in data which can be reasonably compared between cultures. In order to tackle this difficult task, psychiatric research needs to blend both ethnographic and epidemiological methods, emphasizing the unique contribution of both approaches to the understanding of mental illness across cultures.

International psychiatry

Research bias

An important anomaly in cross-cultural psychiatry is that it is largely a speciality of interest to researchers and academics from developed countries. It is not accidental that the recent surge of interest in defining 'culture' within psychiatric research coincides with the spectacular demographic change in the ethnic composition of many developed countries. The majority of research initiated by researchers in developing countries mimics the etic approach and 'culture' is rarely considered adequately as an independent variable. Another major anomaly is that although Western societies are considered 'multicultural' (so that studies need to be conducted for different ethnic groups to ensure findings are 'culturally correct'), developing societies are not offered the same privilege. It is not uncommon to see studies from vast and hugely diverse countries such as India or China being cited in a way which suggests that findings are representative of the entire nation. Such naive assumptions have greatly limited the value of cross-cultural studies where national settings are chosen to represent cultural diversity. Research from Western cultures is considered to be of international significance whereas research from developing countries is of interest for its demonstration of the influence of culture on psychiatric disorders (Patel and Sumathipala 2001). The main limitation of cross-cultural psychiatry, of course, is that it fails to recognize that cultures are dynamic, complex social constructs which defy easy definition or measurement. Cultures are ever-changing, and herein lies the key factor which influences their role in international epidemiology. Globalization has had a phenomenal impact in this respect. No longer do cultures exist in isolation from one another so that attitudes, practices, and beliefs evolve in discrete settings. Instead, cultures are integrating, with values and beliefs from one culture finding new homes in others. While the process of globalization may work in diverse ways, in reality the cultures of industrialized societies are strongly dominant because most mechanisms of globalization, such as the media, are largely controlled by these nations. Societies across the developing world are undergoing dramatic changes and, in the process, differences between cultures are becoming less pronounced. In the face of this reality, one of the key rationales behind cross-cultural psychiatry is becoming increasingly questionable.

Health systems research

In considering methodologies for an international psychiatry, the concept of health systems research is relevant (Box 3.2). Health systems research (HSR) has been adopted as a model for conducting research which is directed to generating practical solutions to public health problems in a community. HSR offers a pragmatic model for investigating world mental health problems because it recognizes that mental illness and mental health care are profoundly influenced not only by culture or biology but also by the complex interaction of numerous social, political, economic, historical, and health service related factors, namely the various components of the health system. An advantage of the HSR approach is that there are likely to be far fewer types of health systems worldwide than different cultures. For example, even though urban Asian and African settings have substantial 'cultural' differences, they may share many health system characteristics, so that research in one setting may inform health services in the other. In contrast, urban and rural Asian settings, even though 'culturally' related, may differ so greatly in their health systems that research in one setting may have little practical relevance to health services in the other.

> ## Box 3.2 **Key principles for health systems research**
>
> - Incorporate a range of variables which describe the health system.
> - Identify priority problems through discussions with service users and providers.
> - Develop problem-orientated objectives for the research programme.
> - Consider the ethical context for the research.
> - Achieve a multi-disciplinary input into the research programme through participatory methodology.
> - Consider the cost-effectiveness of the proposed research programme.
> - Ensure that research findings are adequately communicated to the agencies who will use them.
> - Evaluate the impact of the research.

Objectives for an international psychiatry

Mental illness has acquired considerable global public health attention as a result of recent reports which have focused on the high prevalence and associated disability of mental disorders. However, much of the research on mental illness is derived from a small fraction of the world's population in developed countries (Patel and Sumathipala 2001). In particular, there is a great paucity of relevant health services and interventional research from developing countries. The present state of the psychiatric literature is limiting the growth of the subject itself, since the aetiology of diseases may well be better understood through research carried out in different environments, and innovative treatments are more likely to be discovered by studying practices in a wider global context. From a regional perspective, however, the damage is even greater. Psychiatry as a biomedical discipline has had its roots in Europe and is a relatively young discipline in most countries. Its history in many countries is tainted by its association with colonial-era asylums and terrible abuse of human rights. Many of these abuses continue. Removing stigma from psychiatry will need greater space for research from these countries on international platforms to demonstrate that original and innovative, locally generated programs on mental health care are feasible and successful.

Priorities for international research on mental illness need to move well beyond its current focus on investigating cultural influences, towards action-oriented research which serves to inform regional health policy and practice. Health policy is unlikely to be influenced by research while its findings consist only of the astronomical numbers of persons with mental illness thrown up regularly by surveys, and where no attention has been paid to demonstrating affordable solutions for these problems. Cultural models, pharmacodynamic factors, health service variations and drug availability, are likely to vary substantially throughout the world. A major research priority must therefore be the international evaluation of efficacy and cost-effectiveness with respect to health service interventions and individual-level treatments. These issues have received very little research attention to date (Patel 2000).

A second major research priority is to clarify the relationship between mental disorders and other health priorities. In many developing countries, child development, poverty alleviation, reproductive health, and violence are the major priorities. Mental health issues have obvious relevance for addressing these. For example, learning disabilities are associated with poor school performance and discontinuation of education; poverty is linked to depression and suicide; reproductive health is associated with post-natal depression; and violence is associated with substance abuse and depression. Mental health research, by working within the framework of existing priorities can generate practical information which is of value to existing health programs. In turn, this is likely to make mental health research more amenable to wider acceptance and implementation. Such research is often relatively cheap to implement since it can be 'piggy-backed' on to existing programmes in other fields.

An ethical imperative for international epidemiological research is the empowerment of local health researchers to conduct and lead research programs. Raising capacity must be a core element of all research in developing countries, most of all in the field of psychiatry where these skills are extremely difficult to obtain. A 'dash-in-dash-out' research strategy has dubious ethical standards, where highly skilled researchers from developed countries 'collaborate' with economically and academically weaker colleagues in developing countries to carry out research programs with little local capacity building. Dissemination must be multifaceted: targeting policy makers, health care providers, and the general community. Thus, the objectives of a truly international psychiatry are to establish psychiatry as a relevant medical discipline with strong public health roots in all nations of the world.

Research methodology

The two major academic disciplines at the root of cross-cultural psychiatry are epidemiology and anthropology. The research methods used by these disciplines apply in the same way when studies are conducted in non-Western cultures. Here, we will only consider some key issues to be considered in the method of conducting psychiatric research in different cultures.

General principles of health systems research

The key principles in conducting an HSR investigation (Varkevisser *et al.* 1991) are the following.

(1) *Incorporating a range of health system variables*: An essential component of any epidemiological or health services research investigations is a comprehensive understanding of the variables which define the health system (Fig. 3.1).

(2) *Focusing on priority problems*: Priorities need to be determined in consultation with local health care providers and community leaders. For example, health workers may wish to research how best to manage those persons who consult repeatedly for commonly recognized psychological disorders. Focus group discussions and key informant interviews are useful methods to elicit the priorities and attitudes of stakeholders who will ultimately use the research findings.

(3) *Action-oriented research*: 'Problem-oriented' research aims to take the priorities of health workers and the policy makers and devise action-oriented research questions. For example, what form of treatment at primary care can help reduce the duration and severity of depressive illness? What are the causes of children dropping out of school? What is the impact of postnatal depression on maternal and child health? Answers to these research questions

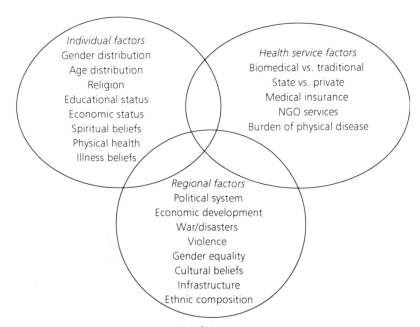

Fig. 3.1 Examples of variables which define a health system.

should lead to ways in which mental illnesses may be more appropriately managed or prevented.

(4) *Multidisciplinary approach*: Academic psychiatrists, particularly in low-income countries, are not representative of mental health care in their societies. Most societies now have a significant private medical sector, particularly general practitioners, who provide the bulk of mental health care. Public health facilities in many countries, particularly in Africa, are manned mainly by nurses. Traditional medical practitioners may outnumber biomedical health workers even in urban areas. Non-governmental organizations (NGOs) play an increasingly important role in community and primary health care initiatives in low-income countries. These agencies tend to focus their activities on communities or groups which are particularly disadvantaged or vulnerable. Rarely do academic psychiatrists take notice of the rich clinical experiences of health workers in these settings—and rarely do non-psychiatric health workers take notice of advances in psychiatric research. The involvement of these different groups of health workers is an essential feature of any successful HSR model.

(5) *Participatory methodology*: Most psychiatric research in developing countries is conceptualized and designed in isolation from the front line of mental health care. The participatory approach involves working from within the health system, by becoming part of it and intimately familiar with all its components and actors. Thus, research objectives arise out of the direct experience and consultations with the users and beneficiaries of the research itself.

(6) *Dissemination*: It is imperative that health systems research is published in local journals, newspapers, and in cheaply produced reports for circulation to the concerned target audience. In this context, researchers should recognize the far greater impact of lay and popular magazines for disseminating findings to the wider community and broaden the scope of their activities to include advocacy for mental health issues through the popular media.

(7) *Evaluation of research*: This is the litmus test of the usefulness of research. Measuring attitudes and practice at various points of a research program is a one method of evaluating the broader impact of the research on actual health care. The implementation of health policy changes in the direction of the research findings is the most potent marker of the success of a HSR program.

(8) *Ethics of research*: This is an extremely important issue, particularly for experimental studies where new interventions are being studied or for invasive studies where biological specimens are to be collected. Ensuring that all research is approved and monitored by a local ethics board should be mandatory.

However, many parts of the world still do not have such systems in place. In such circumstances, the investigator must ensure:

- that participants in the study are not denied treatments known to be effective and which are available to them in the care they receive;
- that all participants are given full information about the project, including a clear statement that their usual care will not be affected in any way by their decision;
- if possible, obtain written consent after such information is provided. However, the participant should not be forced to sign, especially a participant who cannot read or write. In this instance, an independent observer, such as a relative or nurse, could sign the form as a witness to the consent procedure.

Choosing a study setting

In terms of study setting, cross-cultural psychiatric research has adopted two types of study designs.

(1) *International comparative studies*: These are studies which are conducted in different cultures with similar methodologies and pooled analyses. The best examples of these are the WHO sponsored multinational studies. For example, the study on mental disorders in primary care is an excellent example of the multinational study design favoured by the WHO Division of Mental Health with its emphasis on standardization of methodologies in four developing countries to the extent that the same cut-off score was used for case detection for the psychiatric screening questionnaire despite the fact that this score varied widely between the four settings (Harding *et al.* 1980). The International Pilot Studies for Schizophrenia, the reliability studies for various WHO interview schedules and the field studies to validate diagnostic categories are further examples. The strength of these studies lies in the ability for findings from different settings to be compared which, in turn, can be valuable to test aetiological hypotheses. On the other hand, the validity of the findings may be compromised by the emphasis placed on the standardization of methodologies. Furthermore, the studies are most often 'top-down' in their planning and implementation, rarely involving participation of users and field level researchers.

(2) *Studies within one setting*: Two distinct groups of studies are included in this section. First, studies conducted in countries with cultures different to Euro-American culture, such as developing countries. Some of these studies use an ethnographic approach to describe indigenous models or types of mental illness, as discussed later in the chapter. There are several examples of classical epidemiological study designs in single settings. Perhaps the

best-known community survey of psychiatric disorder is Orley and Wing's (1979) work in Uganda which was notable for its setting (one of the few published community studies from rural Africa), its use of structured interviews for psychiatric diagnosis, and its extensive discussion on the various difficulties encountered in using an etic interview in this setting. The case control study by Patel *et al.* (1997*a*) of factors associated with common mental disorders in Harare, Zimbabwe is notable for its sampling of attenders at traditional medical practitioners, general practitioners, and government primary care clinics reflecting the nature of medical pluralism in primary care, and for its use of a locally developed case-detection questionnaire and potential risk factor variables.

A second group comprises studies of different cultural groups in multicultural societies. Good examples of studies of this kind can be found in research from societies where there has been a surge in migration in recent years, notably the USA, Canada, Western Europe, and Australia. Some studies have used the fact that peoples of a specific ethnic origin may now live in different societies to study the aetiology of psychiatric disorders. For example, substantially lower incidence rates of dementia in a Nigerian compared to an African-American population have generated potentially important new aetiological hypotheses (Hendrie *et al.* 2001). The differing rates of diagnosis of schizophrenia in black people in the UK has led to research on the epidemiology of schizophrenia in different communities within the UK and comparisons with rates reported from Caribbean nations. For example, an incidence study from Barbados found that the rates were far lower than those of the emigrant group suggesting that environmental factors, as opposed to genetic factors, were important determinants (Mahy *et al.* 1999). However, while the outcome of psychotic illness is similar in the immigrant group as compared to white Britons, if anything social outcomes and disability seemed better (Goater *et al.* 1999; Harrison *et al.* 1999).

Selecting the variables

Culture is not the only, or even the main, variable which differentiates populations in different parts of the world. The Health Systems Model explicitly recognizes the role of many variables in influencing the aetiology, expression, and management of mental disorders. It is important for a research investigation to be familiar with the distribution of some of these variables and their local significance in planning the investigation and including them in the data collection forms. Examples of the types of variables which should be considered in epidemiological investigations are shown in Fig. 3.1.

Studying indigenous models of illness

One of the key issues in a culturally sensitive psychiatric epidemiology is the recognition that all cultures have indigenous illness taxonomies. By understanding these taxonomies and their relationship to biomedical classifications, it may be possible to evolve a psychiatric epidemiology which bridges the conceptual gap between biomedical and indigenous categories of illness. Typically, the methods used are qualitative and descriptive such as key informant interviews and focus group discussions and case series. There are many such examples of studies of indigenous models of illness.

* Makanjuola (1987) described the symptoms of a category of disorder recognized by Yoruba traditional healers in Nigeria by carrying out in-depth interviews with 30 patients diagnosed to suffer this disorder by healers.

* Patel *et al.* (1995) described local concepts of mental illness using focus group discussions with a range of care providers in Harare, Zimbabwe. Participants in the groups were asked to describe conditions considered as mental illnesses, their causes and treatments.

* Nations *et al.* (1988) described a folk idiom in common use in English-speaking populations and demonstrate its close association with biomedical constructs of anxiety and depression.

* Littlewood (1985) described 'tabanka', an indigenous model of depression which afflicts men in Trinidad, and its sociocultural contexts.

Measurement and diagnosis: using etic instruments

Since epidemiological research relies essentially on the identification of 'cases' of a particular disease or illness, and since psychiatric caseness is entirely determined by scores on interviews or questionnaires, the validity of such measures is an important aspect of a culturally sensitive epidemiology. Perhaps the most difficult issue in psychiatric epidemiology is the lack of a reliable and independent laboratory indicator of psychiatric disorder. In Euro-American cultures where psychiatric classifications originate, standardized interviews such as the Revised Clinical Interview Schedule (Lewis *et al.* 1992) or the CIDI (WHO 1990) are used as the gold standard on the grounds that they closely mirror a full psychiatric examination. However, as discussed earlier, the validity of the concepts of psychiatric classification in other cultures is unresolved and thus the use of such interviews may impose an etic bias. An emic alternative is the use of patient self-assessment or care provider diagnoses as the criterion of caseness. However, a weakness of these criteria are the lack of standardization and reliability. A compromise which bridges the emic and etic approaches would be an agreement between the two sets of criteria for determining the

Box 3.3 **Issues to consider in the translation of etic instruments**

- ◆ Content equivalence (the existence of the measured phenomenon in the second culture).
- ◆ Semantic equivalence (the meaning of individual questionnaire items).
  - • Denotative (their literal meaning).
  - • Connotative (their 'emotional' meaning).
- ◆ Technical equivalence (the appropriateness of the instrument administration in the second culture).
- ◆ Criterion equivalence (relationships with other established criteria).
- ◆ Conceptual equivalence (the extent to which the same underlying construct is being measured in the second culture).

gold standard of caseness. This is often very difficult in practice, and a route which is generally agreed by most researchers in developing countries is the use of etic instruments after careful translation and validation.

Etic studies start with instruments developed in one culture (to date, always a Euro-American culture). These are then translated and applied to another culture. Most cross-cultural studies use this methodology. Given the central importance of language in expressing symptoms, the translation of the instrument is perhaps the single most important step in etic studies (Box 3.3). The translated version should be evaluated on a number of different parameters (Flaherty *et al.* 1988; Sartorius 1993):

(1) *Content equivalence*: Does the phenomenon in question actually occur in the culture and is it noticed by members of the culture? Thus, finding that depression is very common in a society, but that no one seems to recognize it, raises questions about the content validity of the construct itself.

(2) *Semantic equivalence*: Does the meaning of each item remain the same after translation? Both *denotative* and *connotative* equivalence need to be evaluated; the former can be examined by using dictionaries and relies mainly on linguistic analyses, while the latter refers to the 'emotional' meaning and can be studied through ethnographic analysis.

(3) *Technical equivalence*: Does the method of data collection affect results differentially between two cultures? For example, semi-structured interviews such as the Present State Examination in South Africa have been

found to have suboptimal technical equivalence because the Xhosa-speaking people find the direct interviewing style intimidatory (Swartz *et al.* 1985).

(4) *Criterion equivalence:* What is an instrument's relationship with previously established and independent criteria for the same phenomena?

(5) *Conceptual equivalence:* Does the instrument measure the same construct in different cultures? This is difficult to determine, although it may be judged according to the relationships between constructs as measured by the instrument and a comparison with other studies.

Examples of studies which attempt to achieve such validity are few. The following studies are good examples of methodologies used to achieve cultural validation of etic instruments:

- Manson *et al.* (1985) aimed to produce a culturally valid epidemiology of depression among the Hopi Indians of North America. They utilized ethnosemantic techniques to elicit both indigenous categories and symptoms of illness which were then incorporated into the Diagnostic Interview Schedule. As well as using standard techniques of translation and backtranslation, this study was unique in its attempt to take into account Hopi meanings divergent from those of biomedical psychiatry which underpinned the psychiatric interview. Five Hopi categories of illness were included in the instrument and subsequent analysis showed a close relationship between one indigenous category and depressive disorder.

- Bravo *et al.* (1991) adapted the Diagnostic Interview Schedule for use in Puerto Rico by subjecting the interview to a range of tests. Semantic equivalence was evaluated by the translation–backtranslation method; content equivalence was estimated by a bilingual committee and subjecting the interview to a study with case and non-case samples; technical equivalence was achieved by identifying and modifying those items which were poorly comprehended or which failed to convey their psychiatric intent; and criterion and conceptual equivalence were assessed by comparing DIS-generated diagnoses with those of local psychiatrists.

- Mumford *et al.* (1991a) translated the Hospital Anxiety and Depression Scale for use with Urdu speaking patients in the UK. The interview was translated by 6 bilingual translators, backtranslated by another 6, and discrepancies were resolved by a team of 5 bilingual mental health professionals. The English and Urdu versions of the test were administered to a sample of bilingual students in Pakistan; half the students received the English version first whilst the other half received the Urdu version. Both groups were then administered the other language version; this cross-over design ensured that any systematic test–retest discrepancies in the scores were ruled out. Scores were then compared to estimate conceptual equivalence (using rank order correlation), linguistic equivalence (by comparing mean scores) and scale equivalence (by estimating whether the two versions identified the same individuals as high-scorers).

◆ Sumathipala and Murray (2001) describe the use of both quantitative and qualitative methods in the translation of an inventory of somatic symptoms for administration in Sinhala. A panel of nine people individually translated the items and then rated all the available translations for conceptual and semantic equivalence. Translations failing to reach consensus were discussed by the group for modifications and subjected to further discussion to achieve consensus.

Measurement and diagnosis: using emic instruments

Two types of instruments are considered here: instruments developed from within a particular culture to measure mental disorder; and instruments developed to assess the explanatory models of persons with mental disorders. There have been a number of attempts at developing methods of assessment for psychiatric disorder from within a culture. Examples of innovative methodologies are described below:

◆ Studies by Beiser and colleagues with the Serer people of Senegal predate the emic–etic debates by a nearly a decade (Beiser *et al.* 1976). Their methodology closely followed the recommendations of the new cross-cultural psychiatry with ethnographic work setting the stage for eliciting a local taxonomy of mental illness and lexicon of Serer disease terms. A group of patients with 'illnesses of the spirit' were interviewed, showing that these illnesses were closely related to psychiatric concepts of mental illness. The research group then further developed an interview schedule based on a pre-existing questionnaire and the lexicon of disease terms and administered it to a community sample. Factor analysis of the data revealed four dimensions used by the Serer to express neurotic disturbances: physiological anxiety, topical depression, health preoccupation, and episodic anxiety.

◆ Kinzie *et al.* (1982) described the development of a Vietnamese language rating scale for depression. Items were derived from (i) the Beck Depression inventory, (ii) Vietnamese terms elicited from a lexicon generated by bilingual mental health workers, (iii) somatic symptoms frequently presented by Vietnamese patients, and (iv) items designed to tap the behavioural and somatic symptoms of depression. The scale was then administered to samples of cases and non-cases and 15 items were found to distinguish these groups. Of these 15 items, 10 were unrelated to either lowered mood or the Western concept of depression.

◆ The Bradford Somatic Inventory (BSI) developed in the UK for use with patients from the Indian subcontinent (Mumford *et al.* 1991*b*) emphasized the important role of somatic symptoms in the expression of emotional distress. The BSI consisted of somatic symptoms recorded in the case notes of patients in the UK and Pakistan. These items were checked against the case-notes of patients in India and Nepal and over 90% coverage of all somatic symptoms was achieved. The Urdu and English versions were then administered to bilingual students in Pakistan to determine linguistic equivalence. Conceptual equivalence was determined by studying the factor analysis of responses by patients with functional disorders in Britain and Pakistan.

◆ The Chinese Health Questionnaire (CHQ) was developed with the 30-item General Health Questionnaire as a starting point (Cheng *et al.* 1990). An additional 30 items based on the Chinese concepts of illness such as the concern about the heat and coldness of food, were added. The resulting 60-item questionnaire was validated against a standardized psychiatric interview. The final questionnaire consisted of 12 items which discriminated cases best: half originated from the GHQ and the remainder were emic items.

◆ The Shona Symptom Questionnaire: this 12-item questionnaire was developed through a step-wise process in Harare, Zimbabwe (Patel *et al.* 1997*b*). The first step was to elicit ethnographic data on indigenous concepts of mental disorders. This was followed by the generation of a lexicon of idioms of distress through descriptive interviews with patients identified by care providers as suffering from mental illness. These idioms were then evaluated in another study against emic and etic criteria for caseness. The items with the best discriminating ability formed the Shona Symptom Questionnaire. It was noted that most items were similar to those found in Western screening questionnaires. This exercise was a lesson that the symptoms of mental disorder may, indeed, be universal in their diagnostic sensitivity and specificity, and that a valid translation of an etic instrument could be as useful as a home-grown emic instrument (Patel and Todd 1996).

There are several instruments which have been developed to elicit the attributions and beliefs about illness from individual patients. Much of this literature has its roots in sociology of health and illness. Here, we will only consider two such instruments which have been extensively applied to the study of mental illnesses.

◆ The Short Explanatory Model Interview (SEMI). The SEMI is an interview which is derived from Kleinman's explanatory model concept and is aimed to elicit a person's view about their illness. The main advantage of this interview is its simple, open-ended question format and its brevity (a rare asset in the field of medical anthropology!) which enables it to be incorporated as part of ongoing epidemiological studies. This interview can help provide contextual information on symptoms by describing, for example, the patients' views about their cause or outcome (Lloyd *et al.* 1998).

◆ The Explanatory Model Interview Catalogue (EMIC) is a comprehensive interview which explores in depth the explanatory models of illness. Patterns of distress, perceived causes, preferences for help seeking and treatment, and general illness beliefs constitute the framework for the operational formulation of the illness explanatory model (Weiss 1997). The EMIC generates both quantitative and qualitative data which can be cross-referenced in analysis of the explanatory models. The EMIC has been extensively used in developing countries with a wide variety of illnesses.

Conclusion

The study of the epidemiology of mental disorders and their treatments in different cultures and health systems provides an important opportunity for unravelling aetiological factors underlying mental disorders and for discovering new effective treatments. There is a large body of work which serves to guide future research in different cultural settings. This evidence shows that although symptoms of mental disorders can be elicited in most cultures, taxonomies may differ considerably. Instruments developed in one culture may be used in other cultures, but great emphasis needs to be placed on their translation to ensure conceptual validity. Study designs need to incorporate a range of health system variables to ensure the findings are relevant to local health policy. A variety of research methodologies have been used to achieve these goals. Research must be planned in collaboration with potential users and a range of dissemination strategies should be considered. These principles form the basis for the growth of a truly international psychiatric epidemiology.

Practice exercise

You wish to conduct an epidemiological investigation to determine the number of people with dementia in a multi-cultural urban community in a low-income country. The ultimate objective is to use the findings as a guide for the development of services for elderly people with dementia. Develop a study design to conduct this investigation, keeping in mind the principles of health systems research and cultural factors discussed earlier. In particular, consider the following issues:

1. How would you develop the study proposal itself? (i.e. who, for what purpose and how would you consult with?)

2. What variables (and why) would you consider important to measure?

3. How would you ensure the validity of the interview you use for the diagnosis of dementia?

4. What are the ethical issues you would consider?

5. How, and to whom, would the study findings be disseminated?

References

Beiser, M., Benfari, R.C., Collomb, H., and Ravel, J. (1976) Measuring psychoneurotic behaviour in cross-cultural surveys. *Journal of Nervous and Mental Disease*, **163**, 10–23.

Beiser, M., Cargo, M., and Woodbury, M. (1994) A comparison of psychiatric disorder in different cultures: depressive typologies in South-East Asian refugees and resident Canadians. *International Journal of Methods in Psychiatric Research*, **4**, 157–72.

Bravo, M., Canino, G.J., Rubio-Stipec, M., and Woodbury-Farina, M. (1991) A cross-cultural adaptation of a psychiatric epidemiologic instrument: The Diagnostic Interview Schedule's adaptation in Puerto Rico. *Culture, Medicine and Psychiatry*, **15**, 1–18.

Cheng, T.A., Wu, J.T., Chong, M.Y., and Williams, P. (1990) Internal consistency and factor structure of the Chinese Health Questionnaire. *Acta Psychiatrica Scandinavica*, **82**, 304–08.

Eisenbruch, M. (1990) Classification of natural and supernatural causes of mental distress. *Journal of Nervous and Mental Disease*, **178**, 712–19.

Eisenbruch, M. (1991) From post-traumatic stress disorder to cultural bereavement: diagnosis of Southeast Asian refugees. *Social Science and Medicine*, **33**, 673–80.

Flaherty, J.A., Gaviria, F.M., Pathak, D., Mitchell, T., Wintrob, R., Richman, J.A., and Birz, S. (1988) Developing instruments for cross-cultural psychiatric research. *Journal of Nervous and Mental Disease*, **176**, 257–63.

Goater, N., King, M., Cole, E., Leavey, G., Johnson-Sabine, E., Blizard, R., and Hoar, A. (1999) Ethnicity and outcome of psychosis. *British Journal of Psychiatry*, **175**, 34–42.

Harding, T.W., De Arango, M.V., Baltazar, J., Climent, C.E., Ibrahim, H.H.A., Ladrigo-Ignacio, L., Srinivasa Murthy, R., and Wig, N.N. (1980) Mental disorders in primary health care: a study of their frequency and diagnosis in four developing countries. *Psychological Medicine*, **10**, 231–41.

Harrison, G., Amin, S., Singh, S.P., Croudace, T., and Jones, P. (1999) Outcome of psychosis in people of African-Caribbean origin. Population based first episode study. *British Journal of Psychiatry*, **175**, 43–49.

Heggenhougen, K. and Draper, A. (1990) *Medical Anthropology and Primary Health Care*, EPC Publication No. 22. London School of Hygiene and Tropical Medicine, London.

Hendrie, H., Ogunniyi, A., Hall, K., Baiyewu, O., Unverzagt, F.W., Gureje, O., Gao, S., Evans, R.M., Ogunseyinde, A.O., Adeyinka, A.O., Musick, B., and Hui, S. (2001) Incidence of dementia and Alzheimer disease in 2 communities. *Journal of the American Medical Association*, **285**, 739–47.

Kinzie, J.D., Manson, S.M., Vinh, D.T., Tolan, N.T., Anh, B., and Pho, T.N. (1982) Development and Validation of a Vietnamese-Language Depression Rating Scale. *American Journal of Psychiatry*, **139**, 1276–81.

Kirmayer, L.J. (1989) Cultural variations in the response to psychiatric disorders and emotional distress. *Social Science and Medicine*, **29**, 327–39.

Kleinman, A. (1980) *Patients and healers in the context of culture*. University of California Press, Berkeley.

Kleinman, A. (1987) Anthropology and Psychiatry: the role of culture in cross-cultural research on illness. *British Journal of Psychiatry*, **151**, 447–54.

Lewis, G., Pelosi, A., Araya, R., and Dunn, G. (1992) Measuring psychiatric disorder in the community: a standardized assessment for use by lay interviewers. *Psychological Medicine*, **22**, 465–86.

Littlewood, R. (1985) An indigenous conceptualization of reactive depression in Trindad. *Psychological Medicine*, **15**, 275–81.

Littlewood, R. (1990) From categories to contexts: a decade of the 'New Cross-Cultural Psychiatry'. *British Journal of Psychiatry*, **156**, 308–27.

Lloyd, K., Jacob, K., Patel, V., St.Louis, L., and Mann, A. (1998) The development of The Short Explanatory Model Interview (SEMI) and its use among primary care attenders with common mental disorders: a preliminary report. *Psychological Medicine*, **28**, 1231–7.

Mahy, G.E., Mallett, R., Leff, J., and Bhugra, D. (1999) First-contact incidence rate of schizophrenia on Barbados. *British Journal of Psychiatry*, **175**, 28–33.

Makanjuola, R.O. (1987) 'Ode Ori': a culture-bound disorder with prominent somatic features in Yoruba Nigerian patients. *Acta Psychiatrica Scandinavica*, **75**, 231–6.

Manson, S.M., Shore, J.H., and Bloom, J.D. (1985) The depressive experience in American Indian communities: A challenge for psychiatric theory and diagnosis. In *Culture and Depression* (ed. A. Kleinman and B. Good), pp. 331–68. University of California Press, Berkeley.

Mumford, D.B., Tareen, I.A.K., Bajwa, M.A.Z., Bhatti, M.R., and Karim, R. (1991a) The transalation and evaluation of an Urdu version of the Hospital Anxiety and Depression Scale. *Acta Psychiatrica Scandinavica*, **83**, 81–85.

Mumford, D.B., Bavington, J.T., Bhatnagar, K.S., Hussain, Y., Mirza, S., and Naraghi, M.M. (1991b) The Bradford Somatic Inventory: a multiethnic inventory of somatic symptoms reported by anxious and depressed patients in Britain and the Indo-Pakistan subcontinent. *British Journal of Psychiatry*, **158**, 379–86.

Murphy, H.B.M. (1982) *Comparative Psychiatry: The International & Intercultural Distribution of Mental Illness*. Springer-Verlag, Berlin.

Nations, M., Camino, L., and Walker, F. (1988) Nerves: folk idiom for anxiety and depression? *Social Science and Medicine*, **26**, 1245–59.

Orley, J. and Wing, J.K. (1979) Psychiatric disorder in two African villages. *Archives of General Psychiatry*, **36**, 513–20.

Patel, V. (2000) Why we need treatment evidence for common mental disorders in developing countries. *Psychological Medicine* **30**, 743–6.

Patel, V. and Sumathipala, A. (2001) International Representation in Psychiatric Journals: a survey of 6 leading journals. *British Journal of Psychiatry*, **178**, 406–9.

Patel, V. and Todd, C.H. (1996) The validity of the Shona version of the Self Report Questionnaire (SRQ) and the development of the SRQ8. *International Journal of Methods in Psychiatric Research*, **6**, 153–60.

Patel, V. and Winston, M. (1994) The 'universality' of mental disorder revisited: assumptions, artefacts and new directions. *British Journal of Psychiatry*, **165**, 437–40.

Patel, V., Musara, T., Maramba, P., and Butau, T. (1995) Concepts of Mental Illness and Medical Pluralism in Harare. *Psychological Medicine*, **25**, 485–93.

Patel, V., Todd, C.H., Winston, M., Gwanzura, F., Simunyu, E., Acuda, S.W., and Mann, A. (1997*a*) Common Mental Disorders in primary care in Harare, Zimbabwe: associations & risk factors. *British Journal of Psychiatry*, **171**, 60–4.

Patel, V., Simunyu, E., Gwanzura, F., Lewis, G., and Mann, A. (1997*b*) The Shona Symptom Questionnaire: the development of an indigenous measure of non-psychotic mental disorder in Harare. *Acta Psychiatrica Scandinavica*, **95**, 469–75.

Sartorius, N. (1993) SCAN translation. In *Diagnosis and Clinical Measurements in Psychiatry: a Reference Manual for the SCAN system* (ed. J. Wing, N. Sartorius, and T. B. Ustun), Cambridge University Press, London.

Sen, B. and Mari, J. (1986) Psychiatric research instruments in the transcultural setting: experiences in India and Brazil. *Social Science and Medicine*, **23**, 277–81.

Sumathipala, A. and Murray, J. (2001) New approach to translating instruments for cross-cultural research: a combined qualitative and quantitative approach for translations and consensus generation. *International Journal of Methods in Psychiatric Research*, **9**, 87–95.

Swartz, L., Ben-Arie, O., and Teggin, A. (1985) Subcultural delusions and hallucinations: comments on the present state examination in a multi-cultural context. *British Journal of Psychiatry*, **146**, 391–4.

Varkevisser, C.M., Pathmanathan, I., and Brownlee, A. (1991) *Designing and conducting health systems research projects; Vol. 2, Part 1 (proposal development and fieldwork)*, IDRC and WHO, Ottawa and Geneva.

Weiss, M. (1997) Explanatory Model Interview Catalogue (EMIC): framework for comparative study of illness. *Transcultural Psychiatry*, **34**(2), 235–63.

Williams, P., Tarnopolsky, A., and Hand, D. (1980) Case definition and case identification: review and assessment. *Psychological Medicine*, **10**, 101–14.

World Health Organization. (1990) *Composite International Diagnostic Interview (CIDI)*. World Health Organization, Geneva.

Chapter 4

Ethics and research in psychiatry

Anthony S. Kessel and Francesca Silverton

Introduction

This chapter explores ethical issues that arise from research in psychiatry. To a large degree the issues are the same as those generic to other areas of health-care research. Psychiatric research does, however, through the nature of its research participants, direct special attention to issues such as competence and consent. Literature in the field of psychiatric research ethics is not extensive, but growing (Block and Chodoff 1991; Kessel 1998; Roberts *et al.* 1998).

The chapter is structured in the following way. First there is an introduction to ethics and the principles of biomedical ethics. Next the chapter looks at what makes an action morally acceptable and how this relates to healthcare research—an ethical assessment template is provided. The chapter then considers issues of particular pertinence to psychiatry, competence and consent, and finishes by touching upon emerging area of ethical interest in psychiatric research—genetics and confidentiality.

What is ethics?

The word ethics is derived from the Greek word 'ethos', which means custom. In this sense—which is essentially the lay sense—the word ethics refers to the general beliefs, attitudes, or standards that guide customary or community behaviour. As a philosophical term ethics is the branch of philosophy that involves the theoretical study of the principles that guide human conduct. In Socrates' words moral philosophy is the study of 'how we ought to live', and why. Ethical considerations imbue many aspects of our everyday lives, but particular considerations apply to particular circumstances. Biomedical research is one such area.

Ethics, research, and psychiatry

The relationship between ethical aspects of medicine and ethical aspects of medical research is complex. Ethical issues particular to research in medicine are considered by ethics committees, but research can also be viewed as a part of medical practice itself, since clinicians ought to be using research to further medical understanding. This normative claim is strengthened by recognizing that the testing of clinical techniques may be a moral imperative since clinical practices subject to inadequate testing could lead to harmful consequences (Wing 1991).

In psychiatry, new drugs are naturally tested before use. However, this is not necessarily so evident with social treatments, for example the concept of the 'total institution' was accepted into the structure of the psychiatric service with little research. This chapter is an attempt to create a framework for those working in psychiatry to use in addressing possible ethical issues in research.

Principles of biomedical ethics

Biomedical ethics, a term synonymous with medical ethics or healthcare ethics, can be used to create a framework for psychiatric research ethics. Biomedical ethics developed as a discipline of its own in the United States in the 1960s. Within biomedical ethics 'principlism'—first advocated by the American philosophers Beauchamp and Childress (1989)—has emerged as the most popular way of thinking.

Principlism argues that any medico-ethical dilemma can be analysed and discussed with reference to four principles—respect for autonomy, non-maleficence, beneficence, and justice Box 4.1. Principlism makes the claim that whatever our personal beliefs, we should be able to commit ourselves to these principles, which are held to be *prima facie*. This means that that any one of the principles are binding unless the principle conflicts with another principle. If the principles conflict, then we have to choose between them using some other moral theory or belief.

Box 4.1 **Principlism**

Principlism: any medical ethical dilemma can be analysed with reference to the following principles

- Respect for autonomy
- Non-maleficence
- Beneficence
- Justice

The rise of biomedical ethics, as well as principlism itself, has been heavily criticized, and there are several other approaches taken towards medical ethics. In particular, the four principles approach does not provide any method for choosing between conflicting principles. What the approach does provide is a common set of moral commitments, a moral language, and a set of moral issues as a framework for analysing problems. Awareness of the principles, their basic meaning and application is thus useful when thinking about research ethics (Gillon 1994).

The principle of respect for autonomy

Autonomy, or self-rule, is an attribute of all persons. If someone has autonomy, then she can make decisions that are deliberated. The idea of respect for autonomy is the moral obligation to respect other persons. In more detail, autonomy is not only the idea of individual self-rule, but the notion of autonomy extends to include (a) remaining free from both the controlling interference of others and also (b) any inadequate understanding, which could prevent meaningful choices being made. A person of diminished autonomy is restricted in some way of (a) or (b) above. However it is important to note that autonomous persons may make non-autonomous choices such as signing a consent form without reading it.

Some authors prefer to focus on autonomous choices, rather than autonomous persons. This is a choice made intentionally, with understanding, and without controlling influences. Intention is usually considered to be present or absent, while the other two criteria are a matter of degree. Being autonomous and choosing autonomously is not the same as being respected as an autonomous agent. This involves recognising both the person's capacities and perspectives, including his right to hold views, make choices, and to take actions based on personal values and beliefs, and allowing or enabling persons to act autonomously. This means that true respect includes acting to respect others, not the mere adoption of a particular attitude.

In healthcare, the principle of respect for autonomy places a *prima facie* obligation or duty on practitioners to obtain informed consent from patients, keep medical confidentiality, not deceive others (e.g. about diagnosis) and communicate well with patients and research participants.

Non-maleficence and beneficence

The principle of non-maleficence is perhaps best captured in the common maxim *primum non nocere*, which means 'above all (first) do no harm'. The principle of beneficence, or the positive act of helping others, is summed up by the idea that one ought to do or promote good. Beneficence is separate from but does, in some sense, operate together with non-maleficence, as interventions aimed at help others may risk doing harm.

Beauchamp and Childress argue that the obligation of non-maleficence is not only distinct but often more stringent than obligations to take positive efforts to benefit others. Gillon, however, believes we should consider non-maleficence and beneficence together, aiming to produce a balance of benefit over harm. Further, when there is no recognition of need for beneficence to others, we still have an obligation to do no harm.

In order to achieve these moral objectives, Gillon purports that healthcare workers are committed to a range of obligations which include rigorous and effective educational programmes, respect for an individual's autonomy with regard to what constitutes benefit for that patient, and finally clarity about risk and probability in assessment of harm and benefit.

Whether one perceives these principles as separate or not, the concept of harm or injury is central. Injury may refer to harm, disability, death, injustice or wrong. Harm should not be thought of too narrowly but considered as thwarting, defeating or setting back the interests (both mental or physical) of one party by the actions of another party.

Two additional points are of particular importance when considering research ethics. First, duties of non-maleficence relate to the imposition of *risks* of harm as well as the imposition of actual harms. Second, although in medical care there is an assumed beneficent goal in promoting the welfare and health of the patient, in healthcare research the beneficent goal is more complex.

For example, in therapeutic research the participants are likely to benefit themselves with potential parallel benefits to others, but in non-therapeutic research participants are unlikely to gain personally. Ethics committees generally conclude that benefits have to be substantial to justify more than minimal risk in the case of non-therapeutic research.

In medicine, the balancing of beneficence and non-maleficence is particularly difficult in developing areas, where harms and benefits may not be well established (Wing 1991). For example, in the introduction of new medication for schizophrenia and the manic and depressive disorders, what may be harmful and what may be beneficial is often unclear. In these cases decisions have to be made by the doctor and patient together, after a consideration of both the risks and the benefits of treatment.

Typical research projects involve little probability of inflicting harm. However, there is a defined 'minimally acceptable risk' for research to guide researchers (Royal College of Physicians of London 1989). Minimal risk encompasses a range of possibilities from a negligible level of psychological or physical distress, such as a transitory mild headache or feeling of lethargy to a very remote chance of a serious injury or death, if the risk is analogous to that of travelling as a passenger on public transport.

The Medical Research Council specifies in detail the conditions to be met in selecting patients for research trials. Clinical trials should select patients to be representative of the group of interest, and also any allocation of patients between experimental or control groups should be random. Further, patients must be informed and consent to any research. One safeguard for this is that the patient's own doctor should not be involved in the research and should not undertake the discussion necessary to decide consent, if possible. These conditions help to promote beneficence over maleficence (Medical Research Council 1993).

The principle of justice

Justice can be regarded in terms of fairness, desert or entitlement. Distributive justice refers to a fair distribution of society's benefits and burdens. The most obvious area of healthcare to which this is relevant is priority setting or resource rationing, but this principle is also pertinent to healthcare researchers when considering the distribution of research funding.

The principle of justice is not as clear-cut as the former three principles. A single unified theory of justice has proved elusive to philosophy, as indeed has an agreed concept of justice. Modern theories are often based upon Rawls' theory of a fair society being one that maximises the state of the least well off (Rawls 2000). However, whilst these ideas are theoretically rich, their practical relevance to healthcare researchers remains indirect.

These four principles are a foundation for ethical debate and, in addition to these, a consideration of scope and context is important (Gillon 1994). Whilst we may agree on our *prima facie* moral obligations, there may still be differences as to what or to whom our moral obligations are owed. This is the scope of application. For example, we may agree on the principle of respecting autonomy, without agreeing on what counts as an autonomous agent.

Alternatives to principlism

One clear limitation of principlism is that no one principle is overriding when conflicts occur (Kessel and Crawford 1997). Some have argued that this limitation is due to approaching medical ethics as simply the application of principles to health care problems. Suggested alternatives are framed both within bioethics and without. The use of narratives asks questions within bioethics by examining cases themselves. Moral insight is here gained through case studies and not through any principles. This approach contextualizes the nature of morality.

Alternatives from outside the field of bioethics include feminist critiques. These approaches argue that adherence to the principles perpetuates the maleness of language, that is itself a cause of repression in society (Daly 1990). Social science perspectives have rejected ethical theories and concentrated instead on understanding medical–ethical problems in relation to their socio-cultural setting (Hoffmaster 1994).

What makes an action morally acceptable?

Having looked at the principles of biomedical ethics it is useful now to explore the morality of actions generally, before bringing the two together and focusing on healthcare research. Although the common perception of ethics may be of the 'that's just your opinion' variety, in fact ethical analysis needs to be firmly based on rationality and logic. In a morally pluralist society, where competing moral claims are supported by competing ethical theories, there is a need to systematically understand and balance rival positions to come to reasonable conclusions. Broadly speaking there are three different approaches to examining what makes an action morally acceptable. These are outlined below.

A *goal-based approach* considers an action is good if the goal or outcome is good. This consequentialist approach is underpinned by utilitarian theories, is favoured by most economists, and is commonly expressed as 'the ends justify the means'. In this approach, the outcome of actions is what is to be considered and, with a few constraints, good actions can be weighed against bad actions.

Duty-based approaches ask if an action accords with certain principles such as cheating or lying. If so, then the action is wrong, even if the outcome is good. The deontonological approach is underpinned by theories such as Kantianism.

Rights-based approaches stress those individual freedoms and claims protected in a given society by 'rights'. Locke believed, for example, in the right to property ownership, and more extreme rights-based thinkers, such as Robert Nozick promote the importance of the right to liberty (to act freely) as a fundamental necessity for social arrangements (Nozick 1977). In application to health care, we must find out, and respect, the views and feelings of individuals stemming from their personal rights. Tension can develop between the good of protecting and promoting respect for such individual rights, and the good of community benefit.

What makes healthcare research morally acceptable?

Using the three approaches above it is possible to categorize the types of ethical problems which tend to arise in healthcare research. Naturally, depending on the research proposal some areas and questions will be more pertinent than others. As an overview:

Goal-based questions relate to the outcome of research. Questions that are goal based are:

- Is the research designed to achieve its goal?
- Is this the optimal design for the specific research question?
- What is the moral worth of the outcome?
- Does medicine need this research?

The question of moral worth often seems less relevant to researchers, but for funding committees it is highly relevant. Most applications seem to open with a phrase 'This is an important area of research . . .' However, there are very few unimportant questions in medicine, and so the moral worth is relative. With research resources scarce, just distribution is essential.

Duty-based questions relate to research participants. These questions include:

- How will the research participants be treated?
- What risks are they exposed to?
- Are the risks acceptable in the circumstances?

One particular area of difficulty arises in international research when investigators from the developed world collaborate with colleagues in developing countries particularly in therapeutic trials, where an expensive drug may be not be affordable to the country in which the trial is conducted. Recently international researchers have conceded that international declarations, such as the Declaration of Helsinki provide guidance, but need interpretation and there is little definition about what constitutes an acceptable standard of care (Benatar and Singer 2000). The assumption that standards set by the developed world necessarily apply to developing countries has been challenged and researchers are advised to consider the social, economic, and political context in which their work is conducted into ethical considerations (Benatar and Singer 2000).

Finally, rights-based questions relate to informed consent and whether and how informed consent will be sought, as well as issues of human dignity, such as respect for confidentiality. These are returned to later in the chapter.

Equipoise in healthcare research

Before moving on to the ethical assessment template, it is important to mention that in all areas of healthcare research, including psychiatry, therapeutic research can be distinguished from non-therapeutic research by the intention of researchers and the benefit to patients. For example, a clinical trial of a new intervention (therapeutic research) may provide immediate benefit to patients randomised to the new treatment, as well as future patients. In contrast, people participating in a cross-sectional survey obtain no such benefits, although researchers gain a great deal of information which may be used to plan services or study aetiology. In the former example, researchers are directly involved in trying to improve patient care, while the link between research and clinical practice is less direct in non-therapeutic research.

The position of 'equipoise' is necessary in relation to involvement in a therapeutic trial. For this position to be satisfied the researcher must be uncertain whether the new treatment is actually better than the standard, to which it is being compared. Equally, the researcher must be sure the participant is receiving treatment at least as good as that which she would have received had she not been enrolled. In practice this means that placebo-controlled trials are unethical when there is an existing acceptable treatment.

An ethical assessment template for research in psychiatry

The assessment template presented below combines the ethical principles and approaches described above. It draws strongly on a briefing pack developed by the Department of Health (1997) for members of research ethics committees (Box 4.2). The template is meant as a framework to promote thought, rather than as a definitive endpoint. For example, the template does not go into details about how to write a consent form but encourages the thought that should go on beforehand. The ethical principles above lead to three broad question areas that any research project should consider: the areas together

---

Box 4.2 **Assessment of ethical issues in research**

Areas to consider when assessing whether a proposal is ethical or not.
- Validity of the research
- Welfare of the research participants
- Dignity of the research participants
  - Confidentiality
  - Consent

make up the assessment template. The importance of each area will, of course, vary between projects. Corresponding to goal-, duty-, and rights-based approaches to morality, the question areas are: the validity of the research, the welfare of research participants, and the dignity of research participants.

The *validity* of research can be examined with the following questions:

+ How important is the research question?
+ For whom is the research question important?
+ Is it important to future patients?
+ Has the question been answered by someone else, somewhere else? This is the reason why literature reviews should not be included in research proposals to funding committees, but should be done beforehand.
+ Can the research answer the question being asked?
+ Is the research optimally designed methodologically?
+ Are the researchers suitably qualified, with appropriate environment and facilities? Often enthusiasm of researchers can override the need to do the research well, for example, attempts to do qualitative research without appropriate experience. It is usually best to get the 'expert' on board in some way, in this instance by involving a social scientist.
+ Are reporting arrangements in place, so progress can be regularly reviewed? This is especially important, as trials may need to be stopped early for a variety of reasons.

The *welfare* of research participants can be considered with questions such as:

+ What will participating in the research involve?
+ Are any risks to participants necessary and acceptable?
+ Safety and avoiding harm—have regulatory requirements been satisfied for example licensing of research medicines or medical devices?
+ If research is sponsored by a company there may be need for a clinical trial certificate (CTX) or a certificate of exemption (CTE) in accordance with the Medicines Act (1968).
+ There is a need to consider—from the research participants' perspective— viewpoints on matters such as needles, time devoted to the research, numbers of samples to be taken, and so forth.
+ It may be important—particularly if a new treatment or procedure is being used—to involve or provide information, with the participant's permission, to her general practitioner.

The *dignity* of research participants pertains to whether confidentiality is respected, and if consent has been appropriately sought, as described in more detail below.

Confidentiality. Research proposals must pay heed to patient confidentiality (see also section on emerging issues). The United Kingdom General Medical Council used to recognize research as an exception to the rule of confidentiality, stating that information may be disclosed for the purpose of an approved research project without consent as disclosure can be justified by the public interest (General Medical Council 1995; David *et al.* 1998). However this advice has been revised in the light of recent medical scandals, and current guidelines instruct researchers to 'obtain patients' express consent to the use of identifiable data or arrange for the health care team to anonymise records' (General Medical Council 2000).

All efforts should be made to ensure confidentiality of data whenever possible. This may take the form of anonymity of data collection or ensuring that named data is kept securely at all times. As far as disclosure is concerned, it remains most respectful of patient dignity to seek permission.

Consent. The most important aspects of consent are that it must be both voluntary and appropriately informed. It is worth remembering that, when in doubt, it is better to ask. If the researcher is unsure whether it is necessary to explicitly get consent, it is better to err on the side of caution—which is also the side of respect. Doctors in particular have a tendency to make decisions on behalf of patients, including decisions about whether a patient should care about his clinical notes or left over blood sample being used for research purposes. Values differ, and people treated respectfully do tend to want to help.

Achieving completely informed consent is difficult since:

+ the doctor cannot tell everything to the patient;
+ patients can only rarely be as well informed as the doctors, and even with full information will often need advice;
+ telling a patient everything may give an impression of lack of responsibility of the researchers;
+ patients' abilities to understand research projects vary.

Issues for psychiatry—competence and consent

Informed consent (Box 4.3) raises special consideration in the case of psychiatric illness. In particular, there is no provision in English law that allows a proxy to give consent on behalf of an incapacitated individual for either treatment or participation in therapeutic research (Kessel and Meran 1998). Incapacity may be due to various forms of mental illness. Only the doctor can

> ## Box 4.3 **Informed consent**
>
> Consent should be
> - Voluntary/intentional
> - Informed or based on substantial understanding
> - Free from coercion

make a decision on behalf of a patient—taking the patient's best interests into consideration—with regard to treatment or participation in psychiatric therapeutic research.

Seeking consent is underpinned by respect for the principle of autonomy and it is worth referring back to the earlier section. For an action to be self-determined it should be:

(a) *Intentional.* This is more or less self-explanatory. The consent should be voluntary and not fraudulent or inadvertent. Competence is relevant (see the following section).

(b) *Made with substantial understanding.* Clearly comprehensibility is unlikely ever to be complete, but participants should be in a position to make an informed decision. This means that careful consideration should be given to the provision of information sheets and how information will be communicated. It is advisable for participants to be provided with such sheets in advance (generally more than 24 h), so they have an opportunity to think about the research and its implications. These must also be sufficiently extensive, and written using terms and language comprehensible to the general public. Participants should have an opportunity to ask questions, and also must be aware of the option to opt out.

(c) *Made without controlling influences/coercion,* as far as is possible. Here, questions to consider are the method of recruitment, if any payment or other inducement is connected with participation in the research, and how the invitation to participate is presented.

Competence is central to psychiatric research since for individuals to give consent to participate in research, they must be competent. Although the Law Commission has proposed a statutory test and a code of practice for assessing incapacity, uncertainties currently exist over who decides incapacity and using what criteria. In the well known 1994 case of Re C, a person with chronic schizophrenia was held to be mentally competent to give advance refusal to amputation of his gangrenous foot, because he was judged to be able to comprehend and retain treatment information, to believe it in his own way, and to weigh that information, balancing the risks and benefits. It should be noted that it can be particularly difficult to sanction non-therapeutic research on incompetent participants. Indeed, Medical Research Council (1993) guidelines state that individuals unable to consent should be included in non-therapeutic research only if:

♦ the research relates to the individual's condition and this knowledge could not be gained by those able to consent;

♦ approval is gained by the local research ethics committee (LREC);

♦ the individual does not object or appear to object;

♦ an informed, independent person acceptable to the LREC agrees that the individual's welfare and interests have been properly safeguarded; and

♦ there is only negligible risk of harm, and participation is not against that individual's interests.

A similar approach has been recommended by the Law Commission for England and Wales (Nuffield Council on Bioethics 2000).

Emerging ethical issues in psychiatric research

Confidentiality

Psychiatric data may be collected from medical records, may use linked records under local control, or use national and regional databases allowing for record linkage. In all these methods, it is often very difficult for psychiatrists to gain patients' informed consent for each act of data transfer. The possibility of harm coming to patients must be considered at all times, in balance with possible benefits from the research.

In practice, research projects may be subject to problems of carelessness; documents may be left lying around, and attention to security can be inadequate. Identifying data should be removed from confidential documents, and a name-number list kept under secure conditions.

Some guidelines are as follows (Baldwin *et al.* 1976):

♦ name-number lists set up and kept secure;

♦ restriction of access to specified persons;

♦ supervision by a named doctor responsible for confidentiality;

♦ approval by an ethical committee;

♦ data forwarded for collation identified by number only.

Psychiatric research involving genetics

Genetic research in psychiatry may provide knowledge on susceptibility to disorder. Such research involves genetic testing, and creates stores of genetic information. Care must be taken in both obtaining and using this information, especially in the areas described below (Holtzman 1997).

Recruitment

Identifying disorder-related gene loci requires the participation of many people in a few families or a few relatives in many small families. The coercion of patients to participate in research is possible.

Disclosure of research results

Researchers should inform research participants prior to research whether the participants will be informed of results. If participants are given results prior to the completion of research, misleading conclusions may be made using these results. Individuals may then take unnecessary, and even harmful action based on these results. Genetic counselling services should be made available if participants are to be informed of results.

Consent

When DNA is banked for future analysis, consent must be obtained if additional genetic research is performed, and the source's identity is retained. Objections to this may occur when breach of confidentiality is a concern. If identifiers are to be removed, there is usually little disagreement about using this data for research. However, consent should be obtained to anonymise data on grounds of the autonomy of individuals, and this consent must be obtained before the data is anonymised. If a large proportion of people decline this consent, then a special interplay between ethics and epidemiology develops. The group from whom samples have been taken may now be unrepresentative of the wider population, making the results ultimately ungeneralizable and thereby questioning the ethical acceptability of the research (Kessel 2000).

It could be argued that consent is not needed here, as no harm can come to individuals if data is anonymized. Insurance companies, for example, cannot discriminate because they cannot identify individuals. However, individuals may still not wish their data to be used in genetic research, as discrimination may take place to individuals as members of a group, say women or social class (Clayton *et al.* 1995; Kessel 2001). Some individuals may object to the research agenda *per se*, for example, objections may be held to any patenting of human genes, and others may believe the same about research possibly leading to cloning.

Commercialization

Data that is 'commercial' may not be acceptable to be used even if anonymous. Commercial profit from gene patenting and the development of genetic tests has led to the interests of researchers possibly conflicting with patients.

Although not a case specific to psychiatric research, a case in the United States found that doctors must disclose their intention to use tissue for research in advance to the removal of the tissue from any individual. In *Moore v. Regents of the University of California*, Moore had his spleen removed at the University and learned later that his doctor had patented a cell line made from his tissue. Moore sued the hospital, and the court held that the doctor must disclose in advance of removing tissue when there is a chance that scientific or commercial research may be pursued with this tissue (Holtzman 1997).

Conclusions

Embracing the ethical issues that arise in healthcare research is part and parcel of designing and implementing research that is based on sound moral foundations. Researchers should avoid approaching ethical considerations as a hurdle to getting the research done, and should instead think of them in the same vein as making sure the scientific methodology is correct. Similarly, research ethics committees should not be thought of as an obstacle, but as bodies whose role is to facilitate ethically acceptable research.

Most of the issues that arise in research in psychiatry are generic to other areas of healthcare research, and this chapter has outlined the moral bases of these and provided a template through which they can be approached. However, because research in psychiatry inevitably may involve vulnerable participants, it is important to recognise that special attention needs to be paid to competence and ensuring consent is informed.

The research arena in psychiatry is changing, and researchers will need to keep abreast of future developments, which can take the form of new guidelines from relevant bodies and also changes to the law.

Case studies

The following case studies can be tried out using the assessment template and the principles of biomedical ethics. Students should focus on the ethical issues and suggesting how they may be tackled.

Case study 1—Depression in palliative care patients: a longitudinal study

This study will seek to understand better the incidence of depression in terminally ill cancer patients, by means of questionnaires and interviews until the research participants die.

Background to study

While depression among patients with early-stage cancer has been extensively studied, little systematic work has been carried out regarding the nature or response to treatment of depression in those with advanced cancer. Clinical experience suggests that depressed patients often benefit form brief psychotherapy and/or antidepressant drugs, but no controlled trials of either treatment have been reported. Pilot work on 108 new patients at this Hospice showed that 36% obtained high scores for depression and/or anxiety on the Hospital Anxiety and Depression (HAD) scale, and a further 19% obtained borderline scores. Only about 10% were prescribed antidepressant drugs, suggesting that depression is under-diagnosed and under-treated even in this specialized centre.

Purpose of study

To describe the prevalence, symptom pattern, chronology, and response to treatment of depression among 200 cancer patients in the last few months of their lives. The results will improve recognition of depression by medical and nursing staff; delineate the symptom pattern which predicts a good response to drug treatment; and, by identifying factors associated with both high and low vulnerability, may suggest strategies for preventing depression in this population.

Design of study

All new inpatients (up to 200) admitted to this Hospice over a 12-month period will be considered for the study, although some will be too ill to participate and others will die before follow-up interviews. Medical and socio-demographic details, medication and other details will be recorded from notes. A brief interview will include the HAD scale, a self-rating instrument, and inquiry for the symptoms of major depression using the DSM-III-R criteria of the American Psychiatric Association. The same assessments will be repeated fortnightly until death, some patients being followed up at home. The protocol will not include direct initiation of anti-depressant treatment but, given the patient's consent, high HAD scores will be reported to the medical staff who have clinical responsibility and this will be probably lead to increased rates of antidepressant prescribing and psychiatric referral. The outcome of these interventions will be noted.

Case study 2—An open, multi-centre study to investigate and characterise the patients' migraine attacks and their response to Sumatriptan

This study will investigate whether (a) particular symptoms/factors recorded can help build a profile for a migraine attack and (b) whether patients gained relief from the attack by responding to Sumatriptan.

Background

It is apparent that relief from a migraine attack constitutes more than headache severity relief and that for some patients headache may not be the most significant or distressing factor as a whole. It may be that other acute impact factors of a migraine can be more debilitating than the physical symptoms which are commonly associated with a migraine attack. It may also be that some types of migraine are more likely to gain relief from Sumatriptan than others. A new measurement tool, in the form of a diary card to measure global migraine severity and acute impact of migraine on a patient's life, aims to capture the complete improvement experienced by the patient. A therapeutic regime is also evaluated.

Purpose of study

The study objectives are (1) to investigate if different attack profiles respond differently to Sumatriptan and (2) to develop the new tool diary card.

Design of study

(1) The study will involve a total of 250 male and female patients aged 18–65 with severe or moderately severe migraine (international diagnostic criteria), recruited from GP centres in the UK. Many potential participants will be excluded based on their past and current medical history. Over an 8-week period patients will treat two migraine attacks with 50 mg Sumatriptan, then, dependent on the success of the treatment, they will, during a second 8-week period, treat a further two attacks, each with either 50 or 100 mg of Sumatriptan as decided by the patient.

(2) As well as a treatment pack of Sumatriptan, patients will be given diary cards and their use will be explained. Ten symptoms—such as presence of aura, time to useful relief, sleep taken during attack, being sick—will be recorded on a visual analogue scale (VAS) by the patient (physical symptoms and acute impact questions) at time points 0, 1, 2, 3, and 4 h post-dose of Sumatriptan.

Outcomes of the study to be measured are a comparison of individual parameter VAS changes when an attack is and is not successfully treated, the order of distress of physical and impact symptoms, the proportion of attacks which experienced improvement, time to useful relief of migraine symptoms, patients' choice for dose of Sumatriptan, and global assessment of treatment. The study will involve one initial and four follow-up visits, each of 1–2 h.

Acknowledgement

The authors are extremely grateful to the UK Department of Health for kindly allowing adaptation of the assessment template and reproduction of the two cases studies from their 1997 publication *Briefing Pack for Research Ethics Committee Members.*

References

Baldwin, J.A., Leff, J.P., Wing, J.K. (1976) Confidentiality of psychiatric data in medical information systems. *British Journal of Psychiatry*, **128**, 417–27.

Beauchamp, T. and Childress, J. (1989) *The principles of biomedical ethics.* Oxford University Press, New York.

Benatar, S.R. and Singer, P.A. (2000) A new look at international research ethics. *British Medical Journal*, **321**, 824–6.

Block, S. and Chodoff, P. (1991) *Psychiatric ethics.* Oxford University Press, Oxford.

Clayton, E.W., Steinberg, K.K., Khoury, M.J., *et al.* (1995) Informed consent for genetic research on stored tissue samples. *The Journal of the American Medical Association*, **274**, 1786–92.

Daly, M. (1990) *The metaethics of radical feminism.* Beacon Press, Boston.

David, T.J., Wynne, G., Kessel, A.S., Brazier, M. (1998) Child sexual abuse: when a doctor's duty to report conflicts with a duty of confidentiality to the victim. *British Medical Journal*, **316**, 55–57.

Department of Health (1997) *Briefing pack for research ethics committee members.* Department of Health, London.

General Medical Council (1995) *Duties of a doctor (confidentiality).* General Medical Council, London.

General Medical Council (2000) *Confidentiality: protecting and providing information.* General Medical Council, London.

Gillon, R. (1994) Four principles and attention to scope. *British Medical Journal*, **309**, 185–189.

Hoffmaster, B. (1994) The forms and limits of medical ethics. *Social Science and Medicine*, **399/9**, 1155–64.

Holtzman, N. (1997) Ethical and legal issues in genetic epidemiology. *Epidemiological Reviews*, **19**, 163–74.

Kessel, A.S. (1998) Ethics and research in psychiatry. *International Review of Psychiatry*, **10**, 331–7.

Kessel, A.S. (2001). Evaluation of the unlinked anonymous prevalence monitoring programme for HIV in England and Wales: science, ethics and health policy. *Medical Science Monitor*, **7/5**: 1052–10 (full text available on-line: *http://www.MedSciMonit.com*).

Kessel, A.S. and Crawford, M. (1997) Openness with patients: a categorical imperative to correct an imbalance. *Science and Engineering Ethics*, **3**, 297–304.

Kessel, A.S. and Meran, J. (1998) Advance directives in the UK: legal, ethical, and practical considerations for doctors. *British Journal of General Practice*, **48**, 1263–6.

Kessel, A.S. and Watts, C. (2000) Bad blood? Survey of the public's views on unlinked anonymous testing of blood for HIV and other diseases. *British Medical Journal*, **320**, 90–91.

Medical Research Council Working Party on Research on the Mentally Incapacitated (1993) *The ethical conduct of research on the mentally incapacitated.* Medical Research Council, London.

Moore v. Regents of University of California, 793 P.2d 479 (Cal.1990).

Nozick, R. (1977) *Anarchy, state and utopia*. Harvard University Press, Harvard.

Nuffield Council on Bioethics (2000) *Mental disorders and genetics*. The Nuffield Foundation, London.

Re C (adult: refusal of treatment) [1994] 1 WLR 290, 295.

Rawls, J. (2000) *A theory of justice*. Harvard University Press, Harvard.

Roberts, L.W., Solomon, A., Roberts, B.B., and Keith, S.J. (1998) Ethics in psychiatric research: resources for faculty development and resident education. *Academic Psychiatry*, 22, 1–20.

Royal College of Physicians of London (1989) *Research on patients*. Royal College of Physicians, London.

Wing, J. (1991). *Ethics and psychiatric research*. In *Psychiatric ethics* (ed. S. Bloch and P. Chodoff), pp. 415–34. Oxford, Oxford University Press.

General reading

Brazier, M. (1992) *Medicine, patients and the law*, pp. 412–33. Penguin Books, London.

Harris, C.E. (1997) *Applying moral theories*. Wadsworth, Belmont.

Rachels, J. (1993) *The elements of moral philosophy*. McGraw-Hill, New York.

Singer, P. (ed.) (1993) *A companion to ethics*. Blackwell, Oxford.

Section 2

Study design

Chapter 5

Introduction to epidemiological study designs

Tamsin Ford

Importance of study design

Epidemiologists must have a sound understanding of the principles of study design. Ethical considerations naturally prevent us from allocating potentially harmful exposures on an experimental basis in human populations. Observational studies are inherently more vulnerable to the effect of bias and confounding. However, these problems can be minimized by good study design.

The design (and analysis) of a study aspires to maximize the *precision* and *validity* of its findings. The *precision* of an estimate of the prevalence of depression in a population will be reduced by sampling and measurement error. These errors are generally random, that is equally likely to deviate from the truth in either direction. Precision can be improved with larger sample sizes and more accurate measures. Confounding and bias lead to non-random error; that is the effect of the bias or confounder is systematic, tending mainly in one direction, thus reducing the *validity* of a finding. Choices of study design and measurement strategy are key factors in minimizing non-random error and maximizing the validity of the results.

Although the conduct and analysis of epidemiological studies has become increasing sophisticated over time, there are a limited number of basic designs, each with their own advantages and disadvantages. This chapter will provide an overview of study design, illustrated with examples from psychiatric epidemiological studies, while individual types of study will be discussed in greater depth in subsequent chapters.

Classifying study design

Epidemiological studies may be experimental, or observational (Fig. 5.1). Experimental studies can be used to investigate interventions, for example, the effect of family therapy on expressed emotion and relapse in schizophrenia

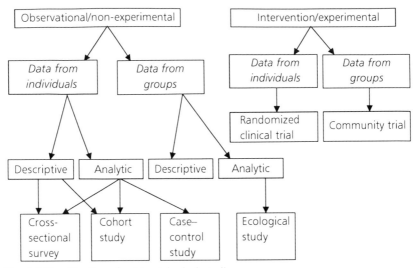

Fig. 5.1 Classification of epidemiological studies.

(Leff *et al.* 1982). In observational studies, epidemiologists try to make inferences about diseases through natural observation of groups of people defined by their exposure or disease status. The key difference between experimental and observational studies is that in the latter, the investigator has no control over the events under investigation.

Observational studies can be descriptive or analytic. A descriptive study illustrates an outcome, such as depression, *or* an exposure, for instance life events, in terms of the characteristics of affected people in a particular place at a particular time. In contrast analytical studies look for associations between outcomes and exposures. However this classification is not rigid and as (Fig. 5.1) suggests, some cross-sectional surveys and cohort studies have both descriptive and analytic elements.

Epidemiological studies may use aggregated data for whole populations, for instance average per capita alcohol consumption in different countries, or they may collect data from individuals, for instance their average personal weekly alcohol consumption.

The brief overview of the common study designs below should be read in conjunction with Table 5.1, which summarizes the main features of each design.

Studies using routine data

Descriptive studies often use routinely collected statistics, such as mortality data, to investigate the occurrence of a disorder, or an exposure.

Table 5.1 Advantages and disadvantages of different types of epidemiological study

	Cross-sectional survey	Case–control	Cohort	Ecological	Clinical trial
Subject selection	Defined population	Caseness	Exposure	Aggregated data	Caseness
Source of bias	Selection Non-response Information (Recall and observer)	Selection Information (Recall and observer)	Information (observer only) Loss to follow up (selection)	Selection of population Ecological fallacy	Selection Information (reduced by blinding)
Probability of confounding	Medium	Medium	Low	High	Very low if randomized
Resources	Quick and cheap	Relatively quick and cheap	Lengthy and expensive	Relatively quick and cheap	Relatively expensive
Applications	Planning services Mapping secular and geographical trends Identifying correlates	Rare outcomes Single outcomes Multiple exposures	Rare exposure Single exposures Multiple outcomes	Rare outcomes Rare exposures Multiple exposures Population exposures such as air pollution	Efficacy of new interventions Effectiveness of new interventions Hypothesis testing Mechanisms
Measures of effect	Prevalence	Odds ratio	Relative risk	Correlation/ regression coefficient	Relative risk/ odds ratio/ difference between means

Accompanying data, for example, on a death certificate, tends to be relatively sparse limiting the potential for the study of co-determinants to simple variables such as age, gender, occupation, region and time period. This is a particularly useful approach for rare disorders, and for outcomes that are relatively completely ascertained for official purposes. Suicide is frequently studied in this manner; data from the UK have suggested an increase in rates among young men in the 1980s and early 1990s (McClure 2000). Descriptive studies can also be used to generate hypotheses, which can then be tested in analytic studies.

The value of routine data may be compromised by incomplete or inaccurate recording. This may complicate secular or regional comparisons, where ascertainment and recording practices differ between geographical areas or over different time periods. For example, the stigma associated with suicide can lead to coroners in some countries tending to return a verdict of misadventure rather than suicide, so that official suicide statistics from these settings are likely to underestimate the true rate in the population.

Ecological studies

Ecological studies examine the evidence for associations by testing for correlations between the average level of an exposure and the prevalence or incidence of an outcome across different populations. The indices of both exposure and outcome are aggregated at the population level. For example, an ecological study suggested that the aluminium content of local drinking water was positively correlated with the incidence of Alzheimer's disease (AD) (Martyn *et al.* 1989). There are three main problems with ecological studies. First, the association can only be applied to populations not individuals. Water supplies, and hence the concentrations of aluminium in the water vary even from house to house in the same street. While districts with high average concentrations of aluminium tend to have higher incidence rates of AD, we do not know that those people drinking water with high concentrations of aluminium are the same people who are suffering from AD. The incautious application of results obtained from data gathered at population level to individuals can therefore result in an 'ecological fallacy'. Second, as ecological studies often use data gathered for reasons other than research, information on potential confounding factors is often lacking. This in the example referenced above we cannot be sure that the association with AD could not be explained by other factors related to high concentrations of aluminium in the water supply. Finally as data on the exposure and the outcome were gathered at the same time, we cannot make any inference about the likely direction of causality.

Cross-sectional surveys

Cross-sectional surveys collect information from a sample of people from a defined base population about the prevalence of an outcome, and exposure to potential risk factors for that outcome. They are quick and relatively cheap to perform and are often used to demonstrate the extent of the disorder, to plan services, and to identify potential risk factors for further study in hypothesis driven analytical studies (see below). As the disorder and the exposure are recorded simultaneously, a cross-sectional survey can never provide direct evidence of causality.

The population under study may be defined by area, for example, all children in Great Britain under 16 (Meltzer *et al.* 2000), or by other characteristics, such all people serving custodial sentences at a particular point in time (Singleton *et al.* 1998). The first step is to identify a sampling frame or list to identify all individuals making up population from which the sample is to be drawn. Administrative lists such as electoral registers are often used, although these can be surprisingly inaccurate. The recent British survey of children's mental health used the child benefit register, as this benefit is drawn for 99% of children, but inaccurate addresses meant that this method achieved only a 90% coverage of the target base population (Meltzer *et al.* 2000). An alternative is for the investigators to compile their own sampling frame by a door-knock census of the area to be surveyed. This obviously becomes impractical in large surveys or those covering extensive areas. If the sampling frame is not representative of the base population the survey may be subject to selection bias; that is, it may either systematically over or underestimate the true prevalence of the disorder in the base population. Explicit inclusion and exclusion criteria, ideally formulated in advance, are an essential component for all cross-sectional surveys. For instance the children's mental health survey excluded children who were in foster care or were 16 or over. Exclusions must be carefully justified on the basis of feasibility, logistics or relevance. Inclusion and exclusion criteria set limits on the generalizability of the survey findings.

A low response rate (less than 80%) will tend to reduce the validity of the surveys findings, as it is likely that non-responders differ from responders in many ways, some of which may be related to either the exposure and/or the outcome under investigation (Market Research Society 1981). However if data is available about those who refused to participate, it may be possible to argue that response bias is relatively unlikely. Conversely, one should not assume that a high response rate necessarily eliminates the possibility of biased estimates (Gerrits *et al.* 2001).

The cross-sectional survey is evidently an inefficient design for investigating rare disorders, for example schizophrenia or autism. A very large sample would need to be investigated in order to study the outcome with any degree of precision. By the same token, it may be necessary to over-sample small but significant sub-populations in order to obtain sufficiently precise information about the distribution of the outcome amongst them. For instance, a survey of mental health in prisoners in England and Wales interviewed 1 in 3 women as they make up less than 5% of the prison population, compared to 1 in 34 sentenced male prisoners who comprised the vast majority of the prison population (Singleton *et al.* 1998).

Case–control studies

Case–control studies are essentially retrospective designs. The aim is to recruit a random sample of cases and non-cases (controls) from the same defined population, and then to inquire about their history of past exposure to possible risk factors. The odds of being exposed are compared between cases and controls. The resulting measure of effect, the odds ratio, should approximate to the relative risk estimated in a cohort study (see Chapter 2) for rare disorders, although this assumption begins to fail as the population prevalence of the disorder rises above 10%.

Case–control studies are relatively quick and cheap to conduct, and are particularly appropriate for the initial investigation of rare disorders. For example, cases of Creutzfeld Jacob disease collected through national surveillance can be compared with suitable controls (van Duijn 1989). They can also be used to study multiple exposures. However they are prone to bias for several reasons. If the chances of being selected as a case or a control are related to your exposure status, the findings of the study will be invalidated due to *selection bias*, which is why it is imperative to define the base population. If cases were collected from prospective referrals to a certain clinic, the controls must be selected from the people who would be referred to the same clinic, were they to develop the disorder under study.

As the data on exposure is sought after the onset of disease, there is a real risk that the information obtained is biased according to disease status. Over-zealous researchers may look harder for evidence of exposure in cases than controls if they are also aware of the hypothesis under investigation and the participant's disease status, creating *observer bias*. Equally people suffering from a disorder are likely to have thought about the potential causes in a way that the controls will not leading to *recall bias*. For example, Lewis and Murray (1987) interviewed the relatives of people with schizophrenia about their birth circumstances using people with other psychiatric diagnoses as a control group. It is possible that the association between obstetric complications and schizophrenia reported by this study could be explained by relatives of schizophrenics being more likely to remember adverse effects, although the association has also been detected in other studies that used obstetric records (Eagles *et al.* 1990). This phenomenon is sometimes referred to as 'effort after meaning'. To minimize *information bias* (both recall and observer bias) it is important to apply the same measures of exposure status to cases and controls and to try and use objective methods such as blood tests and medical records in preference to, or to supplement subjective information. It may also be possible to blind the observer to the outcome status of the participant, and to blind both the observer and the participant to the hypothesis under study.

Cohort studies

There are two essential features of a cohort study:

(1) Participants are defined by their exposure status rather than by outcome (as in case–control design).

(2) It is a longitudinal design: exposure status must be ascertained before outcome is known.

Cohort studies may be descriptive, only illustrating the rates of disease in one particular group (usually an occupational exposure) but more usually compare the rates of a disorder in different exposure groups.

Classical cohort studies start with a group of people defined by their exposure status and compare the incidence of a disorder in these groups over time. If the study is prospective, that is the study commences before the onset of disease and the participants are followed forwards in time, the incidence of the disorder can be directly calculated, information bias is limited and we can ascertain the direction of causality. However due to the number of participants required and the length of time required to accumulate sufficient cases, cohort studies can be prohibitively expensive. If one wanted to investigate the impact of obstetric complications on the incidence of schizophrenia in this manner, one would have to follow the cohort up for 25–30 years and would need an enormous number of people in order to generate a sufficient number of cases. For this reason, cohorts are not the design of choice for studying rare disorders.

A variant of the classical cohort study is the *population cohort study*, in which selection of the participants is not based upon exposure to a single putative risk factor. This permits study of multiple exposures as well as multiple outcomes, and findings are broadly generalizable. For instance, in the Avon Longitudinal Study of Parents and Children (ALSPAC) all children born in Avon during one year are invited for annual assessments. It has gathered information about many disparate issues affecting health and development, from cardiovascular risk factors to allergies in addition to mental health (Golding *et al.* 2001). These children are now 8–9 years old and the study aims to follow them at least through puberty.

The logistical demands and costs of a cohort study can be minimized by using a *historical cohort study* design. The rate of disorder is still compared across exposure groups, but the disease has already occurred at the time of investigation. The essential element is the availability of information on exposure collected for another purpose before the onset of the disorder. Information bias is excluded since as with a classical prospective cohort study, neither the assessors nor the participants under study knew who would develop the disorder at the time when the exposure was ascertained. Thus, Malmberg *et al.* (1998)

linked data routinely gathered about the personality of conscripts to the Swedish army to the National Register of Psychiatric Care in order to investigate the role of personality factors in their future risk of developing Schizophrenia. Jones *et al.* (1994) combined data from the UK National Survey of Health and Development, a representative sample of all babies born in one week in 1946 and the Mental Health Enquiry, a central register of all admissions to psychiatric hospitals. They related various indices of child cognitive, behavioural, social and physical development to the future risk of developing schizophrenia.

Intervention studies

In intervention studies, the experimenter allocates the intervention (exposure) to some individuals or communities and compares the outcome of interest between the treatment groups. By *randomly allocating* participants to the different interventions, the investigator hopes to create groups that are similar in respect to all confounders, both known and unknown. It is also important to ensure, if possible, that both the investigator and the participants do not know which intervention they are receiving, that is to say that trial is '*double-blind*'. This prevents *information bias*, which may otherwise arise where perceptions about the interventions influence self-reported or researcher-ascertained outcome. However, blinding is hard to achieve with psychological interventions and drug effects, such as the Parkinsonism associated with conventional neuroleptics can foil blinding. Asking participants and data collectors which group they thought that they were in at the end of the trial can help investigators to assess the extent to which the double blind was maintained, and also to assess the possible impact of information bias upon the findings.

Spontaneous remission is a particular problem with chronic relapsing and remitting conditions such as depression or schizophrenia. People tend to seek help when their symptoms are most intense, and thus by definition, will tend to improve over time even if placebo treatment is allocated. However, random allocation and blinding minimise the possibility that spontaneous improvement accounts for any observed differences between treatments. If a commonly used intervention for the condition under study is available, it should be used in the comparison group, as it would be unethical to use an inert placebo when an evidence-based treatment existed.

In a rigorously conducted randomized controlled trial, it can be possible to make direct causal and mechanistic inferences from the effects observed. For instance, the efficacy of methylphenidate in suppressing the symptoms of hyperkinetic disorder has lead to the investigation of the involvement of dopaminergic pathways in inattention and overactivity.

Not all intervention trials involve medication. This is particularly true of psychiatry. For instance, anorexia nervosa shows sustained improvement with family therapy in youngsters under the age of 18 and individual therapy in people over 18 (Eisler *et al.* 1997). Some intervention studies involve the application of inventions to groups of people or defined communities such as schools as a point of intervention to prevent bullying among children (Olweus 1997). In community trials it is important that the investigators adjust their design and analysis to account for the fact that, following the example of bullying in schools, the pupils at a particular school, are likely to be more similar to each other than to pupils at other schools. Their observations are *clustered* rather than independent and if this is ignored in the analysis, there is an increased likelihood of detecting erroneous associations where none exist. Similarly, the sample size should be based on the number of schools, as well as the number of children, receiving the intervention.

Quasi-experimental designs

Quasi-experimental designs are opportunistic in that they take advantage of unplanned events to assess the impact of an exposure, or an intervention, on a relatively well-defined group of people who happened to be affected by that event. However, the allocation of the exposure is by definition not random, although the study may be controlled by the addition of a group who were not exposed, or did not receive the intervention.

For obvious reasons a great deal of the work on Post-Traumatic Stress Disorder includes quasi-experimental studies on the survivors of disasters. For example, Yule *et al.* (1990) investigated the impact of trauma on children involved in the sinking of 'the Jupiter' cruise ship which was setting off on an educational cruise of the eastern Mediterranean when it sank. By contacting one of the schools that had sent children on the cruise they were able to compare 25 survivors to 46 girls who had not wanted to go on the cruise and 13 girls who had wanted to go, but had not managed to get places. They also had a control group of 71 girls from a different school, which had not had any involvement with the cruise. The prevalence of emotional disorders was greatest among the survivors.

Practical exercise

Answer the following questions for each of the studies described below:

1. Is the study descriptive or analytic?
2. Is data aggregated or not?
3. What type of study design was used?

4. What is/are the outcome(s)?

5. What is/are the exposure(s)?

6. What measure(s) of effect might be used?

7. What are the types of bias that the investigators will have to guard against?

A. A study was set up to test the predictive validity of the diagnostic category of depressive conduct disorder by examining whether it had different outcomes in terms of psychiatric disorder in adulthood or was more closely related to the adult outcomes of childhood depression or conduct disorder. The investigators contacted three groups of young adults who had attended a psychiatric clinic as children, when they were diagnosed as having depressive conduct disorder, conduct disorder or depression.

B. A study assessed the frequency of childhood eating disorders in the community in a randomly selected population sample of young people aged between 12-21 years of age. Child and family factors were measured at the same time to look for associations with eating disorders.

C. A study examined the performance of young people who regularly used "ecstasy" on a psychometric battery with a group of ecstasy-naïve subjects of the same age.

D. A study compared the rates of suicides among children under the age of 16 between several areas of the country.

E. A study examined frequency of teacher ratings of poor concentration in relation to the food additives in the lunches provided by twelve schools.

References

Eagles, J.M., Gibson, I., Bremner, M.H., Clunie, F., Ebmeir, K.P., and Smith, N.C. (1990) Obstetric complications in DSM III schizophrenics and their siblings. *Lancet*, **335**, 1139–41.

Eisler, I., Dare, C., Russell, G.F., Szmuckler, G., le Grange, D., and Dodge, E. (1997) Family and individual therapy in anorexia nervosa; a five-year follow up. *Archives of General Psychiatry*, **54**, 1025–30.

Gerrits, M.H., Voogt, R., and van den Oord, E.J.C.G. (2001) An evaluation of non-response bias in peer, self and teacher ratings of children's psychological adjustment. *Journal of Child Psychology and Psychiatry*, **42**, 593–602.

Golding, J., Pembrey, M. and the ALSPAC study team. (2001) ALSPAC—the Avon Longitudinal Study of Parents and Children I. Study methodology. *Paediatric and Perinatal Epidemiology*, **15**, 74–87.

Jones, P., Rodgers, B., Murray, R., and Marmot, M. (1994) Child development risk factors for adult schizophrenia in the British 1946 birth cohort. *Lancet*, **344**, 1398–402.

Leff, J., Kuipers, L., Berkowitz, R., Eberlein-Vries, R., and Sturgeon, D. (1982) A controlled trial of Social Intervention in the families of Schizophrenic Patients. *British Journal of Psychiatry*, **141**, 121–34.

Lewis, S. and Murray, R. (1987) Obstetric complications, neurodevelopmental deviance and risk of schizophrenia. *Journal of Psychiatric Research*, **21**, 413–22.

Malmberg, A., Lewis, G., David, A., and Allebeck, P. (1998) Premorbid adjustment and personality in people with schizophrenia. *British Journal of Psychiatry*, **172**, 308–13.

Market Research Society. (1981) Report of the second working party on respondent cooperation: 1977–1980. *Journal of the Market Research Society*, **23**, 3–25.

Martyn, C.N., Barker, D.J., Osmond, C., Harris, E.C., Edwardson, J.A., and Lacey, R.F. (1989) Geographical relation between Alzheimer's disease and aluminium in drinking water. *Lancet*, **351**, 59–62.

McClure, G.M.G. (2000) Changes in suicide in England and Wales 1960–1997. *British Journal of Psychiatry*, **176**, 64–87.

Meltzer, H., Gatward, R., Goodman, R., and Ford, T. (2000) *The mental health of children and adolescents in Great Britain*. The Stationery Office, London.

Olweus, D. (1997) Bully/Victim problems within school; facts and intervention. *European Journal of Psychology of Education*, **12**, 495–510.

Singleton, N., Melzter, H., Gatward, R., Coid, J., and Deasey, D. (1998) *Psychiatric morbidity among prisoners in England and Wales*. The Stationery Office, London.

Van Dujin, C.M., Delasnerie-Laupretre, N., Masullo, C., Zerr, I., de Silva, R., Wientjens, *et al.* (1989) Case–control study of risk factors of Creutzfeldt-Jakob disease inEurope during 1993–5. European Union (EU) Collaborative Study Group of Creutzfeldt-Jakobdisease (CJD). *Lancet*, **351**, 1081–5.

Yule, W., Udwin, O., and Murdoch, K. (1990) The Jupiter sinking: effects on children's fears, depression and anxiety. *Journal of Child Psychology and Psychiatry*, **31**, 1051–61.

Further reading

Jenkins, R., Bebbington, P., Brugha, T., Farrell, M., Gill, B., Lewis, G., Meltzer, H., and Petticrew, M. (1997) National Psychiatric Morbidity Surveys of Great Britain—strategy and methods. *Psychological Medicine* **27**, 765–74.

Kelsey, J.L., Thompson, W.D., and Evans, A.S. (1996) *Methods in observational epidemiology*. Oxford University Press, New York; Oxford.

Lewis, G. and Pelosi, A.J. (1990) The case–control in psychiatry. *British Journal of Psychiatry*, **157**, 197–207.

Pocock, S.J. (1983) *Clinical trials: a practical approach*. John Wiley, Chichester.

Chapter 6

Ecological and cross-level studies

Jan Neeleman

Introduction

Ecological studies differ from other study designs by having *groups* of individuals as their unit of analysis. Studying differences in risk factors between individuals cannot fully explain variations in the health of populations in different regions or over time, and ignores the fact that a population's health impacts on social functioning and collective economic performance (McMichael and Beaglehole 2000). Similarly, there is increasing interest on the impact of social capital, or those aspects of the social environment that promote cohesion and cooperation, which have been associated with improved health and other outcomes. For example, a recent study found higher rates of common mental disorder among British women living in areas of low social capital (McCulloch 2001).

Thus ecological associations can be analysed to gain insight into aetiological mechanisms at the level of individuals (cross-level inference), although there is ongoing debate about whether ecological analyses can add to insights obtained from studies of individual persons. Kasl (1979) stated that 'ecological analyses lead to results which, in themselves, are opaque, unhelpful, potentially misleading'. Others emphasize that population health is more than the sum of the health of individual population members, and that therefore, ecological studies have a separate role alongside individual-level epidemiological research (Rose 1992).

This chapter summarizes the principles and the place of ecological studies in the history of epidemiology, and the distinguishing properties of ecological data. After a description of ecological study designs and their analysis, the chapter argues that ecological data have added value even if individual-level information is available on the associations of interest.

Definition of ecological studies

Individual-level analytical designs are possible only if, of each subject, exposure and outcome status are known, that is, if data are *complete* (Morgenstern 1998). Ecological data are *incomplete* with respect to the individual-level because it is unknown how many *individuals* in each group are ill as well as exposed. Therefore, odds, risk or rate ratios cannot be calculated.

Most ecological studies examine associations of aggregate health indicators, across a number of populations, with overall indices of risk. Three types of ecological exposure index have been distinguished (Morgenstern 1998):

♦ Aggregate measures, summarizing observations on the individuals in the respective groups, for example, the proportion of persons with a religious denomination (Neeleman 1998) or the mean fibre intake (Liu *et al.* 1979).

♦ Environmental measures, like exposure to famine (Susser *et al.* 1996), aluminium in drinking water (Martyn *et al.* 1989) or electromagnetic radiation (Bianchi *et al.* 2000). Their equivalent at the individual level remains unmeasured and is inferred, for instance, from area of residence.

♦ Global measures like the gross national product or the tightness of anti-drug laws (Reuband 1995).

History

Snow and cholera

Snow's (1813–1858) public health interventions during the cholera epidemic in London in 1854 were based on ecological observations (Snow 1854). The 616 cholera cases in Soho during that year clustered around the Broad street water pump, suggesting that its water might be implicated in the transmission of infection. Data on whether cholera patients had in fact drunk from this pump were (mostly) unavailable but their geographical position (home address) with respect to the pump was used as an ecological proxy for exposure.

Durkheim and suicide

The French sociologist Émile Durkheim (1858–1917) studied regional, national, and temporal variations of European suicide rates. He noted an association between suicide rates of 13 Prussian provinces and how many of their citizens were Protestants (Durkheim 1951). Likewise, he linked a peak in the French suicide rate of over 8% in 1878 to the Paris World Exposition in that year. In the last example, a time period is used as an ecological proxy for exposure to risk, in this case, economic upheaval.

The Chicago School

Around 1930 sociologists in Chicago studied the distribution of various morbidity types across neighbourhoods in their city and the term ecological stems from their work. Wirth (1964) summed up their general philosophy in his statement that 'whatever else humans are, they are also animals and as such they exhibit effects of physical aggregation and of their habitat'. Ecological links were found between aggregate local levels of social deprivation and levels of social pathology like psychiatric hospital admission rates (Farris and Dunham 1939).

Geoffrey Rose

Individual-level studies focus strongly on relative risks or risk differences that are assumed to have a certain constancy across populations. However the epidemiologist Rose emphasized that the collective health of groups also affects the health of their individual members (Rose 1992). The link between smoking and ischaemic heart disease will appear non-existent in populations where everybody or nobody smokes. In these extreme cases, the effects of smoking are totally concentrated at the aggregate level.

Ecological data (Box 6.1)

Advantages

Less random error

Random error in exposure or outcome measurement is a problem in individual-level studies resulting in attenuated effect estimates. Ecological data have the advantage that measurement is aggregated over many individuals.

Box 6.1 **The advantages and disadvantages of ecological studies**

Advantages of ecological studies:

- less random error;
- continuous rather than dichotomous data, providing more power to detect associations;
- cheap, quick, and easy data collection.

Disadvantages of ecological studies

- can only demonstrate associations as the researcher is never sure whether those with the exposure are the same individuals as those with the outcome;
- extrapolating results to individuals can be misleading—the ecological fallacy;
- bias such as unbalanced misclassification, auto-correlation, multicollinearity, and non-balanced migration may lead to misleading results.

While individual-level measures may be subject to much random error, group averages may give more precise ecological estimates.

Dichotomous versus continuous measurement

A dichotomous measure at individual-level; exposed yes/no, or outcome yes/no is translated into a continuous measure when aggregated at ecological level; the proportion of the population exposed, or the prevalence of the outcome disorder. Analysis is therefore facilitated and the power to detect associations may be increased.

Data access, ethical issues

Ecological studies can often be conducted cheaply, using existing data collection systems. Joining datasets at the level of individuals is often impossible for ethical and legal reasons but linking at higher aggregation levels like electoral wards is permissible as long as information cannot be traced back to the individual-level (Quinn 1992).

Disadvantages

Unbalanced misclassification

If outcome or exposure classification in individuals is influenced systematically by the grouping variable, unbalanced misclassification results, leading to strongly biased effect estimates. For instance recorded suicide rates are lower in Catholic than Protestant countries (Neeleman *et al.* 1997) but this may be partly due to reluctance in Catholic cultures to record suicides under that label.

Auto-correlation

The level of outcomes and exposures of, for instance, coterminous areas or classes in the same school are not independent and will be more similar than the level of exposure or outcome in areas separated by considerable distance or different schools (Richardson 1992). Autocorrelation can be adjusted for with robust regression or models obtained on the basis of different aggregation levels such as wards and boroughs may be compared (Neeleman and Wessely 1999).

Weighting

Investigators debate whether aggregate exposure or outcome indices should be weighed for the size of the populations from which they are derived. Weighting may be useful when the eventual aim of ecological analyses is to make inferences from ecological data to risk–outcome associations in individuals (Rothman 1986, pp. 304–5). This is less obviously the case when the interest is on the determinants of public health.

Multicollinearity

Exposures tend to be more highly correlated at the aggregate than the individual-level. Thus, multicollinearity may threaten the stability of models especially when there are relatively few units of analysis. The use of multivariate confounder scores has been proposed as a solution (Rothman 1986, pp. 307–9). The outcome is first modelled in a regression equation containing all covariates (confounders) except the covariate of interest. From this model, a multivariate confounder score is calculated for each unit of analysis. Subsequently, this score and the covariate of interest are entered into a model to predict the outcome. However when using this approach, information on the effects of separate confounders is lost.

Non-balanced migration

High socio-economic status is associated with health but also with outward migration so that observed regional links between low socio-economic status and poor health may be due to the healthiest persons having left (Kunst et al. 1990).

Ecological designs

Exploratory studies

The simplest ecological design compares disease rates between populations grouped by their geographical position or the period (time-trend studies) during which they live. These studies often serve to generate theories about aetiology and allow exploration of geographical and temporal variations in disease occurrence. Analyses are mostly adjusted for the age distribution of the outcomes so that standardized mortality or morbidity ratios are compared. For instance, the observation that, in Europe, suicide rates in Hungary and Finland are several times higher than elsewhere has generated the hypothesis that some common Finno-Ugrian ancestry may contribute, genetically, to their high suicide risk (Mogyorosi 1996).

Age-cohort-period studies

These deserve special mention as a separate type of time–trend study. If the interest is on a certain period effect (e.g. changing market conditions, relaxing attitudes towards drug use) on the incidence of problems like depression (Klerman 1988) or drug addiction (Silbereisen et al. 1995), age of onset is an important likely confounder. Sometimes, however, membership of a certain birth cohort (e.g. born during a war, during an influenza epidemic) is also of interest next to age of onset and period effects. However, these three demographic risk factors cannot be separated in ecological designs (see Box 6.2).

Box 6.2 **The relationship between period, age of onset and date of birth**

Period = age of onset + date of birth

Population correlation studies

These studies test hypotheses by using geographical or temporal grouping variables as proxies for aggregate exposures. The aluminium content of local drinking water was the aggregate exposure of interest in a famous ecological study of Alzheimer's disease incidence (Martyn et al. 1989). Many social-epidemiological studies have linked regional (Eames et al. 1993) or temporal (Bunn 1979) indices of social deprivation and poverty with adverse health outcomes.

Ecological (community) intervention studies

These are the (quasi-) experimental variety of population correlation studies. Following findings of negative associations between caries and the fluoride content of drinking water (Dean 1946), an ecological intervention evaluated the effects of adding fluoride to drinking water in one American city (Newburgh) and not another (Kingston) (Ast and Schlesinger 1997). The subsequent reduction in caries may not be due to fluoridation, since actual fluoride exposure in persons with or without caries was unmeasured. Another problem with ecological intervention studies is their low statistical power, as they frequently have no more than two experimental groups. Often, ecological 'interventions' take advantage of natural experiments to evaluate consequences of policy changes or unusual occurrences. For example, a study demonstrating rising rates of suicidal behaviour following the death of Princess Diana (Hawton et al. 2000) suggested that suicidal behaviour is subject to media influence, or the observation that Canadian cirrhosis death rates between 1921 and 1956 were negatively correlated with the price of alcohol (Seeley 1960).

Comparative ecological studies

This powerful and under-utilized design makes detailed comparisons of the average exposure levels between a few (mostly less than four) populations with markedly different rates of disease. The objective is to test whether differences in average levels of exposure could account for the differences in disease rates *in these populations* rather than to look for correlations between exposure and disorder across many populations. These studies can study a large number of exposures, test many hypotheses simultaneously, and can generate new hypotheses for future research.

Ecological analysis

Ecological associations are mostly analysed with linear regression techniques, with the exception of comparative studies. As an example, the link between female suicide and labour force participation rates in 24 OECD countries (Organisation for Economic Cooperation and Development) is examined (WHO 1999; OECD 1998). Figure 6.1 suggests that suicide rates are higher where labour force participation is higher.

The Y-axis denotes the aggregate outcome, X-axis the aggregate predictor, A is the intercept and B the regression coefficient. Such observations feed speculation that changing gender roles may contribute to increasing suicide rates among women of working age.

Cross-level inference from the aggregate level to individuals

In an ideal situation, when

♦ ecological confounders are completely adjusted for;

♦ the base-rate of the outcome is similar across groups;

♦ the risk difference between exposed and unexposed is also similar across the groups;

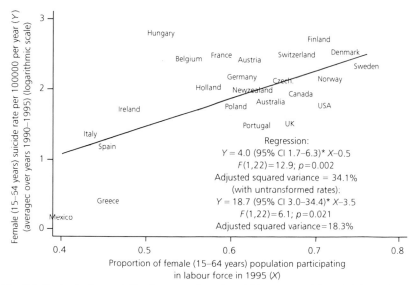

Fig. 6.1 Ecological association between female suicide rates and female labour force participation in OECD countries.

then a relative risk, a measure of effect applicable to individuals, can be derived from an ecological regression line by extrapolation to hypothetical populations with 0% and 100% exposure levels, respectively. This is called a cross-level inference.

As the data in Fig. 6.1 were logarithmically transformed, in the population with 0% exposure $Y = \exp(A + B^*0)$, while in the population with 100% exposure $Y = \exp(A + B^*1)$ which gives a relative risk of

$$\text{Relative risk} = \frac{\exp(A+B)}{\exp(A)} = \exp(B)$$

Applied to the female suicide-labour force participation example; $\exp(B) = 54.6$, suggesting that working women have a suicide rate of approximately 55 times above that of non-working women. This derivation of the relative risk from ecological linear regression was originally described for untransformed outcome data (Beral *et al.* 1979) in which case the extrapolated rate in the 100% exposed population $(A + B^*1)$ relative to the hypothetical population with 0% exposure $(A + B^*0)$ is represented by the formula

$$\text{Relative rate} = \frac{A+B}{A} = 1 + \frac{B}{A}$$

In our example (Fig. 6.1) the coefficient B and the intercept taken from the untransformed data are 18.7 and -3.5, respectively, yielding a negative relative rate. This impossibility arises because the method requires extrapolation of the regression line to values of X well outside the range of observation. In doing so there is an implicit assumption that the relative risk is invariant across the full exposure range, which is unlikely to be the case.

Controlling for confounding at ecological level

Consider an ecological confounder, which increases levels of disorder irrespective of risk factor exposure by a factor of 40.

Ecological confounding often results in strong overestimates of the regression coefficient, as ecological predictors are often strongly correlated. The joint distribution of confounder and exposure may be unknown but if data has been collected on known confounders at aggregate level, adjustment at this level may yield an unbiased ecological effect estimate, as illustrated by Fig. 6.2. An alternative method of adjusting for ecological confounding is to indirectly standardize for the confounders. This is only possible if the outcome distribution with respect to the confounders is known, such as demographic data like age and gender. However many confounders may be unknown or unmeasured.

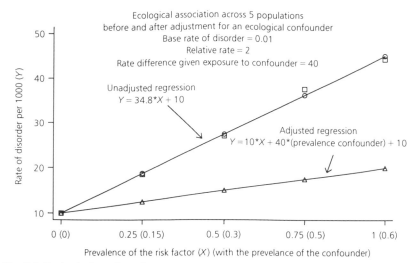

Fig. 6.2 Ecological confounding.

Problems with cross-level inference; ecological bias

In the above example the inferred individual level effect was so strong as to be improbable. Ecological bias refers to the failure of ecological effect estimates to represent a causal association at individual level. Ecological bias can occur under one, other, or both of the following circumstances.

Contextual confounding (confounding by group)

When the base rate of the disease varies in unexposed persons between populations, the ecological regression line can give a biased estimate of individual-level effects. Specifically this occurs where there is an association at ecological level between the prevalence or mean level of the exposure *in the population* and the frequency of the disease outcome in *unexposed individuals*. Clearly the exposure under study cannot have caused the outcome in those who were not exposed, so this association must be spurious. In the example given in Fig. 6.1 we have no way of knowing if the women who committed suicide had been working. It is possible, although unlikely, that all suicides occurred among non-workers. In ecological analyses, as no information is available on the distribution of risk factors among *individuals*, bias due to contextual confounding cannot be remedied with purely ecological data. It can lead to overestimates, underestimates or even reversals of regression coefficients.

Contextual effect modification (effect modification by group)

Contextual effect modification can be said to occur where the *risk difference* between exposed and unexposed differs between populations, specifically where there is an association at the ecological level between the prevalence or mean level of the exposure, or the frequency of the outcome, and the risk difference.

Contextual confounding and effect modification can occur through one or other of three mechanisms.

(a) Third factors, which are true risk factors for the outcome at individual level, are differently distributed between the populations and are associated at ecological level with the exposure under study. Thus in the example in Fig. 6.1, the prevalence of hazardous drinking among women may be associated at country level with female labour force participation, and for individual women there may be an association between hazardous drinking and suicide.

(b) The ecological exposure has a contextual effect separate from any causal effect at individual level. Thus the prevalence of labour force participation in their country may increase individual women's risk for suicide regardless of whether or not they work. Note that this contextual association would be a valid reflection of contextual causation, even though the association is not observed at individual level.

(c) The prevalence of the exposure, or of the disease in the population can modify the strength of the link between individuals' exposure status and their risk of disease. In our example, the difference in the risk of suicide between women who work and those who do not work may be greater in countries with a higher proportion of women working. This would have resulted in an overestimation of the individual relative risk from the ecological correlation. This scenario is probably not uncommon. A good example is found in infectious disease epidemiology, where immunity is often higher when exposure to infection is more prevalent (Koopman and Longini, Jr. 1994). In social epidemiology, unemployment is less strongly linked with morbidity in regions or periods where unemployment is more prevalent, as unemployment becomes less unusual in the population (Platt 1986). The link between membership of given ethnic minority groups and health outcomes depends on the ethnic mix of individuals' neighbourhoods (Neeleman and Wessely 1999). Contextual effect modification has been a longstanding interest of sociologists who have used terms such as density (Rabkin 1979), status integration (Blalock 1967) and risk dilution/concentration effects (Neeleman 1998). The relative risk of disorder, given exposure, varies between individuals according to aggregate features of the groups they are member of, like the risk factor prevalence. In this situation, the shape of the regression line is often curvilinear (Neeleman 1998). As with contextual confounding, contextual effect modification cannot

> ## Box 6.3 **Cross-level inference in ecological studies**
>
> Cross-level inference (extrapolating from ecological studies to the individual level) carries the risk of the ecological fallacy (that ecological associations may differ from individual-level associations in the same population) because they are vulnerable to:
>
> - ecological confounding
> - contextual confounding
> - contextual effect modification.

be remedied with purely ecological data and can result in strongly biased estimates of regression coefficients (Box 6.3).

Conclusion: the ecological fallacy and its individual-level corollary

Contextual confounding and contextual effect modification are responsible for the cross-level bias that invalidates the direct application of aggregate level associations to individuals. Unless stringent conditions are met and there is no bias due to unbalanced misclassification, auto-correlation, multi-collinearity, and non-balanced migration, in addition to no ecological or contextual confounding, or contextual effect modification, authors who apply ecological data to individuals risk committing the *ecological fallacy* (Selvin 1958). It is principally due to this ecological fallacy that ecological studies have acquired their poor reputation.

Does this mean that ecological data do not add anything above and beyond that which can be gleaned from the relative risks as they apply at the individual-level? The mechanisms responsible for cross-level bias, and contextual effect modification in particular, are of great importance to the understanding of the etiology of disease in individuals. Geoffrey Rose first drew attention to the fact that population health is not only dependent on the health of its individual members but that the reverse applies as well. This can be examined only by a combination of individual-level data with ecological exposure indices. Special software may be used for this (Goldstein 1997). However, fitting simple effect functions (Rothman 1986, pp. 233–5) by plotting relative risks against features of study groups like their risk factor prevalence (Neeleman *et al.* 1997) may also demonstrate that the individual-level prediction of disorder is often incomplete when ecological features are not considered.

Practical exercise

An ecological study of suicide rates among prisoners in different countries suggests that countries with high rates of imprisonment also have high suicide rates.

(1) Interpret these results.

(2) What assumptions are made if the investigators state that the ecological regression line and the relative risk can be calculated from each other?

Answer to (2)

(a) Absence of ecological confounding; for instance in this example, it is possible that countries with higher imprisonment rates, also have higher rates of other suicide risk factors like alcohol misuse or social deprivation

(b) Absence of ecological effect modification; for instance, in this example it is possible that imprisonment has a different impact on persons who live in countries where imprisonment is frequent than on persons who live in countries where imprisonment is rare and associated with high levels of (secondary) deviance.

References

Ast, D.B. and Schlesinger, E.R. (1997) The conclusion of a ten year study of water fluoridation. *American Journal of Public Health*, 46, 265–71.

Beral, V., Chilvers, C., and Fraser, P. (1979) On the estimation of relative risk from vital statistical data. *Journal of Epidemiology and Community Health*, 33, 159–62.

Bianchi, N., Crosignan, P., Rovelli, A., *et al.* (2000) Overhead electricity power lines and childhood leukemia: a registry-based, case–control study. *Tumori*, 86, 195–98.

Blalock, H.M. Jr. (1967) Status inconsistency, social mobility, status integration and structural effects. *American Sociological Review*, 32, 790–801.

Bunn, A.R. (1979) Mortality and the business cycle in Australia. *American Journal of Public Health*, 69, 772–81.

Dean, H.T. (1946) Some general epidemiological observations. In (ed. F.R. Moutlon) *Dental caries and fluoride*. AAAS, Washington DC.

Durkheim, E. (1951) *Suicide; A Study in Sociology* (translated by J.A. Spaulding and G. Simpson). Free Press, Illinois.

Eames, M., Ben-Shlomo, Y., and Marmot, M.G. (1993) Social deprivation and premature mortality; regional comparison across England. *British Medical Journal*, 307, 1097–102.

Farris, R.E. and Dunham, H.W. (1939) *Mental disorders in urban areas*. University of Chicago Press, Chicago.

Goldstein, H. (1997) *Multilevel Statistical Models*. Arnold, London.

Hawton, K., Harris, L., Appleby, L., *et al.* (2000) Effect of death of Diana, princess of Wales on suicide and deliberate self-harm. *British Journal of Psychiatry*, 177, 463–6.

Kasl, S.V. (1979) Mortality and the business cycle: some questions about research strategies when utilizing macro-social and ecologic data. *American Journal of Public Health*, 69, 784–8.

Klerman, G.L. (1988) The current age of youthful melancholia; evidence for increase in depression among adolescents and young adults. *British Journal of Psychiatry*, 152, 4–14.

Koopman, J.S. and Longini, I.M. (1994) The ecological effects of individual exposures and nonlinear disease dynamics in populations. *American Journal of Public Health*, 84, 836–42.

Kunst, A.E., Looman, W.N., and Mackenbach, J.P. (1990) Socio-economic mortality differences in the Netherlands in 1950–1984: a regional study of cause specific mortality. *Social Science and Medicine*, 31, 141–52.

Liu, K., Stamler, J., Moss, D., Garside, D., Persky, V., and Soltero, I. (1979) Dietary cholesterol, fat, and fibre, and colon-cancer mortality. An analysis of international data. *Lancet*, 2(8146), 782–5.

Martyn, C.N., Osmond, C., Edwardson, J.A., Barker, D.J.P., Harris, E.C. , and Lacey, R.F. (1989) Geographical relation between Alzheimer's disease and aluminium in drinking water. *Lancet*, 1(8629), 59–62.

McCulloch, A. (2001) Social environments and health: cross-sectional national survey. *British Medical Journal*, 323, 208–9.

McMichael, A.J. and Beaglehole, R. (2000) The changing global context of public health. *Lancet*, 356, 495–9.

Mogyorosi, A. (1996) Is there a Finno-Ugrian suicide gene? *Lancet*, 347, 402–3.

Morgenstern, H. (1998) Ecologic studies. In (ed. K.J. Rothman and S. Greenland), *Modern epidemiology*, pp. 459–80. Lippincott-Raven, Philadelphia.

Neeleman, J. (1998) Regional suicide rates in the Netherlands: does religion still play a role? *International Journal of Epidemiology*, 27, 466–72.

Neeleman, J. and Wessely, S. (1999) Ethnic minority suicide: a small area geographical study in south London. *Psychological Medicine*, 29, 429–36.

Neeleman, J., Halpern, D., Leon, D., and Lewis, G. (1997) Tolerance of suicide, religion and suicide rates; an ecological and individual-level study in 19 western countries. *Psychological Medicine*, 27, 1165–71.

Organization for Economic Cooperation and Development (1998) *Labour Force Statistics*. OECD, Paris.

Platt, S. (1986) Parasuicide and unemployment, *British Journal of Psychiatry*, 149, 401–5.

Quinn, M.J. (1992) Confidentiality. In (ed. P. Elliott, J. Cuzick, D. English, and R. Stern), *Geographical and environmental epidemiology; methods for small area studies*, pp. 132–140. Oxford University Press, Oxford.

Rabkin, J.G. (1979) Ethnic density and psychiatric hospitalization: hazards of minority status. *American Journal of Psychiatry*, 136, 1562–6.

Reuband, K.H. (1995) Drug use and drug policy in Western Europe. *European Addiction Research*, 1, 32–41.

Richardson, S. (1992) Statistical methods for geographical correlation studies. In (ed. P. Elliott, J. Cuzick, D. English, and R. Stern), *Geographical and environmental epidemiology; methods for small area studies*, pp. 181–204. Oxford University Press, Oxford.

Rose, G. (1992) *The strategy of preventive medicine*. Oxford Medical Publications, Oxford.

Rothman, K.J. (1986) *Modern Epidemiology*. Little Brown & Company, Boston.

Seeley, J.R. (1960) Deaths by liver cirrhosis and the price of beverage alcohol. *Canadian Medical Association Journal*, 83, 1361–6.

Selvin, H.C. (1958) Durkheim's suicide and the problem of empirical research. *American Journal of Sociology*, 63, 607–19.

Silbereisen, R.K., Robins, L., and Rutter, M. (1995) Secular trends in substance abuse; concepts and data on the impact of social change on alcohol and drug abuse. In (ed. M. Rutter and D. Smith), *Psychosocial disorders in young people; time trends and their causes*, pp. 490–543. Wiley & Sons, Chichester.

Snow, J. (1854) *On the mode of communication of cholera*, John Churchill, London.

Susser, E., Neugebauer, R., Hoek, H.W., *et al.* (1996) Schizophrenia after prenatal famine. Further evidence. *Archives of General Psychiatry*, 53, 25–31.

Wirth, L. (1964) Human ecology. In (ed. P. Wirth), *On cities and social life, selected papers*. University of Chicago Press, Chicago.

World Health Organization (1999) *Health statistical data collections*. WHO, Geneva.

Chapter 7

Cross-sectional surveys

Martin Prince

Introduction

This chapter considers the strengths and limitations, and the uses and abuses of cross-sectional surveys in psychiatric epidemiology. Certain basic aspects of research methodology; the concept of the base population, sampling strategies, representativeness, the problem of non-response and the practical logistics of population-based research are introduced here, although they are in practice equally relevant to other study designs. The chapter also introduces the problem of bias, arising both from non-response and misclassification. In conclusion, we review major surveys of psychiatric morbidity in a historical context, highlighting methodological developments and discussing the yield of information to be gleaned from them.

Uses and applications of cross-sectional surveys

Cross-sectional surveys can be used to measure the prevalence of a disorder within a population. This may be useful for:

- drawing public and political attention to the extent of a problem within a community;
- planning services—identifying need, both met and unmet;
- describing the impact of a condition within a population; the level of disablement associated with it, the demands on services, and the economic costs.

Such surveys may seek to make comparisons with other populations or regions (in a series of comparable surveys conducted in different populations), or to chart trends over time (in a series of comparable surveys of the same population).

They can also be used to compare the characteristics of those in the population with and without the disorder, thus

- identifying cross-sectional associations with potential risk factors for the disorder;
- identifying suitable (representative) cases and controls for population-based case–control studies.

Findings from population-based cross-sectional surveys can be generalized to the base population for that survey, and to some extent, to other populations with similar characteristics.

The main drawback of cross-sectional surveys for analytical as opposed to descriptive epidemiology is that they can only give clues about aetiology. Because exposure (potential risk factor) and outcome (disorder or health condition) are measured simultaneously one can never be sure, in the presence of an association, which is the cause and which the consequence. The technical term is 'direction of causality'. Thus, in the Gospel Oak Survey (Prince *et al.* 1997), did depression lead to disablement, or disablement to depression?

The design of cross-sectional surveys

The base population

Cross-sectional surveys survey a defined base population, from which the sample for the survey is drawn. The random element of the sampling selection procedure should ensure that the sample is *representative* of this wider population. The findings of the survey should then be *generalizable* to this group.

From the examples given above it should be clear that the base population might be a special sub-population (prisoners, homeless people, hospital inpatients) or the general population (Box 7.1). Whichever, the first step is to identify a sampling frame defining eligibility. Criteria need to be thought through carefully. For population surveys they usually include an age criterion, a place of residence criterion, and a period criterion; thus all residents of a defined area,

Box 7.1 **Examples of base populations taken from the psychiatric literature**

Cross-sectional surveys should have a defined base population such as:

- All children in one or more schools (Patton *et al.* 1996).
- All prisoners in a given country (Brinded *et al.* 2001).
- All residents of a single catchment area, aged 65 and over (Prince *et al.* 1997).
- All residents of several catchment areas taken to be broadly representative of national diversity (Regier *et al.* 1984).
- All adult residents of a country (Jenkins *et al.* 1997; Andrews *et al.* 2001).

The results can be generalized to the base population and also, possibly, to other population.

resident on a particular day or month. Participants may occasionally need to be excluded from the survey because of health or other circumstances that render their participation difficult or impossible. Ideally these exclusion criteria should be specified in advance. Every effort should be made to be as inclusive as possible, in order to maximize the potential for generalizing from the survey findings.

Sampling frames require an accurate register of all eligible participants in the base population. In most countries, such registers are drawn up and updated regularly for general population censuses, taxation, and other administrative purposes, and for establishing voting entitlement in local and national elections. However, there are problems associated with using such registers.

Some may not contain all of the information (e.g. age, sex, and address) that is needed to identify and contact a sample with a specified age range. Many governments will either not allow researchers to have access to these registers, set limits on the information that can be gleaned from them, or will limit the way in which the data is used. Also many administrative registers are surprisingly inaccurate, particularly in the case of highly mobile urban populations. Thus people move address without informing the relevant agency, or move or die in the interval between regular updates of the register. For government censuses this problem is referred to as undercounting. If a socio-demographic group (ethnic minorities or older people), or people with a health condition under study (depression) are particularly likely to be underrepresented this can lead to significant biases. Because of these deficiencies, some population-based surveys draw up their own register by carrying out a door-knock census of the area to be surveyed. While this is practical for a small catchment area survey, a survey of a larger base population such as the population of a whole country would need a different strategy. Often investigators draw a random sample of households, which are then visited by researchers who interview either all eligible residents, or individuals selected at random from among the eligible residents in the household.

Sampling strategies

It is clearly not necessary to interview every resident of a country to estimate the prevalence of major depression with reasonable precision. Sample size calculations may be carried out to determine the minimum sample size required to measure a given prevalence with a given precision (e.g. ±1%). Sampling is guided by two overriding aims:

- to achieve the maximum precision for a given outlay of resources;
- to avoid bias.

Bias in sampling arises when

+ the sampling is non-random;

+ the sampling frame (list, register or other population record) does not cover the population adequately, completely or accurately;

+ some sections of the intended population are difficult to find or are likely to refuse to co-operate.

There are several different possible sampling strategies. Note however that each of these involves random selection.

Simple random samples	for example, 1 in 5 residents of an area.
Stratified random samples (with a fixed sampling fraction)	for example, 1 in 5 selected at random from each age group, or both genders, or each housing district. This eliminates between strata sampling error
Stratified random samples (with a variable sampling fraction)	for example, 1 in 10 of those aged 65–74, 1 in 5 of those aged 75–84 and 1 in 2 of those aged 85 and over. The aim is to over-sample strata with low numbers, or high standard errors in order to ensure adequate precision in each subgroup. When the final prevalence estimate for the whole population is calculated, the over-sampling of the sub-groups will have to be taken into account. Estimates for sub-groups are *weighted back* to their distribution within the whole population by using *weights* that are calculated according to the different *sampling fractions* applied.
Cluster random sample	for example, a random sample of schools in the UK, a random sample of classes within the selected schools, and a random sample of children within the selected classes. A simple random sample of all UK school-children would necessitate negotiating access to and visiting a much larger number of schools. As long as the cluster sampling is truly random and the analysis is appropriately weighted, unbiased and generalizable estimates should result.

Response rates/representativeness

The size of the achieved sample (those who have been interviewed and contributed data) will differ from that of the target sample because of non-response. Some participants will refuse to be interviewed, others will have died or moved away since the register or sample was established. In establishing the sample or register, some data (usually at least age and gender) is available on all potential participants. It is therefore possible to check the representativeness of the achieved sample. Systematic differences between the characteristics

---

Box 7.2 **Factors that can influence the response rate**

Certain characteristics of the study may affect the response rate and should be considered in the survey design:

- ♦ the manner of the initial approach to the participant;
- ♦ the burden imposed on the participant by the survey;
- ♦ the medium for the administration of the research interview.

---

of those who were interviewed and those who were not can lead to biased estimates of prevalence, and bias in investigations of aetiological associations. One way to limit non-response bias is to ensure the highest response rate possible, and factors that can influence the response rate are discussed below and should be considered in the design of the survey (Box 7.2).

Approaching the participant

The first contact is of vital importance. This will usually be by mail, or by direct contact. The project should be described honestly and comprehensively, but in simple and non-threatening terms. The potential value of the project should be stressed, together with a description of any burden that will be placed on participants in terms of time or discomfort. The layout of printed material should be clear, and should be of a professional appearance. It can sometimes be helpful to include a letter of introduction from some person known to the participant, such as their general practitioner, or some locally prominent person. It is unethical to carry out any kind of biomedical research on humans without their informed consent. Participants will need to read, or have read to them, an information sheet describing the research and their role in it. An investigator should be available to answer any questions the potential participant may have. It should be made clear that the choice, whether or not to participate, is for them alone, and that they are free to decline, or to pull out after first agreeing, at any time, without giving reasons and with no adverse consequences. Those who wish to participate should sign a consent form. The investigator and the participant should both keep a copy of the consent form.

The burden imposed on the participant

Potential participants are likely to be put off by lengthy, unwieldy interviews. Special care should be taken if it is proposed to enquire into culturally sensitive areas such as sexual behaviour or marital relationships. Physical examinations and procedures such as taking blood samples may also reduce the response rate. The incorporation of biological measures into epidemiological research poses particular difficulties. However recent well-designed studies have demonstrated the feasibility of collecting blood, cheek scrapes for genetic material, saliva for cortisol, and even carrying out carotid artery ultrasonography on large population-based samples (Hofman *et al.* 1997). Epidemiological surveys inevitably involve some element of compromise between the depth and breadth of the data that investigators might ideally wish to gather, and that which can be pragmatically achieved. There is no point in developing a complex survey protocol that achieves a response rate of only 30%. Simpler less sophisticated measures may be nearly as precise while achieving a much higher response.

The medium for the administration of the research interview

Questionnaire-based measures can be administered in a face-to-face interview, over the telephone, or by post. The postal method can obviously only be used for self-completion questionnaires. It may seem appealing at first sight because of the apparent savings in personnel time, cost, and efficiency. However, response rates can be very low, typically only 30–40% on first mailing. Non-responders tend to have lower socio-economic status and lower educational level (there is evidently a particular problem with the illiterate) than responders; hence this is likely to lead to bias. Postal methods will thus only be acceptable if the questionnaire is exceptionally simple and clearly laid out, and if considerable resources can be allocated to pursuing non-responders by postal reminders, and if need be, with telephone calls or home visits.

Telephone interviews may be an acceptable alternative that still offers economies in terms of time saved taken to travel to a participant's home. Repeated telephone calls can be made to gain access to those who are rarely at home. Response rates can therefore be quite high, and many instruments have been shown to be both feasible and valid when administered in this way. Evidently this method can only be used in settings where a substantial proportion of the population have a telephone in their home, effectively limiting its use to certain developed countries. The telephone system can even be used to generate representative samples for population surveys, using the technique of random digit dialling (Breslau *et al.* 1999).

Face-to-face interviews offer the participant the convenience of being interviewed in their own home, by an interviewer who should

- be polite,
- be neatly and appropriately dressed,
- carry identification,
- be sensitive to their position as guests in the participant's home.

Some participants may prefer to be interviewed in a research centre rather than in their own homes, and provision should be made for this eventuality.

The resources committed to following up non-response

Eligible participants who state clearly that they do not wish to participate in the survey should not be pressured or otherwise induced into changing their minds. They may however be invited to provide some basic data (e.g. age, gender, social class, smoking behaviour) that can be used later to check whether their non-response is likely to have led to bias. However, much non-response arises from eligible persons who have not replied at all to the request for an interview, as opposed to having actively refused participation. Many of these may agree to participate if they are approached again. Most researchers would make it their practice to approach such 'passive non-responders' on at least two, and possibly up to four further occasions before accepting that their failure to respond indicates a positive wish not to participate. Initial approaches by letter can be supplemented by telephone calls or even home visits. Home visits may reveal another reason for non-response; the register may be inaccurate and the person has moved away or died. Following-up non-response can be time consuming and costly, so provision needs to be made for this in the survey budget and time schedule.

Interviews/assessments

All instruments need to be valid and reliable. The concepts of validity and reliability are dealt with in more detail in the chapter on measurement in psychiatry. Validity refers to the extent to which an instrument measures what it purports to measure. Instruments should be validated *for the population in which they are being used*. Some instruments have been validated for clinical populations, but not for community samples. Others have been validated for one culture (e.g. a developed country setting) but not another (e.g. a developing country setting). Establishing validity for an instrument may necessitate pilot work, which may include

- translation and back translation
- checking conceptual validity using ethnographic procedures
- field trialling for feasibility, and for criterion validity against a local gold standard.

In cross-sectional surveys of psychiatric morbidity, it is often necessary to assess large numbers of participants. For this reason, assessments tend to be made by lay interviewers rather than by psychiatrists. Great reliance is placed on highly structured diagnostic instruments that are validated for lay administration. Reliability is achieved partly through the highly structured nature of the assessments, and by rigorous training of lay interviewers, with continuing monitoring during the course of the survey for quality control. The two most widely used instruments are the CIDI and the CIS-R (see Jenkins *et al.* 1997, and Chapter 2). These have been demonstrated to be capable of identifying a range of psychiatric disorders in the community with reasonable sensitivity and specificity. However, concerns have been raised regarding the validity of these diagnoses against the gold standard of semi-structured assessments administered by experienced clinicians. These have revealed generally poor concordance for common mental disorders (Brugha *et al.* 1999*a,b*). There have also been particular problems in the rating of symptoms of psychosis that require some degree of interviewer judgement as to the pathological significance of the behaviour or experience described (Cooper *et al.* 1998). Much more work is required to validate lay administered structured assessments in general population samples, and to identify the source and significance of discrepancies with clinician semi-structured diagnoses. One promising approach is to train experienced lay survey interviewers in semi-structured, clinical, diagnostic interviewing (Brugha *et al.* 1999*c*). An alternative approach is to use lay interviewers with a structured interview, but to collect verbatim accounts from participants about areas of difficulty that can then be reviewed by experienced clinicians. This approach minimizes misclassification due to the respondent misunderstanding the question, and allows identification of disorders that are non-symptomatic as they are being actively treated (Meltzer *et al.* 2000). Whatever approach is used, there will be some misclassification. This may either be random (not related to actual caseness or exposure) or systematic. Systematic misclassification may bias the estimate of prevalence, and may also bias investigations of aetiological associations.

Two-phase surveys

For rare conditions, such as schizophrenia, a two-phase diagnostic procedure may be indicated. The lay instrument is used as a screen. Those with a high probability of being a case are then given a more extensive and definitive second stage clinical assessment, often carried out by a psychiatrist. A similar two stage approach is used in the diagnosis of dementia, in which a cognitive test is used as a screening instrument; those performing badly receive a more detailed neuropsychological assessment, a clinical interview, a physical examination and an informant interview to establish a definitive diagnosis. These designs are superficially attractive, providing diagnostic precision, but with considerable economies of research effort. The rarer the condition, the greater the economy. However, they should be used with extreme caution given several significant caveats and disadvantages (Dunn *et al.* 1999):

(1) The screening measure should have high sensitivity and specificity.

(2) For a rare condition, the positive predictive value of the screening instrument will tend to be low, even when specificity is high. Most of the screen-positive participants will be false positives, and significant resources may need to be allocated to the second phase.

(3) Unless (and this is most unusual) one can be confident that the screening measure has 100% specificity, that is, there are no false negatives, one must interview a sufficient number of randomly selected false negatives to assess the false negative rate with reasonable precision.

(4) The analysis of the data is greatly complicated, particularly with respect to estimates of standard errors (and confidence intervals) and in testing for statistical significance of differences between prevalences observed in sub-groups (see below under analysis for further details).

(5) Further more serious complications arise where, as is usual there is non-response in the more burdensome second phase, and this non-response, whether it arises from deaths, refusals or moving away is non-random with respect to the exposure and the outcome had it been measured (informative censoring).

Although most of these problems have been recognised for some time (Deming 1978) two-phase surveys are enduringly popular but often incorrectly designed, analysed and inferenced.

Data processing

Interviewers may record data on to a paper questionnaire, which should be clearly laid out with variable names and coding boxes for each item of data to be recorded. Data coded on the questionnaires then needs to be entered into a computerized database. Many errors can occur in this process. The data entry clerk may misread the coding on the questionnaire, or their finger may slip on the computer keyboard. Errors can be considerably reduced by double entering data. When the data is entered a second time the computer identifies discrepancies between the first and second entry and requests clarification. Errors can be further reduced by validity checks. These can be incorporated into the data entry program. Thus the entry field for the variable gender could be set to accept 1 (for male) 2 (for female) and 9 (for missing value), but to reject all other values. Double data entry and computerized validity checks are available with a variety of data entry software packages. The EPI INFO package is public domain software developed by the WHO and CDC Atlanta, and can be downloaded from *http://www.cdc.gov/epiinfo/*. Validity checks can also be run after all the data has been entered. Frequency distributions can be run for all variables to check that all recorded values are sensible. Cross-tabulations may be used to establish, for instance, that all pregnancies are recorded as occurring in women.

Increasingly surveys are using lap-top computers for questionnaire administration and data recording. The script of the questionnaire is contained on a computer file. The interviewer reads the question from the screen of the laptop and enters the data directly onto the computer. The data that is entered can then be retrieved in the form of a data spreadsheet. This facility is also available within the EPI INFO package, although more sophisticated programs are available commercially (e.g. Microsoft Access). Computer administered questionnaires offer considerable advantages in terms of flexibility. Complex branching structures can be built into the questionnaire. Thus different sections of the questionnaire can be administered to men and women. Lengthy detailed sections can be omitted unless a particular combination of screening items is endorsed. Data transfer errors are eliminated.

Data management is a crucially important component of any well-conducted survey. However it is often neglected, and few reports give adequate descriptions of the procedures that were followed. Data handling is an important source of random error for many studies.

Analysis of data from cross-sectional surveys

The frequency of the mental health condition in the population is generally expressed as in terms of prevalence. Prevalence refers to the proportion of persons in a defined population that has the condition at the instant of the survey. Some mental health conditions (e.g. depression) are relapsing and remitting disorders, and for that reason period prevalence rates are sometimes quoted. A period prevalence (e.g. 12 months prevalence) is the proportion of those in a defined population, who *either* have the condition at the instant of the survey *or* have had it at any time over the previous 12 months. Several standard assessments (e.g. the CIDI and the SCAN) enquire after lifetime experience of mental disorders, and generate lifetime prevalence estimates. The validity of this approach is understandably controversial, relying as it does upon accurate recall of symptoms experienced many years previously (Parker 1987; Wittchen *et al.* 1989).

Cross-sectional surveys tend by their very nature to be descriptive and exploratory rather than being driven by specific hypotheses. The strategy for analysing cross-sectional surveys should nevertheless be closely linked to prior research objectives. The following are some basic principles.

(1) Start with simple description, univariate comparison between groups and classical stratified analysis. Proceed to more complex analyses, for example multivariate modelling with caution, and only when strictly indicated.

(2) Prevalence estimates should be weighted back to the composition of the base population, taking account of the sampling fractions applied in a two-phase survey. This is not a straightforward matter. Although point estimates can be calculated accurately by simple algebra (the Horvitz–Thompson estimator) standard errors will be underestimated, and require the application of special techniques. Dunn provides an excellent overview (Dunn *et al.* 1999). It is also not appropriate to test for the statistical significance of observed differences between proportions in subgroups (e.g. the prevalence of depression in men and women) using standard χ^2 tests. SPSS will not help, and only certain more specialized statistical software packages (e.g. STATA (StataCorp 1997)) provide appropriate techniques. From all of the above it should be evident that the evident economies of two-phase designs are to a considerable extent offset by the complications implicit in the correct analysis of these complex data sets. Expert statistical advice *must* be sought in the planning of such studies, and will almost certainly be required to assist in their analysis.

(3) Prevalence estimates should be accompanied by 95% confidence intervals, giving an indication of the precision of the estimate given the sample size (see above for the special circumstances of the two-phase survey). This may not be appropriate or necessary in catchment area surveys where the whole population has been surveyed (e.g Prince *et al.* 1997). Sampling error cannot occur when there has been no sampling.

(4) Potential risk factors for the main outcome disorder can be investigated by comparing the characteristics of cases and non-cases. In the first instance these comparisons should be univariate, for example *t*-test for differences in the mean age of cases and non-cases, or χ^2 test for differences in the proportions smoking.

(5) Bear in mind that the risk of making one or more Type 1 errors increases with the number of statistical comparisons being made. It is important to be judicious in the way in which you explore the data, and honest in the way in which you report the conduct of your analysis. Thus if you make 60 statistical comparisons it would be wrong to report the two 'statistically significant' differences without referring to the 58 'non-significant' tests.

(6) As in analytical epidemiology, multivariate modelling can be used to control for confounding and to test for interaction (effect modification). See Chapters 8 and 9 on case–control and cohort studies for more details.

Major psychiatric morbidity surveys—A historical review of methodological developments, scope, and achievements

The USA's NIMH Epidemiologic Catchment Area study

The Epidemiologic Catchment Area (ECA) survey was the first large scale attempt to estimate the prevalence of psychiatric morbidity in a nationwide survey (Regier *et al.* 1984). This was a governmental initiative developed during the presidency of Jimmy Carter (1976–1980) to inform future mental health policy in the USA. Five catchment area communities were selected for study, to represent broadly the ethnic, socio-economic and geographic diversity of the nation. A probability sample of over 18,000 adults was drawn from these sites. The survey interview was the comprehensive, lay administered, fully-structured Diagnostic Interview Schedule (DIS) (Robins *et al.* 1981). The principal focus of the ECA was upon one year and lifetime prevalences of diagnoses according to the then current Diagnostic and Statistical Manual of Mental Disorders-III (DSM-III) criteria, for example (Weissman *et al.* 1988). Aspects of the ECA have been criticized, particularly the validity of the DIS lifetime diagnoses (Burvill 1987; Parker 1987), the appropriateness of lay interviews, the applicability of the diagnostic ascertainment for older people and its failure to assess the findings of the survey in the context of the existing epidemiological data (Burvill 1987).

The US National Comorbidity Survey

The National Comorbidity Survey (NCS) was the second major national survey conducted in the USA. It differed from the ECA in its sampling methodology; a truly representative national sample was drawn of 8098 persons 15–54 years of age (Blazer *et al.* 1994). On this occasion the survey interview was a modified version of the World Health Organisation's Composite International Diagnostic Interview (CIDI), a fully structured, lay administered interview generating diagnoses according to DSM-IV criteria. The focus of the survey was to measure prevalence and to identify the extent of comorbidity between major and minor mental disorder and alcohol and substance use disorders (Blazer *et al.* 1994; Kendler *et al.* 1996; Kessler *et al.* 1997). Extensive analyses were conducted of lifetime experience of mental disorders using reported ages of onset, and sequence of onset of co-morbid disorders to identify windows of opportunity for preventive interventions in younger adults (Kessler *et al.* 1998). A further feature of the NCS was the investigation of possible aetiologic factors for mental disorders. Certain of these investigations were limited by the problem of attributing direction of causality to the observed associations, for example, between social support and depression (Zlotnick et al. 2000) and smoking and mental disorder (Lasser et al. 2000). Other reported associations, for example, that between child sexual abuse and adult mental disorder (Molnar et al. 2001), are more likely to reflect causal processes because of the latency between the reported exposure and the outcome, although recall bias may still be a problem. The remarkably prolific published output from the NCS may be explained in part by the decision to archive the data set in the public domain, making it available to the whole scientific community. This is now a standard procedure for surveys funded by the US National Institutes of Health.

UK National Psychiatric Morbidity Survey

In another governmental initiative the UK Department of Health commissioned its Office of Population Censuses and Surveys (OPCS) in 1993 to conduct a survey of psychiatric morbidity in a nationally representative household sample of 10,108 adults aged 16–65 (Jenkins et al. 1997). The survey interview was the Clinical Interview Schedule—Revised (CIS-R) (Lewis et al. 1992). This generated diagnoses of common mental disorders (i.e. excluding psychoses) according to ICD-10 criteria, and a scalable score allowing exploration of the impact of psychiatric morbidity as a continuum in the general population. Psychoses were assessed using a two-stage method in which participants reporting psychotic disorders or symptoms suggestive of psychotic disorders or responding positively to items from the Psychosis Screening Questionnaire were subsequently interviewed with the comprehensive semi-structured clinical assessment SCAN. The National Psychiatric Morbidity Survey (NPMS) was repeated in 2000, using essentially the same methodology. On this occasion the upper age limit was extended to 74 years. There was also a major focus for the first time upon the prevalence and impact of personality disorder assessed using the SCIDII. Both surveys also included assessment of alcohol and substance use disorders.

The UK National Surveys were part of a wider UK policy-driven initiative to estimate the extent and impact of mental disorders with particular reference to implications for service delivery. This acknowledged the limitations of household surveys, which might miss vulnerable and dependent persons with mental disorders. To compete the picture, several complementary surveys of special settings, using comparable methods, were therefore conducted by ONS over the 1990s (Jenkins et al. 1997):

(1) A sample of residents of institutions caring for the mentally ill ($N = 1191$); hospitals, nursing homes, residential care homes, hostels, group homes and supported accommodation.

(2) A sample of homeless people ($N = 1166$) accessed through hostels, night-shelters, private sector leased accommodation and day centres (Gill *et al.* 1996).

(3) A supplementary sample of patients with psychosis, known to services and living in private households ($N = 350$) (Foster *et al.* 1996).

(4) Prisoners (Singleton *et al.* 1998).

(5) A sample of 10,438 Children and Adolescents aged 5–15 accessed through the child benefit register. All those with disorder and a one in three sample of those without disorder were followed up at 18 months and again at 3 years. A survey of children looked after by local authorities has just been completed.

The Australian National Survey of Mental Health and Wellbeing

The Australian mental health survey drew a nationally representative probability sample of Australian households. The sample size was 10,641 adults, and the survey interview was the CIDI version 2.1. In addition to reports of the prevalence of mental disorders (Andrews *et al.* 2001), a major area of investigation has been the burden of mental disorders in terms of associated disability, both comparing individual mental disorders (Sanderson and Andrews 2002), and comparing mental disorders with major chronic physical health conditions (Vos *et al.* 2001). The investigators have also focussed upon unmet need (Parslow and Jorm 2001) and access to services, drawing attention, for example, to the particularly low levels of help-seeking from primary care services of people with common mental disorders (Andrews and Carter 2001), with the practical suggestion that a system of registration with a local family physician might help to remedy this problem. Conversely they identified relatively high rates of help-seeking among persons with suicidal ideation, particularly among those who had gone on to make an attempt (Pirkis *et al.* 2001), with obvious implications for targeted preventive interventions.

The World Mental Health 2000 surveys

The World Mental Health 2000 (WMH 2000) initiative, coordinated by the World Health Organization's International Consortium in Psychiatric Epidemiology (ICPE), is the most ambitious attempt yet to generate data on the prevalence and impact of mental disorders that will permit valid comparisons between countries and regions worldwide (Kessler 1999). The core instrument for the surveys is the WHO Composite International Diagnostic Interview (CIDI). The investigators hope eventually to complete 160,000 interviews in 24 countries including all major continents. A particular feature is the goal to validate the CIDI in every centre with clinical interviews (SCAN) of all CIDI cases and a random sub-sample of all CIDI non-cases. Impact will be assessed in terms of associated impairment and disability, using the WHO's new Disability Assessment Scale (WHODAS II). The Global Burden of Disease Report (1996) has identified mental disorders as a hitherto unremarked major contributor to disease burden in developed and developing countries alike. WMH 2000 will build upon the findings of the GBD report by estimating associated disability directly, rather than relying upon applying disorder specific disability weights derived from consensus groups. As the principal investigator of the initiative, Ron Kessler notes 'valid and representative general population epidemiological data on patterns, predictors and adverse consequences of psychiatric disorders are needed as a foundation for public health initiatives. Formidable methodological and logistical challenges arise in implementing this agenda, but we are confident that these challenges can be met'.

Dissemination of findings from cross-sectional surveys

In addition to publication in peer-reviewed scientific journals, investigators should always consider alternative methods to reach the target audience, the consumers for their research. Findings from cross-sectional surveys may be of relevance to:

◆ politicians

◆ health policymakers

◆ non-governmental organisations and mental health advocacy groups

◆ public health physicians

◆ health practitioners

◆ community leaders

◆ the wider community

◆ participants taking part in the survey.

Action research will be firmly orientated toward the public health and policy priorities for the population under study. It should gauge its success by the impact that it achieves in terms of raising awareness, altering priorities, and informing better preventive and treatment interventions. Achievement of these goals will certainly depend upon well-designed and focussed research, but equally upon an effective and balanced dissemination strategy (Box 7.3). This should certainly extend beyond publications in high quality peer-reviewed publications, and presentations at research conferences (which will

> ### Box 7.3 **A balanced dissemination strategy for action research**
>
> - High impact publications in peer-reviewed scientific journals.
> - Research presentations at national and international conferences.
> - Special local and national workshops including policymakers, clinicians, and community leaders.
> - Community meetings.
> - Fact sheets.
> - Press releases.
> - Media interviews.

influence the academic community, but may be relatively ineffective in other respects).

Practical

(1) How might you set about drawing a representative sample for a cross-sectional survey measuring the prevalence of DSM-IV major depression in each of the following four settings (think of the example of your own country)?

- All inpatients in a general hospital
- All general hospital inpatients in the whole country
- All residents of a particular city borough aged 65 and over
- All residents of the whole country (aged 18–65).

(2) (a) How did the investigators in the two background reading papers (the National Psychiatric Morbidity Survey, Jenkins *et al.* 1997, and the Gospel Oak Project, Prince *et al.* 1997) define their base populations? What are the advantages and the disadvantages of the contrasting approaches of the two surveys?

(b) How did these two surveys establish their register/sampling frame?

(c) What efforts were made in the two surveys to maximize response?

(d) How might misclassification bias have caused problems in the two surveys?

(e) What do you think is the practical usefulness of the Gospel Oak Survey?

(3) Discuss, critically the following paper

Hendrie, H.C., Osuntokun, B.O., Hall, K.S., Ogunniyi, A.O., Hui, S.L., Unverzagt, F.W., Gureje, O., Rodenberg, C.A., Baiyewu, O., Musick, B.S., *et al.* (1995) Prevalence of Alzheimer's disease and dementia in two communities: Nigerian Africans and African Americans. *American Journal Psychiatry*, 152(10), 1485–92.

This paper reports striking differences in the prevalence of Alzheimer's disease between Nigerians and African Americans.

(1) What are the possible explanations for this finding?

(2) Were methodologies, particularly dementia diagnostic procedures adequately standardized between Nigeria and the US?

(3) Life expectancy is much higher among African-Americans than among Nigerians—could this have accounted for the finding?

(4) Does a difference in prevalence imply that there is also a difference in incidence? If not why not?

(5) If there is a genuine difference in disease frequency between the two settings what might that imply?

(6) What further studies might you wish to see carried out?

(7) How might the study findings from Nigeria be disseminated to benefit the local community?

References

1996, *The Global Burden of Disease. A comprehensive assessment of mortality and disability from diseases, injuries and risk factors in 1990 and projected to 2020.* The Harvard School of Public Health, Harvard University Press.

Andrews, G. and Carter, G.L. (2001) What people say about their general practitioners' treatment of anxiety and depression, [see comments] [erratum appears in *Med J Aust* (2001) Nov 19; 175 (10): 560]. *Medical Journal of Australia,* 175 (Suppl), S48–S51.

Andrews, G., Henderson, S., and Hall, W.(2001) Prevalence, comorbidity, disability and service utilisation. Overview of the Australian National Mental Health Survey. [erratum appears in *Br J Psychiatry* (2001) Dec; 179: 561–2.]. *British Journal of Psychiatry,* 178, 145–53.

Blazer, D.G., Kessler, R.C., McGonagle, K.A., and Swartz, M.S. (1994) The prevalence and distribution of major depression in a national community sample: the National Comorbidity Survey. *American Journal of Psychiatry,* 151(7), 979–86.

Breslau, N., Chilcoat, H.D., Kessler, R.C., Peterson, E.L., and Lucia, V.C. (1999) Vulnerability to assaultive violence: further specification of the sex difference in post-traumatic stress disorder. *Psychological Medicine,* 29(4), 813–21.

Brinded, P.M., Simpson, A.I., Laidlaw, T.M., Fairley, N., and Malcolm, F. (2001) Prevalence of psychiatric disorders in New Zealand prisons: a national study. *Australian and New Zealand Journal of Psychiatry,* 35(2), 166–73.

Brugha, T.S., Bebbington, P.F., and Jenkins, R. (1999a) A difference that matters: comparisons of structured and semi-structured psychiatric diagnostic interviews in the general population. *Psychological Medicine,* 29(5), 1013–20.

Brugha, T.S., Bebbington, P.E., Jenkins, R., Meltzer, H., Taub, N.A., Janas, M., and Vernon, J. (1999b) Cross validation of a general population survey diagnostic interview: a comparison of CIS-R with SCAN ICD-10 diagnostic categories. *Psychological Medicine,* 29(5), 1029–42.

Brugha, T.S., Nienhuis, F., Bagchi, D., Smith, J., and Meltzer, H. (1999c) The survey form of SCAN: the feasibility of using experienced lay survey interviewers to administer a semi-structured systematic clinical assessment of psychotic and non-psychotic disorders. *Psychological Medicine*, 29(3), 703–11.

Burvill, P.W. (1987) An appraisal of the NIMH Epidemiologic Catchment Area Program. [Review] [56 refs]. *Australian and New Zealand Journal of Psychiatry*, 21(2), 175–84.

Cooper, L., Peters, L., and Andrews, G. (1998) Validity of the Composite International Diagnostic Interview (CIDI) psychosis module in a psychiatric setting. *Journal of Psychiatric Research*, 32(6), 361–8.

Deming, W.E. (1978) An essay on screening, or two-phase sampling, applied to surveys of a community. *International Statistical Review*, 45, 28–37.

Dunn, G., Pickles, A., Tansella, M., and Vazquez-Barquero, J.L. (1999) Two-phase epidemiological surveys in psychiatric research. *British Journal of Psychiatry*, 174, 95–100.

Foster, K., Meltzer, H., Gill, B., and Hinds, K. (1996) *OPCS Surveys of Psychiatric Morbidity in Great Britain, Report 8: Adults with a psychotic disorder living in the community.* HMSO, London.

Gill, B., Meltzer, H., Hinds, K., and Petticrew, M. (1996) *OPCS Surveys of Psychiatric Morbidity in Great Britain, Report 7: Psychiatric Morbidity among homeless people.* HMSO, London.

Hofman, A., Ott, A., Breteler, M.M.B., Bots, M.L., Slooter, A.J.C., van Harskamp, F., van Duijn, C.N., Van Broeckhoven, C., and Grobbee, D.E. (1997) Atherosclerosis, apolipoprotein E, and prevalence of dementia and Alzheimer's disease in the Rotterdam Study. *Lancet*, 349, 151–4.

Jenkins, R., Bebbington, P., Brugha, T., Farrell, M., Gill, B., Lewis, G., Meltzer, H., and Petticrew, M. (1997) The National Psychiatric Morbidity surveys of Great Britain—strategy and methods. *Psychological Medicine*, 27(4), 765–74.

Kendler, K.S., Gallagher, T.J., Abelson, J.M., and Kessler, R.C. (1996) Lifetime prevalence, demographic risk factors, and diagnostic validity of nonaffective psychosis as assessed in a US community sample. The National Comorbidity Survey. *Archives of General Psychiatry*, 53(11), 1022–31.

Kessler, R.C. (1999) The World Health Organization International Consortium in Psychiatric Epidemiology (ICPE): initial work and future directions—the NAPE Lecture 1998. Nordic Association for Psychiatric Epidemiology. *Acta Psychiatrica Scandinavica*, 99(1), 2–9.

Kessler, R.C., Olfson, M., and Berglund, P.A. (1998) Patterns and predictors of treatment contact after first onset of psychiatric disorders [see comments]. *American Journal of Psychiatry*, 155(1), 62–9.

Kessler, R.C., Zhao, S., Blazer, D.G., and Swartz, M. (1997) Prevalence, correlates, and course of minor depression and major depression in the National Comorbidity Survey. *Journal of Affective Disorders*, 45(1–2), 19–30.

Lasser, K., Boyd, J.W., Woolhandler, S., Himmelstein, D.U., McCormick, D., and Bor, D.H. (2000) Smoking and mental illness: A population-based prevalence study. *Journal of the American Medical Association*, 284(20), 2606–10.

Lewis, G., Pelosi, A.J., Araya, R., and Dunn, G. (1992) Measuring psychiatric disorder in the community: a standardized assessment for use by lay interviewers. *Psychological Medicine*, 22(2), 465–86.

Meltzer, H., Gatward, R., Goodman, R., and Ford, T. (2000) *Mental Health of Children and Adolescents in Great Britain*. The Stationery Office, London.

Molnar, B.E., Buka, S.L., and Kessler, R.C. (2001) Child sexual abuse and subsequent psychopathology: results from the National Comorbidity Survey. *American Journal of Public Health*, 91(5), 753–60.

Parker, G. (1987) Are the lifetime prevalence estimates in the ECA study accurate? *Psychological Medicine*, 17(2), 275–82.

Parslow, R.A. and Jorm, A.F. (2001) Predictors of partially met or unmet need reported by consumers of mental health services: an analysis of data from the Australian National Survey of Mental Health and Wellbeing. *Australian and New Zealand Journal of Psychiatry*, 35(4), 455–63.

Patton, G.C., Hibbert, M., Rosier, M.J., Carlin, J.B., Caust, J., and Bowes, G. (1996) Is smoking associated with depression and anxiety in teenagers? *American Journal of Public Health*, 86(2), 225–30.

Pirkis, J.E., Burgess, P.M., Meadows, G.N., and Dunt, D.R. (2001) Suicidal ideation and suicide attempts as predictors of mental health service use [see comments]. *Medical Journal of Australia*, 175(10), 542–5.

Prince, M.J., Harwood, R., Thomas, A., and Mann, A.H. (1997) Gospel Oak V. Impairment, disability and handicap as risk factors for depression in old age. *Psychological Medicine*, 27, 311–21.

Regier, D.A., Myers, J.K., Kramer, M., Robins, L.N., Blazer, D.G., Hough, R.L., Eaton, W.W., and Locke, B.Z. (1984) The NIMH Epidemiologic Catchment Area program. Historical context, major objectives, and study population characteristics. *Archives of General Psychiatry*, 41(10), 934–41.

Robins, L., Helzer, J.E., Croughan, J., and Radcliff, K.S. (1981) National Institute of Mental Health Diagnostic Interview Schedule: its history, characteristics and validity. *Archives of General Psychiatry*, 38, 381–9.

Sanderson, K. and Andrews, G. (2002) Prevalence and severity of mental health-related disability and relationship to diagnosis. *Psychiatric Services*, 53(1), 80–6.

Singleton, N., Meltzer, H., Gatward, R., Coid, J., and Deasy, D. (1998) *Psychiatric morbidity among prisoners in England and Wales*. The Stationary Office, London.

StataCorp (1997) *Stata Statistical Software: Release 5.0*.

Vos, T., Mathers, C., Herrman, H., Harvey, C., Gureje, O., Bui, D., Watson, N., and Begg, S. (2001) The burden of mental disorders in Victoria, 1996. *Social Psychiatry and Psychiatric Epidemiology*, 36(2), 53–62.

Weissman, M.M., Leaf, P.J., Tischler, G.L., Blazer, D.G., Karno, M., Bruce, M.L., and Florio, L.P. (1988) Affective disorders in five United States communities [published erratum appears in Psychol Med 1988 Aug;18(3):following 792]. *Psychological Medicine*, 18, 141–53.

Wittchen, H.U., Burke, J.D., Semler, G., Pfister, H., Von Cranach, M., and Zaudig, M. (1989) Recall and dating of psychiatric symptoms. Test-retest reliability of time-related symptom questions in a standardized psychiatric interview. *Archives of General Psychiatry*, 46(5), 437–43.

Zlotnick, C., Kohn, R., Keitner, G., and Della Grotta, S.A. (2000) The relationship between quality of interpersonal relationships and major depressive disorder: findings from the National Comorbidity Survey. *Journal of Affective Disorders*, 59(3), 205–15.

Chapter 8

The case–control study

Matthew Hotopf

Imagine an investigator wants to test the hypothesis that obstetric complications are more common in schizophrenia than in the general population. There are two main approaches to this problem. The first involves identifying babies who have had a complicated birth and following them up to see whether they have a higher risk of schizophrenia in later life than babies with an uncomplicated births. This would be a cohort study—the 'ticket of entry' into the study is the exposure status of the individual. Under these circumstances, a well-designed cohort study would undoubtedly give the answer, but it would be a very long time in coming, require a huge sample, and be extremely expensive. This is because schizophrenia is a rare disorder, which develops in early adulthood. Therefore large numbers of individuals would have to be followed over many years in order to find each case of schizophrenia.

The alternative approach is to use the case–control design. This involves identifying cases with schizophrenia and comparing them with controls who are unaffected. The investigator would then use some method to *look back* and determine the exposure status of cases and controls.

The rationale for the case–control study

The decision on whether to use a case–control or cohort study depends on a number of considerations, which this example illustrates. Case–control studies are most appropriate when the disorder under study is (i) rare (ii) takes a long time to develop after the exposure (sometimes referred to as the latent period) and (iii) where the exposure is common. Cohort studies are more appropriate when the disorder is (i) common (ii) it does not take long to develop and (iii) the exposure is rare.

This may be illustrated using a series of hypothetical sample size calculations. Table 8.1 shows the sample sizes required for cohort studies where equal sized cohorts (exposed and unexposed) are compared over a 10 year period. The investigator sets the power at 80% and the confidence at 95% and looks for a two-fold increase in risk in the exposed group. For a condition with an

Table 8.1 Sample sizes required to detect a two-fold risk in a cohort study run over 10 years with 80% power, and 95% confidence

Incidence rate of disorder	Sample size
10/100,000/year	52,000
100/100,000/year	5300
1000/100,000/year	650

incidence rate of 10/100,000/year, the investigator will require 52,000 subjects in all. Important psychiatric outcomes such as suicide, and schizophrenia have incidences of approximately this order. Therefore cohort studies would have to be very large and expensive to cope with such conditions.

Table 8.2 shows the same power calculation for a case–control study. Instead of varying the incidence of the disorder, the frequency of the exposure has been changed. This illustrates when the prevalence of the risk factor is very low, case–control studies have to be very large.

Some additional points are worth making in relation to these tables. First, note that for the cohort study, the frequency of the exposure was not mentioned. This is because in cohort studies the investigator manipulates exposure status by selecting individuals into the study on the basis of their exposure experience. This means that rare exposures can be studied. In Table 8.2, the prevalence of the illness under study was not mentioned, because in case–control studies this is what the investigator manipulates. Thus, in each study design the investigator has control over either the frequency of the exposure (cohort) or the outcome (case–control).[1]

Second, although the sample sizes for the examples in Tables 8.1 and 8.2 may *look* similar, Table 8.1 relies on a 10 year follow up, whilst for Table 8.2,

---

[1] These remarks apply to classical cohort study designs, however, as discussed in Chapter 9, many cohort studies assessing psychiatric outcomes have used *population cohort* (sometimes called *panel*) *designs*, where a detailed cross sectional study assessing both exposures and outcomes has been performed at time 1, and the entire population has been followed at one or more time points. This design is useful for common exposures and outcomes (such as socio-economic factors in the development of common mental disorders). They are usually established to determine the prevalence, incidence and risk factors for a wide range of disorders, including psychiatric disorders. Examples in the UK involve the Health and Lifestyle Survey, the British Household Panel Study, and the three national birth cohort studies.

Table 8.2 Sample sizes required to detect a two-fold risk in a case–control study with 80% power, and 95% confidence

Frequency of the exposure	Sample size case–control study
0.1%	52,000
1%	5,200
10%	620

the results are—at least theoretically—available immediately. Cohort studies, by virtue of their longitudinal component are time-consuming. (The exception to this is the retrospective or historical cohort study, where participants are still identified according to exposure status, but the exposure is ascertained using historical records see Chapter 9.)

Case–control studies may assess the role of *multiple* exposures on a *single* disorder. In contrast, cohort studies assess the role of a *single* exposure on *multiple* disorders. In the example of obstetric complications, a cohort study would not just be able to look at their impact on schizophrenia, but could also investigate other psychiatric disorders of physical diseases. A case–control study would not be able to do that, but would be able to investigate a wide range of risk factors.

Risk, odds, and the relationship between cohort and case–control studies

In both cohort and case–control studies the main purpose is to determine the relationship between an exposure and an outcome. This is expressed as the risk or rate ratio in cohort studies and the odds ratio in case–control studies. The relationship between these parameters is important to understand, and in describing this relationship one can gain a better grasp of the assumptions underlying case–control studies.

Cohort studies and risk

Cohort studies follow individuals who are free from a disorder to determine their risk of developing that disorder over a particular period of time. The *risk* is a proportion, namely the number of individuals who develop the disorder divided by the number studied. In cohort studies risks are calculated separately for those exposed and those who are unexposed to the factor under study. The relative risk is derived from Table 8.3.

Table 8.3 Derivation of risks and odds in a cohort study

| | Disorder | | Risk of disorder | Odds of disorder |
	Yes	No		
Exposure				
Yes	a	b	a + b a/(a + b)	a/b
No	c	d	c + d c/(c + d)	c/d
Total	a + c	a + d		
Odds of exposure	a/c	b/d		

Table 8.3 describes the situation in a cohort study when two groups (exposed and not exposed) are followed to determine the number who develop a disorder over a fixed length of time. The risk of the disorder in those exposed is:

$$p_1 = a/(a + b)$$

and in the unexposed is

$$p_2 = c/(c + d)$$

The risk ratio is simply calculated as the proportion of these two fractions:

$$RR = p_1/p_2$$

The odds and odds ratio

The odds ratio may be calculated in a cohort study in a similar fashion. The odds is simply the proportion calculated by dividing the number of the times the event happens by the number of times it does not happen, so from Table 8.3, the odds in the two groups is:

$$\text{Odds of disorder in exposed} \quad = a/b$$
$$\text{Odds of disorder in unexposed} = c/d$$

The odds is an intuitively difficult concept to grasp, but has some mathematical advantages over the risk. The risk is by definition a fraction with a value from between zero and one. The odds can take any value from zero to infinity, and this makes it an easier parameter to manipulate. Another important feature of the odds is its relation to the risk. Provided the disorder under study is rare, the odds will very closely approximate to the risk. In other words, if a is small in relation to b (i.e. many more people do not develop the disorder than do develop it) the odds will approximate to the risk. This is the basis of the so called *rare disease assumption* which states that if a disease or disorder is sufficiently rare the odds will approximate to the risk.

The next step is to calculate the odds ratio, which is simply:

$$OR = (a/b)/(c/d)$$

which can be simplified algebraically to the 'cross products' of Table 8.3

$$OR = ad/bc$$

A worked example

The following example is taken from a cohort study on the effects of unemployment on depression (Weich and Lewis 1998). This was a prospective cohort study of 7726 individuals who were interviewed at baseline and one year later. Depression was measured on the General Health Questionnaire. The main analysis used individuals who were not depressed at baseline, and recorded depression at follow up according to employment status at baseline (Table 8.4).

$$RR = 0.206/0.181 = 1.14$$
$$OR = 53*3102/686*204 = 1.17$$

Note that as the disorder (depression) is quite common, the risks and odds are slightly different, and the odds ratio is bigger than the risk ratio.

Odds ratios in the case–control study

So far, we have worked from the perspective of the cohort study, in defining the risks and odds of developing the disorder according to exposure status. However, if we were to turn the problem on its head it would be possible to

Table 8.4 Risk of depression according to employment status

	Depressed		Total	Risk of depression	Odds of depression
	Yes	No			
Exposure					
Unemployed	53	204	257	0.206	0.260
Employed	686	3102	3788	0.181	0.221
Total	739	3306			
Odds of exposure to unemployment	0.077	0.066			

calculate the odds of *having the exposure according to disorder status.* Returning to Table 8.1 we see that:

$$\text{Odds of exposure if develop disorder} = a/c$$
$$\text{Odds of exposure if do not develop disorder} = b/d$$

Once again we can determine the odds ratio, which will be

$$OR = (a/c)/(b/d) = ad/bc$$

This value is identical to the odds ratio calculated previously. In other words, the odds ratio is symmetrical—it is the same whichever way it is calculated, this mathematical property makes the odds ratio easier to manipulate than the risk ratio.

We can now consider the same example from the perspective of a case–control study, where individuals were identified not on the basis of their exposure status, but on the basis of whether or not they developed the disorder under study. In the unemployment and depression example we would need to define cases as individuals with a recent onset of depression, and controls as individuals who were not depressed. Returning to the data presented in Table 8.4, let us assume that we identified *all* the cases of depression, and selected one control who had not developed depression for each case who had. The table would look something like Table 8.5.

The cells for the cases are identical to those in Table 8.4, but for the controls we have attempted to keep the odds of exposure to unemployment as close to the value in Table 8.4 as possible (in order to get it identical we would have had to give fractions of people). Note now that we are unable to calculate the risk of depression in the two exposure groups. Because of the case–control design we have no denominator data with which to calculate the risk or odds

Table 8.5 Case–control study of depression and unemployment

	Depression		Total	Risk of depression	Odds of depression
	Yes (cases)	No (controls)			
Exposure					
Unemployed	53	46	99	NA	NA
Employed	686	693	1379	NA	NA
Total	739	739			
Odds of exposure to unemployment	0.077	0.066			

of depression according to exposure status. However, what we are still able to do is calculate the odds of exposure according to disorder status, and we are therefore able to calculate the odds ratio:

OR = odds of exposure in cases/odds of exposure in controls

= 0.077/0.066 = 1.17

We can see that this is identical to the odds ratio calculated from the cohort study data. Any differences here would arise from the approximation used to avoid having fractions of people in Table 8.5.

Steps to take in conducting a case–control study

Define a problem

Unlike cohort studies, which can give estimates of the incidence of a disorder, and cross-sectional studies, which can give estimates of the prevalence of a disorder, the sole purpose of case–control studies is to explore relationships between exposures and outcomes. Schlesselman (1982) distinguished the exploratory and the analytic case–control studies. In an *exploratory* study the starting point is often a new problem—for example, a clustering of new cases of a disease—and the investigators seek to identify the cause from a wide range of candidate exposures. Because the disorder may be new (or described in a novel group), too little may be known to narrow the search for exposures, so a wide range of possibilities is explored. The problem with this unfocussed approach is that if a high number of possible associations are explored, there is a strong chance that some will turn out 'positive' by chance (so called type one error). Therefore, exploratory studies should usually be followed by analytic studies, where the list of candidate exposures is reduced to allow fewer hypotheses to be tested.

Identifying cases

Definition of cases

As full a definition of cases as possible should be included in the protocol. In psychiatry this will usually be based on operational criteria using ICD, or DSM systems. However, such systems are not necessarily the most appropriate means of defining cases: for example, if one was studying minor psychiatric disorder in its broadest sense, it would be valid to use a predetermined level of severity on a psychiatric questionnaire or interview, and compare those who fell above the cut off with those who fell below it. Similarly one might want to describe risk factors across entire groups of disorders such as psychotic illness or somatoform disorders.

Source of cases

The source of cases should be defined. The key decision is usually whether cases are to be recruited from known clinical samples, or whether they should come from the community. For example, cases of schizophrenia could be identified from secondary care. A clinical service would be used, and all individuals with schizophrenia within that service would be identified. This is usually a much easier and cheaper approach than defining a community or catchment area, and trying to identify all cases of schizophrenia within that area.

An important consideration is whether cases identified from health care settings are *representative* of the broader population of individuals with the disorder, or whether they are a selected group. How much this matters depends on the disorder under study and the nature of the healthcare system: when dealing with psychosis in a developed country, a high proportion of patients will have been admitted to hospital or been under the care of a community mental health team at some time in their illness. Thus identifying patients from secondary case will probably lead to a reasonably representative sample of the population of people with psychosis being identified. For depression or anxiety, the vast majority of patients never reach psychiatric care, and therefore secondary care samples are likely to be very unusual. Patients who reach secondary care are likely to have more severe illness, greater comorbidity, more treatment failures and so on.

In developing countries, where psychiatric services are scarce, many patients with psychosis may never be treated in secondary care, and those who are may be an unusual group. For example, they may have wealthy relatives who can afford psychiatric care, or they may have displayed violent behaviours which have led them to come to the attention of services. If there are specific risk factors which predict whether an individual with the disorder under study is referred to the setting they are recruited into, this can cause selection bias.

A further consideration is the ease of using recruitment from a wider community. It is difficult to screen communities to identify patients with psychosis—unless one is prepared to administer lengthy and costly psychiatric interviews to very large numbers of individuals. In close knit communities it may be possible to use key informants to identify individuals with psychotic illness, but this approach is likely to be much less feasible in big cities.

Prevalent or incident cases?

Most illnesses have a number of potential outcomes: patients may get better; they may have fluctuating symptoms; they may remain chronically ill; or they may die. For example, many patients with depression recover, at least in the short term. Some go on with a chronic illness, a few die from suicide or other causes, and many have a relapsing and remitting course. It is usually most convenient to select cases from a population who are *currently* unwell. However, the problem with this is that the sample of cases selected may no longer be representative of the wider population of individuals who develop the disorder. This means that the study may end up finding risk factors for *chronicity* of the condition, instead of its cause. This is sometimes referred to as prevalence bias. A way around this problem is to use only new or *incident* cases of the disorder.

This approach may not always be practical, especially in psychiatric epidemiology. Many psychiatric disorders have an insidious onset, and run a relapsing and remitting course. Depression may have gone unrecognized for some months or even years before it is detected. 'Incident' cases of depression identified from a general practice or psychiatric outpatient clinic may therefore be no such thing, but instead represent individuals who have had several previous episodes of depression that went undetected.

Defining the controls

Defining the controls is one of the most difficult problems in designing case–control studies. The best way to answer this is to ask: 'If this individual (who I have called a control) were to get the condition under study, would he/she been included as a case?' If the answer to this question is 'no' then the control group is probably invalid. Thus if a list of exclusion criteria is used for the cases, the same list should be applied to the controls.

Source of controls

This depends largely on how the cases were defined. If they are a population-based sample of all new cases with the disease over a one-year period, then it would make sense to draw controls directly from the same population. If cases came from clinical samples gathered from a general hospital serving a defined area, it would be reasonable to pick controls living in the same population who would also be likely to be treated in the same hospital were they to get ill. However, if cases were gathered from a highly specialized hospital, which attracts referrals from all over the country, the population of controls is much less easy to define. There may also be all sorts of factors independent of the disease which lead to patients being referred to a specialist units, including social class and educational level. This introduces the possibility of *selection bias* (see below). Some approaches to the selection of controls are shown in Box 8.1.

Matching

Matching is a method of avoiding confounding (see below for a definition of confounding). In a case–control study it is desirable to have cases and controls

> ## Box 8.1 **Some sources of controls in case–control studies**
>
> - Hospital (or clinic) controls: Individuals with other disorders presenting to the same hospital or community mental health service as the cases.
>
> - Primary care: In UK and some other health services, a high proportion of the population are enrolled with a general practitioner. It is often possible to identify controls who attend the same general practitioner as the case, even if the case is identified from secondary care.
>
> - Electoral or other population registers: Electoral registers provide a sampling frame of adults. This method may under-estimate certain groups (e.g. young, mobile individuals, or those who are disaffected and disinclined to vote).
>
> - Dead controls: For suicide research it may be reasonable to select controls who have died by other means.
>
> - Random digit dialling: If cases all have telephones in their homes, another method is to contact controls by random dialling of telephone numbers with the same area codes.

who differ only in terms of disease status, therefore matching is one way to ensure that cases and controls are of similar age, gender, ethnic group, and so on. Although matching is intuitively appealing, it may cause a number of problems including:

(1) *Logistical difficulties.* Potential controls may be lost in order to find one which matches the cases. If cases and controls are to be matched on several variables (age, gender, social class, ethnic group) one may have to exclude many potential controls because they do not exactly match the case.

(2) *Problems in the analysis of data.* Matched designs require matched analyses which are somewhat more complex and less easy to follow than unmatched analyses.

Modern statistical techniques or alternative methods of controlling confounding in the design of studies may be more suitable methods to avoid confounding. Box 8.2 describes some approaches to manage confounding in the design and analysis stages of case–control studies. One approach in the design is to sample the controls in such a way that they are broadly similar to the cases on certain key variables such as gender and age.

Box 8.2 **Mechanisms for avoiding confounding in case–control studies**

Design

- Restriction: Individuals with the confounder are excluded from the study. For example, a case–control study of anorexia nervosa might exclude male patients, as this is an unusual subgroup, and gender could be an important potential confounder.

- Matching: Controls are matched to cases on several key potential confounding variables, for example, gender, age group, or setting from which they are recruited.

- Sampling: Rather than individually match, controls may be selected such that they are broadly similar to cases as a group. If 30% of cases are male, the controls can be selected to ensure that 30% of controls are male.

Analysis

- Stratification: The analysis is effectively done separately according to the presence or absence of the confounder, and a summary odds ratio taking this into account may be calculated.

- Logistic regression analysis: The odds of being a case or control are modelled according to the presence of a number of exposure variables simultaneously. This allows for independent effects of the exposure to be estimated, corrected for the presence of confounders.

How many control groups should be used?

An investigator may want to test the hypothesis that childhood sexual abuse is a risk factor for bulimia. He or she could either use healthy controls, or controls with different psychiatric diagnoses. The choice of control group changes the question being asked. If cases with bulimia had much more reported sexual abuse than healthy controls, the conclusion might be that sexual abuse causes bulimia. However if an additional control group with depression was included, and they were found to have the *same* rate of childhood sexual abuse, it could be argued that abuse was a risk factor for both conditions, and was not *specifically* associated with either.

How many controls per case?

If we imagined that a disorder was so rare, it was only possible to recruit 30 patients. One way to increase statistical power in this situation would be to

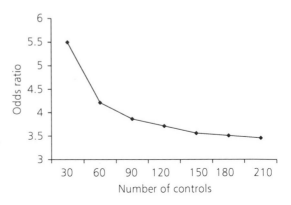

Fig. 8.1 With 30 cases, the relationship between the number of controls and the odds ratio which may be detected at 80% power and 95% confidence, given an exposure with 20% prevalence.

have more controls than cases. Figure 8.1 demonstrates that by having more than one control per case, it is possible to increase statistical power. With one control per case (i.e. 30 in each group), and assuming that the exposure was present in 20% of the control population, the study could only detect a relatively big odds ratio of 5.5. By doubling the number of controls to 60 the odds ratio falls to 4.2 and by having four controls per case it falls to 3.7. However, after this there is a law of diminishing returns and having 210 controls (i.e. 7 : 1) allows an odds ratio of 3.45 to be detected.

Selection bias

The main point of much of the previous discussion on the definition of cases and controls is to avoid selection bias. This is probably the most challenging aspect of designing a case–control study. Selection bias occurs when the exposure status of cases or controls influences the likelihood that they are entered into a study.

This is well illustrated by the example of post-infectious fatigue syndrome. In UK and USA, there has been growing interest in fatigue syndromes which were considered to have been caused by viruses (Wessely *et al.* 1998). A number of papers suggested that individuals with such fatigue syndromes had more antibodies to certain viruses in their blood than healthy controls. However, many of the studies were performed by physicians or virologists who recruited patients referred to their clinics. But these patients were often referred because general practitioners had noticed they had raised viral antibodies, and wanted a virological opinion. Thus the exposure (prior viral infection) and the outcome (chronic fatigue) were not independent in the way cases were selected. These problems could have been resolved by identifying cases of chronic fatigue syndrome from primary care and comparing with controls from within the same setting—the process of referral often involves subtle processes which can lead to selection bias.

Estimating exposure status

Once cases and controls have been defined, the task is to estimate their exposure to the risk factor under study. This may be done by giving the subjects or their relatives questionnaires, using historical records, taking blood or measuring other biological markers. The main aim is to avoid *information bias*.

The procedure by which cases and controls are approached and interviewed should be as similar as possible. They should receive the same interview schedule, and the same questions. If an informant is used to elicit information about cases, an informant should also be used for controls.

Recall bias

There are two important forms of information bias which are pertinent to case–control studies. The first is *recall bias*. This occurs when the experience of having a disease in itself affects the process of recalling prior exposures. One example is in dementia: patients with dementia have global cognitive deficits, including memory problems, therefore they are unlikely to be able to recall prior events. If the question under study was whether prior head injury causes dementia, asking sufferers from dementia would clearly cause problems, as they may well have forgotten past events. One would instead have to use con-temporaneous records (e.g. hospital notes) or ask an informant who knew the patient well.

A more common problem is that the illness being studied *increases* the recall of prior exposure. Most individuals when they get ill may want to make sense of their suffering and think of many different prior events which could be implicated. This *effort after meaning* may mean that when asked about prior events they put more effort into recall than someone without the illness. For example, the parent of a patient with schizophrenia may spend considerably more effort recalling past exposures like obstetric complications than the parent of healthy individuals. This also is a potential problem for life events research, where individuals with existing depression are asked to recall life events over the previous 6 months or year, and events are contextualized in order to determine how severe was their impact. Individuals with depression often have distortions in their thought processes which may lead them to preferentially recall negative events.

Recall bias may be reduced by:

♦ using alternative sources of information which do not depend upon the memory of subjects (e.g. previous hospital records);

- disguising the hypothesis from the subject by nesting questions related to the exposure of interest in an interview which covers other aspects of lifestyle;
- using controls who have another disorder. (This may change the nature of the question being asked, because many risk factors in psychiatry are not specifically related to individual diagnoses, but increase the risk of a wide variety of psychiatric disorder.)

Observer bias

The second form of information bias is observer bias. This occurs when the interviewer's knowledge of the subject's disease status affects the way he or she asks them questions. This could either be conscious cheating on the part of the interviewer, or more commonly a subtle process by which the interviewer is more diligent when asking cases than controls.

Observer bias may be overcome by the following techniques:

- 'blinding' the interviewer to the hypothesis under study, by nesting key questions about the exposure in a more extensive interview about other aspects of lifestyle;
- 'blinding' the interviewer to the disease status of participants (this may be very difficult to achieve in psychiatric epidemiology);
- using highly structured interviews which force the interviewer to ask each participant the same question in an identical manner;
- using questionnaires or computerized interviews which the participants complete themselves.

Examples of case–control designs in psychiatric epidemiology

The following section describes a number of recent well-conducted case–control studies in psychiatry.

Case–control studies nested in a cross-sectional surveys

We have already seen that selection bias is a major problem for case–control studies. One way around this is to perform a case–control study within an existing cross-sectional study. Cross-sectional studies aim to identify all cases of a disorder within a given population—they therefore provide a ready-made sampling frame for the case–control study. Whilst cross-sectional studies are often able to assess risk factors, when a detailed ascertainment of risk factors is required, it is usually unnecessary to apply this to all participants in the cross sectional study. Instead a nested case–control study can be performed.

An example of this is a study of life events in elderly individuals with depression (Brilman and Ormel 2001). Cases of depression were identified in a cross-sectional study. Controls were selected randomly from non-depressed participants in the same study. Cases and controls were then given a detailed interview (the Life Events and Difficulties Schedule, Brown and Harris 1978). The main rationale for this approach is that the LEDS is a long interview, and it would have been wasteful to have administered it to the entire population studied in the cross-sectional study. The use of a population-based sampling frame radically reduced the possibility of selection bias in the case–control study.

Case–control studies nested within cohort studies

The term 'nested case–control study' more usually refers to a sub-study of a larger cohort study, where information on specific exposures may be expensive to obtain on all participants at baseline. For example, one might be interested in the relationship between conjugal loss and depression, and perform a cohort study to compare rates of onset of depression in individuals who recently lost a spouse, compared to those who were still married. The quality of the marital relationship might be considered to be a key additional risk factor, which might nevertheless be prohibitively expensive and time consuming to ascertain through a structured interview on every cohort member at baseline. One might instead select all those who develop depression (the cases) and compare them with a proportion of randomly selected individuals who did not develop depression (the controls). This would change the design to a *nested* case–control study, as the selection of participants now would depend on their outcome status in the cohort study. The ascertainment of exposure is now retrospective, and information bias may be a problem. The nested case–control study is a particularly efficient design for genetic exposures. Blood samples may be taken and stored on all participants, but the expensive DNA extraction and genotyping need only be performed on incident cases and suitable controls. Information bias is evidently not a problem. Two or three controls per case can be shown to provide near equivalent power for the comparison as if the whole cohort had been genotyped.

In the section on risk and odds, we showed how cohort studies and case–control studies can be thought of as related. Rothman (1986) has argued that all case–control studies can be thought of as being 'nested' within either real or theoretical cohort studies. A good example is a case–control study assessing the school performance cases with schizophrenia and controls without schizophrenia (Cannon *et al.* 1999). The authors set out to test the hypothesis that individuals with schizophrenia have difficulties in childhood (which might reflect problems in neurodevelopment) which manifest as poorer school performance.

The study was 'nested' within a birth cohort, namely all individuals born within Helsinki between 1951–1960. It is important to note that this was in effect a 'virtual' cohort—it existed as a theoretical entity, but no one had previously collected data from all its members. This nesting, however, allowed the researchers to define a population base to recruit into the case–control study. Cases were identified from national databases which allowed all known cases of schizophrenia to be identified. The researchers linked these records with child health cards in Helsinki, which determined whether they had been educated in that city. Controls were identified as the next individual to appear on the child health cards, who was also born in Helsinki between 1951 and 1960 and who did not grow up to develop schizophrenia. Cases and controls were then compared according to school performance by going back to school records. The main result was that whilst academic performance and behaviour at school were no different in the children who developed schizophrenia and those who did not, individuals who developed schizophrenia had poorer performance on other non-academic activities.

The psychological autopsy study

Suicide is an especially difficult area to study. It is a rare outcome, whose definition may vary over time, and between countries, according to legal and cultural factors. Obviously, once suicide has happened the 'participant' is by definition dead. Case–control studies of suicide have therefore tended to use the 'psychological autopsy' approach, where a detailed interview is administered to a relative of the suicide victim. This presents difficulties for ascertaining the same information in the controls—if living controls are used, it is necessary to use the same technique. Information bias would result from any approach where the information was being gathered differently on controls as opposed to cases—hence there is a need to ensure that information on controls is gathered by asking an informant rather than directly asking the control. A recent example is a study from New Zealand (Beautrais 2001) which used this method to compare risk factors for suicide and severe deliberate self with a control population drawn from an electoral register. Suicides were defined from routine death registrations. Severe deliberate self-harm cases were identified from local hospitals. Relatives of the two groups of cases and controls were asked to provide information on risk factors over the lifetime of the participants. This approach is probably the closest one can get to an unbiased estimate of risk factors in suicide, however there are still major problems with potential recall bias. Suicide is frequently associated with powerful feelings of guilt in the relatives of the victim, and such feelings may act to emphasize or de-emphasize risk factors.

Analysis of case–control studies

Once the data have been collected on cases and controls it is entered onto a statistical software package and analysed.

The first step should be a description of the population from which cases and controls came, how many potential cases and controls were excluded, and how many refused to participate. For example, the suicide autopsy study described above, gave participation rates for cases and controls. This gives the reader a view of the representatives of the sample. Key features of the case should be described: for example, how long had they been ill? How many were in-patients? What was the severity of their illness?

The next step should be a comparison of the main socio-demographic characteristics of cases and controls. The reader should be able to see any major differences in terms of their age, gender, social class, occupational group and so on. There are two main reasons for this. It may be that these socio-demographic variables are to be studied as risk factors in their own right. Alternatively, the study may aim to examine other risk factors, and it is important to know whether any relationships could be due to confounding by these socio-demographic variables.

Statistical tests are frequently reported to demonstrate that differences between cases and controls are 'non-significant'. However it should be emphasized that when statistically non-significant differences are found between cases and controls, the variables involved can still act as a confounder. It is more important to look for the *size of the difference* between the two groups.

The relationship between exposure and outcome: the odds ratio and 95% confidence interval

Subsequent tables should show how the exposures of interest may be distributed throughout cases and controls. The odds ratio is the basic measure of relative risk in the case control study, and has been described in detail above. Ideally odds ratios should be presented with their 95% confidence intervals (CIs). This gives an indication of the precision of any effect size determined. Returning to Table 8.5, we can calculate the confidence interval for the odds ratio as follows. First the standard error is calculated:

$$\text{SE} = \sqrt{\left(\tfrac{1}{a} + \tfrac{1}{b} + \tfrac{1}{c} + \tfrac{1}{d} \right)}$$

This is then multiplied by 1.96 (to get 95% CI).

And then exponentiate this term to get an error term (ET).

$$ET = e^{1.96SE}$$

The 95% CI are derived by multiplying and dividing the odds ratio by the error term. From the example shown in table y the standard error is:

$$SE = \sqrt{\left(\frac{1}{53} + \frac{1}{46} + \frac{1}{686} + \frac{1}{693}\right)} = 0.209$$

$$ET = e^{1.96 \times 0.209} = 1.51$$

The odds ratio was 1.17 so the upper boundary of the 95% CI is:

$$1.17 \times 1.51 = 1.77$$

and the lower boundary of the 95% CI is:

$$1.17/1.51 = 0.77$$

This gives us an odds ratio of 1.17 with a 95% CI of 0.77–1.77. This indicates that we can be 95% confident that the true odds ratio lies somewhere between 0.77 and 1.77. As the null value for the odds ratio is one (i.e. an odds ratio of one indicates no difference) and these 95% confidence intervals include one, we can infer that the relationship is not statistically significant at $p < 0.05$. More importantly, these confidence intervals would indicate the degree of precision of this estimate.

More than one level of exposure

Many exposures have more than one level of severity. For example, individuals may have experienced no life events, one life event, two events, or more than three events. This may be handled by making a table like this:

Sample	Cases	Controls
No life events	a	b
One event	c	d
Two events	e	f
Three or more events	g	h

The odds ratio for each level of exposure may be calculated on its own *using* 'no life events' as the reference:

- for those with three or more events it would be: ah/bg
- for those with one event it would be ac/db.

The 95% CIs are calculated by pretending that there are a series of 2 × 2 tables for each exposure compared with the no life event group.

Controlling for confounding

The main issue in the analysis of case control studies is to control for potential confounders. Confounders are defined as variables which are causally related to the *outcome*, and are associated with the exposure of interest, but are not simply on a causal pathway between exposure and outcome (see Fig. 8.2).

Stratification. Here the 2 × 2 table shown above is broken down (or *stratified*) according to the presence or absence of the confounder. If controlling for gender, there would be a 2 × 2 table for men and another for women. The odds ratios for each could then be compared, and using Mantel Haenszel techniques a combined odds ratio controlled for gender may be derived.

Modelling. Logistic regression techniques model the odds of being a case according to the presence of one or more additional variables simultaneously. The computer derives an odds ratio for each of these variables. Logistic regression may be used to control for multiple confounders simultaneously.

The analysis of the matched case–control study

These comments on the analysis of case–control studies have focussed on unmatched designs. When cases and controls have been matched, different statistical methods are required. A detailed discussion of such techniques is outside the scope of this chapter. The main difference is that all statistical tests should take into account the matching (so instead of performing independent t tests, paired t tests should be used, and instead of using the χ^2 test, the McNemar test is used). For modelling in matched case–control studies, conditional logistic regression, which takes into account the clustered nature of each matched pair, should be used.

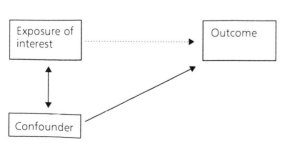

Fig. 8.2 Illustration of the mechanism of confounding. The confounder causes the outcome under study, and is also associated with the exposure of interest. Thus the confounder can confuse the investigator into believing that the exposure is causal.

Interpretation of case–control studies

Once the analysis has been performed, the results must be interpreted. As always in epidemiological studies five possible explanations for an association exist:

- reverse causality
- bias
- confounding
- chance
- causality.

The role of bias and confounding have been explored in this chapter and elsewhere in some detail. However it is worth considering how reverse causality and chance may be especially relevant in case–control studies.

Reverse causation

Case–control studies are usually unable to rule out this possibility, since by definition the illness has already occurred when the cases are recruited. Thus it is always possible that the illness led to the exposure and not vice versa. This is especially true in social psychiatry, where exposures such as unemployment, and life events may arise directly from the effects of the illness on behaviour. This is less of a concern if previous records can be used in order to ascertain the exposure. In the literature on schizophrenia and obstetric complications, for example, it has been possible to determine the presence of obstetric complications from hospital records, which were recorded long before the individual developed the illness.

Chance

Statistical testing, and the use of confidence intervals are the techniques most widely used to deal with chance in studies. One advantage of case–control studies is that they can assess the role of *multiple* exposures simultaneously. If the level of significance is set at 95%, this means that a *p* value of 0.05 or less may be detected one time in 20 *just by chance*. If the investigators have assessed the role of 40 exposures, one would expect that two of these would come up as having an association *by chance alone*. This is one reason why it is important for findings in exploratory case control studies to be replicated in subsequent more rigorous analytic studies.

Conclusions

The case–control study, if well conducted, is able to give unbiased estimates of effect sizes between exposures and outcomes. They are a particularly efficient design—and this efficiency makes them a more viable approach in the study of rare disorders than cohort studies.

Practical

This practical involves using two examples of case–control studies, and discussing some of the advantages and disadvantages of the approaches used in these papers.

Paper 1 (Yousef *et al.* 1988): This paper describes a case control study assessing the relationship between chronic enterovirus infection and a fatigue syndrome. Consider the following questions:

1   How were the cases identified and selected? Is there adequate information?

2   How were the controls selected? Are there any possible problems with this method?

3   Was this a matched case–control study? If so, was a matched analysis performed?

4   Were confounding variables considered?

5   What alternative explanations might there be for the reported association?

6   What improvements could be made to the design which would address these concerns?

Paper 2 (Dalman *et al.* 2001): This is a population-based case–control study assessing the relationship between obstetric complications and schizophrenia.

1   Describe the main advantages of the design chosen. What particular features of the design make this a good study?

2   What was the main problem with their use of obstetric records?

3   How could observer bias be minimized in this study?

Answers

Paper 1:

1   There is no information on the selection of cases for this study. The authors worked in a general hospital, and it is possible that some of the patients had been referred to see a virologist. This leads to selection bias, because the exposure under study is a virus—it is likely that individuals suffering from fatigue were preferentially selected into the study because of their history of viral illness.

2   Controls were nominated by cases. This is an unsatisfactory approach to selection of controls because it is likely that exposure status (viral illness) also plays a role in determining whether the control is selected. If the cases were aware of the question under study, it is possible that they were *less likely* to select controls who had a recent history of viral illnesses.

3   It was a matched design, but the analysis appears to have been unmatched. Note that there was a major imbalance between the numbers of cases and controls, which is curious in a matched case–control study—usually one would expect the same number of controls as cases, or that the number of controls would be a multiple of the number of cases.

4   No confounding variables were considered.

5   The most likely explanation for the association is selection bias, caused by the method of selection of cases.

6   The use of a population-based case–control design would have been preferable, in which cases could have been identified from general practice, or cross-sectional surveys. Alternatively, this question may be better addressed using a cohort design.

Paper 2:

1   This paper had a number of strengths: The investigators used a population based design, which minimized the chances of selection bias. They used obstetric records, which removes the possibility of recall bias. The study was large, so it had adequate statistical power to address the main questions under study, and the authors used both matching and conditional logistic regression in order to control for confounders.

2   The main problem with the use of obstetric records was that many of the records did not contain an Apgar score (which is a method of recording asphyxia at birth). They therefore had to rely on entries into the notes about the various items of the Apgar score (heart rate, breathing, colour, tone, and the excitability of the infant). This introduces the possibility of misclassification (i.e. some of the infants who might have been had a low Apgar score, might have been categorised as healthy, and vice versa). Another possibility is observer bias—as the information gathering depended to some extent on the researcher's judgement, the researcher may have been more thorough when assessing the notes of the cases (who later developed schizophrenia) compared with the controls.

3   Observer bias could be avoided (and in this paper was avoided) by asking midwives to rate the notes without any knowledge to the case control status of individuals in the study.

References

Beautrais, A.L. (2001) Suicides and serious suicide attempts: two populations or one? *Psychological Medicine*, **31**, 837–45.

Brilman, E.I. and Ormel, J. (2001) Life events, difficulties and onset of depressive episodes in later life. *Psychological Medicine*, **31**, 859–69.

Brown, G.W. and Harris, T.O. (1978) *Social origins of depression: a study of psychiatric disorder in women.* Tavistock Publications, London.

Cannon, M., Jones, P., Huttunen, M.O., Tanskanen, A., Huttumen, T., Rabe-Hesketh, S., and Murray, R.M. (1999) School performance in Finnish children and later development of schizophrenia. A population-based longitudinal study. *Archives of General Psychiatry*, **56**, 457–63.

Dalman, C., Thomas, H.V., David, A.S., Gentz, J., Lewis, G., and Allebeck, P. (2001) Signs of asphyxia at birth and risk of schizophrenia. Population-based case–control study. *British Journal of Psychiatry*, **179**, 403–8.

Rothman, K.J. (1986) *Modern epidemiology*, 1st edn. Little, Brown and Company, Boston.

Schlesselman, J.J. (1982) *Case–control studies*, 1st edn. Oxford University Press, New York.

Weich, S. and Lewis, G. (1998) Poverty, unemployment, and common mental disorders: population based cohort study. *British Medical Journal*, **317** (7151), 115–9.

Wessely, S., Hotopf, M., and Sharpe, M. (1998) *Chronic fatigue and its syndromes*, 1st edn. Oxford University Press, Oxford.

Yousef, G., Bell, E., Mann, G., Murgesan, V., Smith, D., McCartney, R., and Mowbray, J. (1988) Chronic enterovirus infection in patients with postviral fatigue syndrome. *Lancet*, **1**, 146–50.

Chapter 9

Cohort studies

Scott Weich and Martin Prince

Introduction

A cohort study is one in which the outcome (usually disease status) is ascertained for groups of individuals defined on the basis of their *exposure*. At the time exposure status is determined, all must be free of the disease. All eligible participants are then followed up over time. Since exposure status is determined before the occurrence of the outcome, a cohort study can clarify the temporal sequence between exposure and outcome, with minimal information bias.

The historical and the population cohort study (Box 9.1) are efficient variants of the classical cohort study described above, which nevertheless retain the essential components of the cohort study design.

The exposure can be dichotomous [i.e. exposed (to obstetric complications at birth) vs. not exposed], or graded as degrees of exposure (e.g. no recent life

---

Box 9.1 **Types of cohort study**

- Classical cohort study: The groups to be studied are selected on the basis of exposure, and are followed up to estimate and compare the incidence of one or more outcomes of interest in each.

- Population cohort study: The population (panel) to be studied is selected on the basis of convenience or circumstance. Multiple exposures are ascertained at baseline and related to multiple outcomes of interest over an often lengthy period of follow-up.

- Historical cohort study: An exposure or exposures of interest were measured years before the commencement of the study, *for other purposes*. Those upon whom these assessments were completed can be traced to the present day in order for the outcome or outcomes of interest to be ascertained.

events, one to two life events, three or more life events). The use of *grades of exposure* strengthens the results of a cohort study by supporting or refuting the hypothesis that the incidence of the disease increases with increasing exposure to the risk factor; a so-called *dose–response relationship*.

The essential features of a cohort study are:

- participants are defined by their exposure status rather than by outcome (as in case–control design);
- it is a longitudinal design: exposure status *must* be ascertained before outcome is known.

The classical cohort study

In a classical cohort study participants are selected for study on the basis of a single exposure of interest. This might be exposure to a relatively rare occupational exposure, such as ionizing radiation (through working in the nuclear power industry). Care must be taken in selecting the unexposed cohort; perhaps those working in similar industries, but without any exposure to radiation. The outcome in this case might be leukaemia. All those in the exposed and unexposed cohorts would need to be free of leukaemia (hence 'at risk') on recruitment into the study. The two cohorts would then be followed up for (say) 10 years and rates at which they develop leukaemia compared directly. Classical cohort studies are rare in psychiatric epidemiology. This may be in part because this type of study is especially suited to occupational exposures, which have previously been relatively little studied as causes of mental illness. However, this may change as the high prevalence of mental disorders in the workplace and their negative impact upon productivity are increasingly recognized. The UK Gulf War Study could be taken as one rather unusual example of the genre (Unwin *et al.* 1999). Health outcomes, including mental health status, were compared between those who were deployed in the Persian Gulf War in 1990–91, those who were later deployed in Bosnia, and an 'era control group' who were serving at the time of the Gulf war but were not deployed.

There are two main variations on this classical cohort study design: they are popular as they can, depending on circumstances, be more efficient than the classical cohort design.

The population cohort study

In the classical cohort study, participants are selected on the basis of exposure, and the hypothesis relates to the effect of this single exposure on a health outcome. However, a large cohort or *panel* of subjects are sometimes recruited and followed up, often over many years, to study *multiple exposures and outcomes*. No separate comparison group is required as the comparison group is generally an unexposed sub-group of the panel. Examples include the British Doctor's Study in which over 30,000 British doctors were followed up for over 20 years to study the effects of smoking and other exposures on health (Doll *et al.* 1994), and the Framingham Heart Study, in which residents of a town in Massachusetts, USA have been followed up for 50 years to study risk factors for coronary heart disease (Wolf *et al.* 1988). The Whitehall and Whitehall II studies in the UK (Fuhrer *et al.* 1999; Stansfeld *et al.* 2002) were based again on an *occupationally defined* cohort, and have led to important findings concerning workplace conditions and both physical and psychiatric morbidity. Birth cohort studies, in which everyone born within a certain chronological interval are recruited, are another example of this type of study. In birth cohorts, participants are commonly followed up at intervals of 5–10 years. Many recent panel studies in the UK and elsewhere have been funded on condition that investigators archive the data for public access, in order that the dataset might be more fully exploited by the wider academic community.

Population cohort studies can test multiple hypotheses, and are far more common than any other type of cohort study. The scope of the study can readily be extended to include mental health outcomes. Thus, both the British Doctor's Study (Doll *et al.* 2000) and the Framingham Heart Study (Seshadri *et al.* 2002) have gone on to report on aetiological factors for dementia and Alzheimer's Disease as the cohorts passed into the age groups most at risk for these disorders.

A variant of the population cohort study is one in which those who are prevalent cases of the outcome of interest at baseline are also followed up effectively as a separate cohort in order (a) to study the natural history of the disorder by estimating its maintenance (or recovery) rate, and (b) studying risk factors for maintenance (non-recovery) over the follow-up period (Prince *et al.* 1998).

Historical cohort studies

In the classical cohort study outcome is ascertained prospectively. Thus, new cases are ascertained over a follow-up period, after the exposure status has been determined. However, it is possible to ascertain both outcome and exposure retrospectively. This variant is referred to as a historical cohort study (Fig. 9.1).

A good example is the work of David Barker in testing his low birth weight hypothesis (Barker *et al.* 1990; Hales *et al.* 1991). Barker hypothesized that risk for midlife vascular and endocrine disorders would be determined to some extent by the 'programming' of the hypothalamo-pituitary axis through foetal

Past	Present (initiation of study)	Future
Prospective cohort design	Ascertainment of exposure	Follow-up ⟶ Ascertainment of outcome
Retrospective (historical) cohort design Historical ascertainment of exposure 'Follow-up' ⟶ for example another study (birth cohort), birth records, school records, etc.	Ascertainment of outcome	

Fig. 9.1 Prospective and retrospective (historical) cohort designs.

growth in utero. Thus 'small for dates' babies would have higher blood pressure levels in adult life, and greater risk for type II diabetes (through insulin resistance). A prospective cohort study would have recruited participants at birth, when exposure (birth weight) would be recorded. They would then be followed up over four or five decades to examine the effect of birth weight on the development of hypertension and type II diabetes. Barker took the more elegant (and feasible) approach of identifying hospitals in the UK where several decades previously birth records were meticulously recorded. He then traced the babies as adults (where they still lived in the same area) and measured directly their status with respect to outcome. The 'prospective' element of such studies is that exposure was recorded well before outcome even though both were ascertained retrospectively with respect to the timing of the study.

The historical cohort study has also proved useful in psychiatric epidemiology where it has been used in particular to test the neurodevelopmental hypothesis for schizophrenia (Jones *et al.* 1994; Isohanni *et al.* 2001). Jones *et al.* studied associations between adult-onset schizophrenia and childhood sociodemographic, neurodevelopmental, cognitive, and behavioural factors in the UK 1946 birth cohort; 5362 people born in the week 3–9 March 1946, and followed up intermittently since then. Subsequent onsets of schizophrenia were identified in three ways:

(a) routine data: cohort members were linked to the register of the Mental Health Enquiry for England in which mental health service contacts between 1974 and 1986 were recorded;

(b) cohort data: hospital and GP contacts (and the reasons for these contacts) were routinely reported at the intermittent resurveys of the cohort;

(c) all cohort participants identified as possible cases of schizophrenia were given a detailed clinical interview (Present State examination) at age 36.

Milestones of motor development were reached later in cases than in non-cases, particularly walking. Cases also had more speech problems than had non-cases. Low educational test scores at ages 8, 11, and 15 years were a risk factor. A preference for solitary play at ages 4 and 6 years predicted schizophrenia. A health visitor's rating of the mother as having below average mothering skills and understanding of her child at age 4 years was a predictor of schizophrenia in that child. Jones concluded 'differences between children destined to develop schizophrenia as adults and the general population were found across a range of developmental domains. As with some other adult illnesses, the origins of schizophrenia may be found in early life'.

Jones' findings were largely confirmed in a very similar historical cohort study in Finland (Isohanni *et al.* 2001); a 31 year follow-up of the 1966 North Finland birth cohort ($n = 12,058$). Onsets of schizophrenia were ascertained from a national hospital discharge register. The ages at learning to stand, walk and become potty-trained were each related to subsequent incidence of schizophrenia and other psychoses. Earlier milestones reduced, and later milestones increased, the risk in a linear manner. These developmental effects were not seen for non-psychotic outcomes. The findings support hypotheses regarding psychosis as having a developmental dimension with precursors apparent in early life.

There are many conveniences to this approach for the contemporary investigator.

♦ The exposure data has already been collected for you.

♦ The follow-up period has already elapsed.

♦ The design maintains the essential feature of the cohort study, namely that information bias with respect to the assessment of the exposure should not be a problem.

♦ As with the Barker hypothesis example, historical cohort studies are particularly useful for investigating associations across the life course, when there is a long latency between hypothesized exposure and outcome.

Despite these important advantages, such retrospective studies are often limited by reliance on historical data that was collected routinely for other purposes; often these data will be inaccurate or incomplete. Also information about possible confounders, such as smoking or diet, may be inadequate.

Advantages and disadvantages of cohort studies (Box 9.2)

Advantages

1 Cohort studies are always longitudinal, and are therefore appropriate for studying the *temporal sequence* between exposure and outcome.

2 Cohort studies are ideal for studying *rare or opportunistic exposures*, since subjects are recruited on the basis of their exposure status. Examples in psychiatry include maternal perinatal exposures such as the Dutch wartime famine (Susser *et al.* 1996), and influenza and the risk for schizophrenia (Cannon *et al.* 1996). (It is for this reason that the cohort study is especially suited to the study of occupational exposures.)

3 Unlike case control studies, cohort studies can assess *multiple outcomes* associated with a single rare or opportunistic exposure.

4 Cohort studies *minimize information bias (observer and subject or informant recall) in ascertainment of exposure status*, since this is recorded before the outcomes in question have occurred.

Box 9.2 **Advantages and disadvantages of cohort studies**

Advantages

1 Cohort studies can study the *temporal sequence* between exposure and outcome.

2 Cohort studies are ideal for studying *rare or opportunistic exposures*.

3 Unlike case–control studies, cohort studies can assess *multiple outcomes*.

4 Cohort studies *minimise information bias*.

5 Unlike case–control studies, cohort studies permit the *direct estimation of disease incidence rates*.

Disadvantages

1 Classical cohort studies are restricted to the study of a *single exposure*.

2 If prospective, cohort studies can be very *time consuming*, and *expensive*.

3 Cohort studies are generally *unsuitable for the study of rare outcomes*.

4 Cohort studies are prone to *selection bias* arising from incomplete follow-up, and *confounding*.

5   Unlike case–control studies, cohort studies permit the *direct estimation of disease incidence rates* in subjects exposed and those not exposed to specific risk factors. They can also distinguish between factors associated with the onset of a disorder and those that influence its duration. This is generally difficult to achieve in a cross-sectional survey or case–control study.

Disadvantages

1   Unless undertaken as part of a longitudinal follow-up of a whole population, cohort studies are restricted to the study of a *single exposure.*

2   If prospective, cohort studies can be very *time-consuming*, and *expensive.* Definitive results may not be available for many years.

3   Cohort studies are generally *unsuitable for the study of rare outcomes.* On the other hand, a cohort study might still be suitable for an outcome which is rare in the general population but which is hypothesised to be common in those exposed to a specific risk factor.

4   Cohort studies are prone to *selection bias* arising from incomplete follow-up, and *confounding.*

Important aspects of cohort study design

Choosing the study population

In common with all epidemiological studies, the aim of any cohort study is to estimate the magnitude of association between risk exposures and outcomes. The study groups should be as similar as possible in every respect *except for* exposure to the risk factor of interest. There is no such thing as a perfect epidemiological study. The choice of study population often represents a compromise between *validity* and *generalizability.*

A primary purpose of any epidemiological study is to produce findings that can be generalized to populations of interest. But study findings cannot be generalized if they are not valid. The effects of smoking on health were studied among British doctors not because this was the only group in whom the results were of interest, but because, it was logistically possible to undertake an unbiased study using this group. Thus validity was maximized, potentially at the expense of generalizability. However, although doctors differ in some respects from the general population, these differences were not thought to be sufficient to prevent associations between smoking and lung cancer, observed among doctors, being generalized to the rest of the population of Britain. There are no statistical tests to indicate whether results can be generalized and this remains wholly a matter of judgement.

It is important also to consider the likelihood of securing participation in the study and compliance with follow-up. For this reason, stable occupational groups with professional registers that allow participants to be traced if they move job, such as doctors, nurses or trade union members can also be used for investigation of common exposures, such as smoking and cardiovascular risk factors, which are not confined to any particular occupational group.

Selecting the exposed group

The choice depends in part on the exposure in question. Occupational or geographical cohorts are commonly used for rare exposures (e.g. asbestos workers, uranium miners, rubber workers or those living near nuclear power stations).

Selecting an external comparison (unexposed) group

This is as important, and as difficult, as selecting a control group for a case–control study. As with case–control studies, comparison groups in a cohort study must be carefully chosen to minimize *confounding* and *selection bias*.

The cardinal rule for selecting a comparison group for a cohort study is that this group should be as *similar as possible to the exposed group with respect to all factors other than the exposure under study*. This is not always an easy task, and it is not uncommon for researchers to 'hedge their bets' by recruiting more than one comparison group. For example, workers in nuclear power stations might be compared with another local occupational group, and with a general local population sample for their risk for developing leukaemia. While attractive, this option is risky: it is costly and the findings may be difficult to interpret if the results based on different comparison groups are inconsistent. For the Gulf War Study, British service personnel deployed to the Persian Gulf were compared first with those deployed to Bosnia on peace-keeping duties. In both deployments there was the anticipation that those deployed would see action, and in many cases they did. However, in Bosnia service personnel were not exposed to many of the hypothesized causes of 'Gulf War Syndrome; burning oil wells, multiple vaccinations, nerve agent' prophylaxis. However, those designing the study identified a problem with this comparison. The Bosnian deployment occurred several years after the Persian Gulf deployment. Secular changes in the health of British service personnel might therefore have biased the study of the effects of Gulf War exposure. It was therefore decided to include an 'era control' group of service personnel serving in the UK military at the time of the Gulf War, but not deployed. Here again there may have been problems, but of a different kind. Units not deployed might have been less combat ready, and fit, than those that were deployed.

In general, two types of comparison are most commonly used in cohort studies.

(1) The general population living in the same region, and of the same age and sex, as the exposed group. This approach is limited in three respects:

(i) It is only feasible where the relevant outcome data for the comparison population are routinely available. In practice, this is likely to be restricted its use to studies of mortality and the incidence of notifiable diseases such as cancer. Data on potential confounding variables will also generally not be available.

(ii) Those who are employed tend to be healthier than those not in work. This so-called 'healthy worker effect' means that that any occupational cohort is likely to experience less morbidity and mortality than the general population, and may lead to an underestimate of the effects of the exposure under study, when the general population is used as a comparison group.

(iii) Those in the exposed group will also be included in any data on the general population. This will not much affect the study findings if the exposed group is small in comparison with the size of general population used for comparison.

(2) Individuals living in the same small area (such as a neighbourhood) or working in the same setting as the exposed group. Examples would include employees working in different occupation from the exposed group in same factory, those doing similar tasks in a different factory, or individuals living in the same geographical area as the exposed group but not employed in the factory. This approach has one important limitation. It is often impossible to exclude the possibility that those in the comparison group have been exposed to the risk factor under study. They may be 'contaminated' by their geographical proximity to the source of exposure, or by living with others who have been exposed. Misclassification of this nature would bias results towards the null.

Data collection

General principles

The aim of any study is to collect complete, unbiased and comparable data on all study subjects. To this end a number of general principles applied:

(1) To minimize both observer and subject bias (collectively called information bias), information must be collected from all study participants in the same way, regardless of whether they are in the exposed or comparison groups.

(2) In cohort studies information bias arising from misclassification of outcome (differentially with respect to exposure) is much more likely to

occur than that arising from misclassification of exposure (differentially with respect to outcome). To minimize this possibility, assessment of outcome should be undertaken blind to exposure status and preferably blind to the study hypothesis. This may be a serious problem since many cohort studies are prompted by concern about the effects of specific exposures, where widely publicized theories and lay attributions about the potentially damaging effects of the exposure are well known among those who are exposed. Examples include the 'Gulf War syndrome' experienced by some combatants in the 1991 Gulf War, and the Camelford incident in which a copper compound inadvertently introduced into the local water supply turned some local residents' hair green, and was widely suspected to have caused a neuropsychiatric syndrome.

(3) The definitions of all exposures and outcomes must be operationalized (i.e. made explicit), and the presence or absence of each must be assessed using standardized measures with established psychometric properties.

(4) Where bias can be excluded, the greatest remaining threat to validity is confounding. In other words, that any difference in outcome between exposed and unexposed groups is due not to the exposure being studied, but rather to some other difference between these groups. The confounding variable is thus associated independently with both the exposure and the disease outcome. While many such differences can be measured at the time that exposure is determined and controlled for in the analysis, there is always the danger that these groups might differ in ways which are *unknown, unanticipated and not measured*. Measurement of potential confounders must therefore be as comprehensive and accurate as possible.

(5) The completeness of data is crucial to the success of a cohort study.

Collecting exposure data

Exposures cannot be measured with perfect accuracy. Nevertheless, *misclassification* must be kept to a minimum, and its effects given careful consideration when interpreting study findings. Misclassification can be either random or non-random. These occur for different reasons, and affect the study findings in different ways.

Random misclassification is said to occur where exposure is misclassified to the same degree in each of the study groups, and often arises out of the inherent difficulties of measuring certain sorts of exposures. The effect of random misclassification is to make the exposed and unexposed groups more alike, thereby biasing associations between exposure and outcome(s) towards unity (or the null). This is the more likely phenomenon in cohort studies, and can never lead to over-estimates of associations.

Non-random misclassification occurs when exposure status is systematically under- or over-reported in those who do or do not develop the outcome. This is very unlikely in true prospective cohort studies, since in recalling, ascertaining or recording the exposure, neither subject nor investigator can be influenced by the outcome, which has not yet occurred. It can (in theory at least) be a problem for retrospective cohort studies, where historically recorded exposure data may be 'contaminated' or biased by the modern investigators' knowledge of the outcome.

Minimizing misclassification. The first consideration is whether exposure data can be collected from routine (or pre-existing) data sources, or whether this will have to be obtained from the study participants themselves. In some cases the answer will be self-evident. While it may be argued that individual responses about personal behaviours such as smoking, alcohol consumption and diet are likely to be biased by social desirability, it is unlikely that accurate data is available from any source. Direct interview of participants means that information can also be collected about a range of other exposures and potential confounding variables.

There are certain types of exposure that the exposed will not know about, particularly those arising in the external environment such as electromagnetic radiation, or radon gas. Environmental exposures such as these pose real difficulties for epidemiologists. Direct measurement (e.g. using measuring devices attached to clothing) may not be feasible or acceptable, and indirect measures are often used. Such measures include occupation or job description, area of residence or distance from the putative exposure source. These are all insensitive to variation of intensity of exposure over time (and hence to the effective dose of an exposure).

Collecting outcome data

There are three potential sources of outcome data:

1. routine data, for example, death certificates or cancer registrations;
2. self-report data from subjects (either by questionnaire or by interview);
3. standardized assessments or examinations (e.g. measuring blood pressure, blood lipids or psychopathology).

Each of these has their strengths and weaknesses, and will be more or less appropriate for different types of outcome. Cancer epidemiology relies heavily upon the first of these. In psychiatric epidemiology, it is rare for outcomes of interest, with the exception of suicide, to be readily available from pre-existing data sources. However this approach has been widely used for schizophrenia, which is considered so striking and serious that those affected will soon seek medical care. Thus treated incidence is considered to be a reasonable and unbiased approximation to population incidence. This approach will not work for conditions with relatively low rates of help seeking and/or identification (for instance, dementia and depression). Use of routine service-based incidence data will lead to identification of factors associated with seeking help or being screened for the disorder. Under these circumstances there is no alternative other than to attempt to keep the whole cohort under regular surveillance using standardized assessments or examinations.

A further complication for psychiatric epidemiology is that, unlike many physical diseases (such as cancer), many psychiatric disorders (such as depression) run a remitting and relapsing course. In a classical cohort study, participants are free of the disease under study at baseline, when exposure status is ascertained. In a cohort study of risk factors for depression, should those with previous episodes of depression (but currently well) be included or excluded? If there is to be a second assessment of mood status after a fixed interval, say one year, participants may have experienced an episode of depression during this period but recovered. Will it be possible to capture such episodes? Given that participants may experience a number of transitions (both remission and onset or relapse) over a period of a year or so, perhaps it is some other parameter such as the proportion of time spent with depression that should be used as the outcome? Perhaps the course should be characterized in more than two categories, for example, continuously well, continuously ill, onset with remission, onset with no remission, etc. Whichever approach is selected, it is likely that repeated assessments of outcome status will be required, and that some information will need to be gathered regarding status of participants in the intervals of time between assessments. Past history of mental illness, including the particular disorder under study, should also be ascertained and included in the analysis where appropriate (perhaps as an effect modifier, or as a confounder).

For other psychiatric disorders, the concept of disease 'onset' itself may have dubious validity. For example, dementia is distinguished from mild cognitive impairment by the degree to which general function has been compromised. This relies heavily on the subjective judgement of the interviewer and is likely to be influenced by a number of factors (e.g. cultural expectations of function, level of family support) besides the degree of cognitive impairment. Furthermore, most forms of dementia are known to have a long 'prodromal' period from the earliest detectable pathological changes to the emergence of the clinical syndrome. Unless a cohort study has a longer follow-up period (i.e. greater than 10–20 years), the disorder cannot be claimed to be absent at baseline and the direction of causation between exposure and outcome may therefore be difficult to infer. Schizophrenia is a disorder with similar problems for shorter-duration follow-up studies. The onset may be ascertained with reasonable validity (at least in some cases) but it may be difficult to distinguish short-latency risk factors from prodromal symptoms.

In cohort studies, outcome data are more prone to non-random misclassification than are exposure data. The exposure has already happened, and knowledge of exposure status may influence ascertainment, recall or recording of outcome. Thus the outcome must be operationalized and ascertained using standardized measures of proven reliability and validity. Procedures for determining outcome must be the same in *all* study subjects, who along with the assessors should ideally be blind to exposure status and the study hypotheses.

Non-participation and loss to follow-up

Non-participation and loss to follow-up are by far the most important sources of bias in any cohort study. Perhaps the single greatest challenge in any cohort study is to maximize the participation of all those who are eligible, and to ensure that outcome is ascertained for as many study subjects as possible. Given the nature of the outcomes studied this is a particular problem for psychiatric epidemiology.

Non-participation

Those who participate in research studies are likely to differ from those who refuse to participate in ways that are not random with respect to exposure. Non-participants are, in general, likely to be less well educated, less affluent, less healthy and more likely to be out of work than participants. Fortunately, the estimate of the association between the exposure and the outcome will only be biased if non-participation is related to outcome differentially with respect to exposure, for example if among smokers but not among non-smokers, those who participate are more likely to develop lung cancer. Usually, non-participation does not affect the validity of the study findings, but it often poses a serious challenge to their generalizability. If, for example, heavy drinkers were much less likely than moderate or non-drinkers to participate in a study of the effects of alcohol on the incidence of cognitive impairment, then any study findings could not be generalized to the population of *all* drinkers.

As much information as possible should be collected on non-participants. It is usually possible to construct a 'minimum data set' on all those invited to participate, including age and sex. The availability of other data will depend on the nature and setting of the study in question. It is usually possible to compare participants and non-participants, and to identify any substantial differences between these groups.

Loss to follow-up

As with non-participation at the outset of a study, loss to follow-up over the course of the study can reduce the generalizability of study findings, but may also undermine their validity. Loss to follow-up may result in under- or over-estimates of outcome (usually disease incidence) in the population of interest. The strength of the cohort design is that this will not bias estimates of associations between exposures and outcomes unless it is related to both outcome and exposure. For example, in a study of schizophrenia and obstetric complications (OCs), the association between exposure and outcome would only be biased if loss to follow-up was *differentially associated* with *both* the onset of schizophrenia *and* a history of OCs. Thus, findings would only be biased if those with OCs and schizophrenia were more likely to drop out than those with OCs but no schizophrenia, or those with schizophrenia but no OCs.

Although loss to follow-up rarely leads to bias in estimates of association between exposures and outcomes of interest, this type of attrition (and all non-participation in general) may undermine the *generalizability* of the study findings. Non-response will also lead invariably to bias in the estimated prevalence of exposures and outcomes. For example, if those who experienced OCs are especially unlikely to take part in research, studies will under-estimate the prevalence of OCs in the populations under investigation. Likewise the incidence of schizophrenia may be under-estimated if this is associated with significant non-participation. While the association between OCs and schizophrenia may remain relatively free from bias *in the study population*, it will prove difficult to generalize the study findings if, for example, only those from the highest social classes agree to take part in the research. Loss to follow-up can also be disastrous if a particularly high proportion of those who develop the outcome are not followed, and the outcome, for example, schizophrenia is rare. Under these circumstances it is a major threat to power.

Unlike non-participants at baseline, much more is usually known about those lost to follow-up, and about the ways in which they differ from those for whom follow-up data is complete. Thus the effects of loss to follow-up can be studied in more detail. Nevertheless it is essential that loss to follow-up should be kept to a bare minimum. Tracing all eligible participants is inevitably expensive and time-consuming, but necessary. Contact with can be maintained over the follow-up period with Christmas or Birthday cards, and relatives or friends can be identified who could inform the investigators of the whereabouts of subjects who had moved. Regular information can be passed on to participants about the progress of the study. Those who do not actively express a wish *not* to participate further should be approached *tactfully* at least three or four times, by post, telephone or home visits. It is always worthwhile considering alternatives to follow-up by face-to-face interview, which can be time consuming for participants. Alternatives include postal questionnaires and telephone interviews.

Analysis of cohort studies

Data from a cohort study are used to estimate rates of outcome in both the exposed and unexposed samples. One of two types of incidence measure can be used, depending on the nature of the study and the outcome.

Measures of incidence

An incidence risk is defined as the number of disease onsets observed divided by the number of persons in the cohort at risk at the beginning of the study. Such rates are typically expressed as *x* per 1000 (or 10,000 etc.) per annum. Loss to follow-up is treated in one of two ways, either by simply ignoring it or by a crude adjustment of the denominator. One such adjustment involves subtracting half the number of subjects lost to follow-up from the number of those who were at risk at the beginning of the study.

An incidence rate is the number of disease onsets divided by the *person-years at risk*. The denominator 'person-years at risk' is defined as the number of subjects at risk multiplied by the interval over which they remained at risk. Participants contribute time at risk until they are *censored* either because they die, are lost to follow-up or because they develop the outcome condition. The concept of person-years at risk really comes into its own where there are repeated assessments of outcome. Such studies have the advantage of being able to quantify the denominator with much greater precision, which in turn increases the accuracy with which outcome rates can be estimated. This precision arises from measuring the *exact* amount of time each study participant remains at risk.

Figure 9.1 gives an example of how to calculate incidence risks and incidence rates from just 10 people followed up for 10 years. The outcome of interest is dementia.

Measures of effect

Associations between exposure(s) and outcome(s) are then estimated, most often by calculating absolute and relative differences in outcome rates between the exposed and unexposed groups. The risk ratio (or rate ratio depending on

Participant	Year										PYARS contributed
	1	2	3	4	5	6	7	8	9	10	
1					×		+				5
2			+								3
3											10
4											10
5									×		9
6						+					6
7											10
8				×	+						4
9											10
10											10

× = dementia onset.

+ – death.

Note that censoring occurs at the first censoring endpoint, that is, for participant 1 at the onset of dementia after 5 years, and not at the time of death 2 years later:

Total incident cases = 3

Total at risk = 10

Period at risk = 10 years

Incidence risk = 3/10 per 10 years = 30/1000 per year

Total incident cases = 3

Total person years at risk = 77

Incidence rate = 3/77 = 39/1000 person years

which incidence measure is used) is the measure of relative difference, and is defined as the incidence in the exposed divided by the incidence in the unexposed. The attributable risk (AR) is the simplest measure of absolute difference, and is defined as the incidence risk in the exposed minus the incidence risk in the unexposed. The attributable risk percent (AR%) is the proportion of outcomes among the exposed attributable to the exposure.

In formulaic terms

$$\text{Relative risk} = \frac{IR^{exp+}}{IR^{exp-}}$$

$$\text{Attributable risk} = IR^{exp+} - IR^{exp-}$$

$$\text{Attributable risk percent} = \frac{IR^{exp+} - IR^{exp-}}{IR^{exp+}}$$

The different information conveyed by these three measures of effect is clearly demonstrated in a classic example from a classic study, the British Doctor's Survey. Although the principal aim of this cohort study was to test the hypothesis that smoking was associated with lung cancer, several other outcomes were studied.

Mortality rates (per 100,000 men per year) from three conditions:

Condition	Exposure (smoking)				
	Never	Ever	RR	AR	AR%
Lung cancer	10	83	8.3	73	88
Ischaemic heart disease	413	554	1.3	141	25
Suicide	21	31	1.5	10	33

In relative terms smoking is more strongly associated with lung cancer, than with ischaemic heart disease or suicide (an eight-fold increase in lung cancer risk for smokers, compared with a less than two-fold increase for the other two conditions). However, lung cancer is a rare condition and heart disease is common. Thus, in terms of absolute risk, nearly twice as many deaths from heart disease (141 per 100,000) are attributable to smoking as deaths from lung cancer (73 per 100,000). The AR% provides a useful index of potential for prevention. If 88% of onsets of lung cancer among smokers are attributable to smoking, then these deaths might have been prevented had none of these doctors had smoked. Note that the AR% gives an index of potential for prevention only among those exposed to the risk factor. If the exposure is quite rare then the potential for prevention in the general population may be limited, even if the AR% is high. The population attributable fraction (PAF) gives an index of potential for prevention at the population level, taking into account both the prevalence of the exposure and associated relative risk

$$PAF = \frac{IR^{\text{total population (exp+ and exp-)}} - IR^{\text{exp-}}}{IR^{\text{total population (exp+ and exp-)}}}$$

which can be shown to be equivalent to:

$$PAF = p\,(RR - 1/RR)$$

where p is the prevalence of the exposure in the general population and RR is the observed relative risk associated with the exposure. The population attributable fraction signifies the proportion of incident cases *in the population* which would be prevented if a causal exposure were removed, assuming an unconfounded causal association.

Conclusions

The cohort study is a powerful epidemiological tool for evaluating the size of associations between certain exposures and outcomes. As a longitudinal study, the cohort design can be used to elucidate the chronological sequence between exposure and outcome, and is especially well suited to the study of rare exposures. A further strength of the cohort design is the capacity to study multiple outcomes. Cohort studies are less prone to certain types of bias, particularly recall bias, than cross-sectional studies.

Cohort studies are an inefficient way of studying rare outcomes, and (unless designed as the follow-up of an entire population) are limited to the study of a single exposure. Cohort studies can be expensive, and invariably take far longer to complete than a cross-sectional study. Though susceptible to selection bias arising from non-participation and loss to follow-up, this usually limits the generalizability of the study findings but not their validity so far as estimating associations between exposure(s) and outcome(s) is concerned. Like all observational studies, the results of any cohort studies are subject to confounding not only by exposures that are known about and measured, but also by those that remain unknown to investigators.

Suggested classroom practical exercise

Part I: Design a study to investigate the effect of unemployment on depression.

1. What is the exposure?
2. What is the outcome?
3. What type of study would you recommend, and why?
4. If you have opted for a cohort study, what are the reasons for not choosing either a cross-sectional or case–control study?
5. Who would you include in the exposed group, and how would you go about recruiting subjects? What factors must you take into account? What difficulties might you encounter?
6. Who would you include in your comparison group?
7. What are the most important sources of bias in your study? How might these affect your results?
8. What are the most important confounders?

Part II: Consider the following cohort study by Weich and Lewis (1998). Subjects were not depressed at baseline. Results at 12 month follow up were:

9. What are the incidence rates for depression among (a) the unemployed and (b) the employed?

	Depressed		Total
	No	Yes	
Employed	3102	686	3788
	81.89	18.11	100.00
	64.13	66.99	64.63
Unemployed	204	53	257
	79.38	20.62	100.00
	4.22	5.18	4.38
Not working	1531	285	1816
	84.31	15.69	100.00
	31.65	27.83	30.98
Total	4837	1024	5861
	82.53	17.47	100.00
	100.00	100.00	100.00

10. Calculate the (a) relative risk, (b) attributable risk, and (c) odds ratio for depression among the unemployed, compared with the employed. Why do the results of (a) and (c) differ?

Answers

1. It is probably simplest to think about three employment categories, namely those in paid employment, those unemployed and looking for work, and those not working but not seeking work. The latter are often referred to as 'economically inactive' and include students, the retired and those not working for reasons of ill-health. In the UK, about 6% of the general population are unemployed, and a further 30% are economically inactive.

2. A large number of simple, standardized measures of 'depression' are readily available, many of which can be administered by lay interviewers. The prevalence of depression in the adult population of the UK is between 5% and 15%.

3 and 4. The study of unemployment and depression lends itself to a cohort design. Both the outcome and exposure are common. Perhaps the greatest challenge is elucidating the chronological sequence between unemployment and depression, since depression itself can cause people to lose their jobs. Neither cross-sectional nor case–control studies could exclude the possibility of reverse causality.

5 and 6. There are no 'correct' answers here. The exposed group should probably be restricted to the unemployed (rather than the economically

inactive, who will include people not working because of mental health problems). The important factors to bear in mind are

* the population to whom it is hoped to generalise the study findings,
* the logistics of recruitment.

Identifying and recruiting unemployed subjects is difficult. Several previous studies have followed up adolescents of school leaving age, comparing outcomes for those who do and those who do not find jobs. Elsewhere, researchers have recruited subjects in an opportunistic fashion following factory closures, or large-scale redundancies. Perhaps for this reason, the effects of unemployment have often been studied as part of population-based cohort studies. Duration of unemployment is important; the long-term (>6 months) unemployed are a highly select group. Once an exposed group has been identified, a comparison group can be identified following the principles set out in the lecture notes. It is particularly important that the two groups are as similar as possible in terms of age, sex, socio-economic status.

7. Selection bias arising from non-participation and loss to follow-up. These are most likely to bias estimates of the rate of unemployment and the incidence of depression, but probably not the size of the association between them.

8. Important confounders include age, sex, education, and socio-economic status. Those who are unemployed are likely to experience more financial hardship than those in work. Other confounders include ethnicity, physical health, and recent life events. The recently unemployed have been exposed to a major life event which may account for an increased incidence of depression.

9. (a) 18.11%, (b) 20.62%.

10. (a) RR = 1.14, (b) AR = 2.51%, (c) OR = 1.17.

Results (a) and (c) differ because depression in this study violates the rare disease assumption; ORs are therefore numerically greater than RRs.

References

Barker, D.J., Bull, A.R., Osmond, C., and Simmonds, S.J. (1990) Fetal and placental size and risk of hypertension in adult life [see comments]. *British Medical Journal*, 301 (6746), 259–62.

Cannon, M., Cotter, D., Coffey, V.P., Sham, P.C., Takei, N., Larkin, C., Murray, R.M., and O'Callaghan, E. (1996) Prenatal exposure to the 1957 influenza epidemic and adult schizophrenia: a follow-up study [see comments]. *British Journal of Psychiatry*, 168 (3), 368–71.

Doll, R., Peto, R., Wheatley, K., Gray, R., and Sutherland, I. (1994) Mortality in relation to smoking: 40 years' observations on male British doctors [see comments]. *British Medical Journal*, 309 (6959), 901–11.

Doll, R., Peto, R., Boreham, J., and Sutherland, I. (2000) Smoking and dementia in male British doctors: prospective study [see comments]. *British Medical Journal*, 320 (7242), 1097–102.

Fuhrer, R., Stansfeld, S.A., Chemali, J., and Shipley, M.J. (1999) Gender, social relations and mental health: prospective findings from an occupational cohort (Whitehall II study). *Social Science and Medicine*, 48 (1), 77–87.

Hales, C.N., Barker, D.J., Clark, P.M., Cox, L.J., Fall, C., Osmond, C., and Winter, P.D. (1991) Fetal and infant growth and impaired glucose tolerance at age 64 [see comments]. *British Medical Journal*, 303 (6809), 1019–22.

Isohanni, M., Jones, P.B., Moilanen, K., Rantakallio, P., Veijola, J., Oja, H., Koiranen, M., Jokelainen, J., Croudace, T., and Jarvelin, M. (2001) Early developmental milestones in adult schizophrenia and other psychoses. A 31-year follow-up of the Northern Finland 1966 Birth Cohort. *Schizophrenia Research*, 52 (1–2), 1–19.

Jones, P., Rodgers, B., Murray, R., and Marmot, M. (1994) Child development risk factors for adult schizophrenia in the British 1946 birth cohort. *Lancet*, 344 (8934), 1398–402.

Prince, M.J., Harwood, R.H., Thomas, A., and Mann, A.H. (1998) A prospective population-based cohort study of the effects of disablement and social milieu on the onset and maintenance of late-life depression. The Gospel Oak Project VII. *Psychological Medicine*, 28, 337–50.

Seshadri, S., Beiser, A., Selhub, J., Jacques, P.F., Rosenberg, I.H., D'Agostino, R.B., Wilson, P.W., and Wolf, P.A. (2002) Plasma homocysteine as a risk factor for dementia and Alzheimer's disease [see comments]. *New England Journal of Medicine*, 346 (7), 476–83.

Stansfeld, S.A., Fuhrer, R., Shipley, M.J., and Marmot, M.G. (2002) Psychological distress as a risk factor for coronary heart disease in the Whitehall II Study [see comments]. *International Journal of Epidemiology*, 31 (1), 248–55.

Susser, E., Neugebauer, R., Hoek, H.W., Brown, A.S., Lin, S., Labovitz, D., and Gorman, J.M. (1996) Schizophrenia after prenatal famine. Further evidence [see comments]. *Archives of General Psychiatry*, 53 (1), 25–31.

Unwin, C., Blatchley, N., Coker, W., Ferry, S., Hotopf, M., Hull, L., Ismail, K., Palmer, I., David, A., and Wessely, S. (1999) Health of UK servicemen who served in Persian Gulf War [see comments]. *Lancet*, 353 (9148), 169–78.

Wolf, P.A., D'Agostino, R.B., Kannel, W.B., Bonita, R., and Belanger, A.J. (1988) Cigarette smoking as a risk factor for stroke. The Framingham Study. *Journal of the American Medical Association*, 259 (7), 1025–29.

Chapter 10

Randomized controlled trials

Sube Banerjee

There are three main questions in health care: 'what is going on?', 'why?' and 'what do we do about it?'. 'What is going on?' forms the basis for clinical assessment including history taking, examination, and diagnosis. The question 'why?' underlies all aetiological research from laboratory science to epidemiology. The cross-sectional, case–control and cohort methodologies discussed in other chapters in this book provide the methodology for addressing 'why?' questions. However, just as medicine is more than diagnosis it also covers treatment, medical research is more than aetiology: it also necessarily extends to the evaluation of interventions.

Aetiological research which cannot be translated into health benefits through new or improved interventions is at best sterile and at worse self-indulgent, begging another important question: 'so what?'. Flawed evaluations of interventions can be even more problematic since these may harm rather than help. Intervention studies (of which randomized controlled trials (RCTs) are the most important type, on the basis of quality of evidence available from them) take aetiological insights into action and provide the best evidence upon which to found clinical practice.

In this chapter we will consider some of the more important factors in the design, conduct, analysis, and interpretation of RCTs.

What is an RCT?

Last (1995) defines an RCT as:

> An epidemiologic experiment in which participants in a population are randomly allocated into groups, usually called 'study' and 'control' groups, to receive or not to receive an experimental, preventative or therapeutic procedure, manoeuvre or intervention. The results are assessed by rigorous comparison of rates of disease, death, recovery, or other appropriate outcome in the study and control groups respectively. Randomized controlled trials are generally regarded as the most scientifically rigorous method of hypothesis testing available in epidemiology.

> Box 10.1 **The elements of a randomized controlled trial (RCT)**
>
> - Define the research question
> - Identify and recruit the sample
> - Apply the intervention at random
> - Measure the outcome and compare between intervention groups
> - Summarise and disseminate findings

An RCT therefore sets out to find out the effect of an intervention. Stages in this process are summarized in Box 10.1. While this process may be clear it is not necessarily simple. RCTs require a substantial investment of resources in terms of time, expertise, personnel, and finance. This is not to say that the constituent components of assessment, intervention, reassessment, analysis, and interpretation need themselves be complex. Indeed much of the rigour in trial design revolves around ensuring that these components are simple, meaningful, and explicit before the start of the experiment.

What are RCTs for?

Treatment is fundamental to health care and we need information to decide what treatment to give, and to invest in. At its simplest, an RCT answers the question 'does Treatment A work?'; one level of complexity higher is the design which answers the question 'does new Treatment B work better than established Treatment A?'. Studies that simply observe the effects of treatment without randomization or control groups are difficult to interpret, in particular with respect to the size and direction of effect. The use of historical controls (e.g. comparing two case series, one before a new drug and one after) is also problematic (Altman and Bland 1999), generally resulting in an overestimation of the effect of the new intervention (Sacks *et al.* 1982).

The orthodoxy for the past 40 years has therefore been that RCTs rather than observational studies are the best way to judge the effect of an intervention. Two recent studies have challenged this (Benson *et al.* 2000; Concato *et al.* 2000), these compared data from observational studies and RCTs studying the same questions and concluded that observational studies yielded very similar odds ratios to RCTs with less variability of response. Ioannidis *et al.* (2001) in an editorial response questioned these findings, in particular highlighting: (a) the relatively small degree of actual overlap between the two methods; (b) some major negative correlations not quoted; (c) reconsideration of the data showing a lower level of agreement than was presented; and (d) the potential problems of pooling data. The authors concluded with a sensible statement of the particular values and roles of the two study types. They state that where observational studies have shown large harmful effects RCTs are likely to be unethical, as may also be the case where large beneficial effects have been demonstrated (e.g. risk ratios less than 0.4). Interventions with modest effect sizes (risk ratios from 0.4 to 0.9) are particularly suited to RCTs, while for those with very small effect sizes (0.9–1.0), or for very rare outcomes, RCTs may be difficult to perform and observational evidence may be the best data available. On balance there is a role for both study types. However for the majority of disorders and interventions RCTs potentially provide the most clear and unbiased evaluation of effect.

The methodology and practice of RCTs cannot be divorced from their impact upon clinical practice and health policy, and the wider financial and industrial context. There are increasing moves worldwide to base clinical practice on good quality evidence. This is a reaction to the realization that practice has often varied widely and doctors of all specialties have very often been unable to support their actions with anything other than protestations of established practice, anecdote or peer group consensus. Quality of evidence for clinical effectiveness forms a hierarchy with consistent findings from several well conducted RCTs at the top.

So on one level the purpose of RCTs is to allow clinicians to select the best treatment for a patient and to allow patients to receive the treatment with the best benefit to risk ratio for their condition. However there are other agencies interested in the data produced by RCTs. Those who purchase health care, be they health insurance agencies or governmental health authorities use evidence of effectiveness to focus or ration care within a limited financial envelope. These agencies therefore factor an assessment of the financial and political costs of sanctioning treatment into their interpretation of RCTs.

The pharmaceutical industry has a particularly strong interest in the findings of RCTs. Billions of dollars are spent in research and development of novel compounds by drug companies each year. It is they who design, conduct, analyse, and promote the vast majority of RCTs, albeit within a framework of governmental control agencies. While the betterment of humanity may occasionally be a by-product, the data from RCTs are the primary channel through which an experimental compound can be turned into a marketable commodity, so that investment can be turned to income and profit. The complex and competing inter-relationships of clinicians, patients, researchers, health purchasers, and drug companies is of profound importance in any consideration of an RCT. Occurrences such as the discontinuation of the FAME trial of a lipid lowering statin in older adults for purely commercial reasons raise both scientific and ethical issues (Evans and Pocock 2001; Lievre *et al.* 2001).

Fundamental design issues

As with all other epidemiological studies, primary objectives in the design of RCTs are to exclude bias and to measure confounding so that its effect can be controlled for in the analysis. Important aspects in the design are summarized in Box 10.2. Lind's elegant mid-eighteenth century comparative trial of different treatments for scurvy contains many of these methodological components (Lind 1753; Bull 1959; Lilienfield 1982). In this study he took 12 patients with scurvy on board the *Salisbury* who were 'as similar as I could have them', he gave them a common diet, divided them into six intervention groups and supplemented the groups' diets in different ways. The two people in each group received either: a quart of cider a day; '25 gutts of elixir vitriol'; two spoonfuls of vinegar; a course of sea water; 'the bigness of a nutmeg'; or two oranges and a lemon. After six days the group on the oranges and lemon had recovered to such an extent that one returned to duty and the other became the nurse for the remaining patients. However the translation of research findings into clinical practice was just as much of a problem in the eighteenth century as it is in the twenty first, and it took a further 50 years before the Royal Navy provided its sailors with lemon juice (Pocock 1983).

Box 10.2 **Fundamental design issues**

- ◆ Thorough review of existing evidence
- ◆ Clear hypothesis formulation and statement of objectives
- ◆ Informed consent
- ◆ Random allocation of intervention
- ◆ Use of placebo or active control
- ◆ Accurate and careful measurement of potential confounding factors
- ◆ Accurate and careful measurement of outcome
- ◆ Maximization of follow-up
- ◆ Blinding
- ◆ Intention to treat analysis
- ◆ Unbiased dissemination of findings

One way to understand the particular challenges posed by the carrying out of an RCT is to set up a perfect scenario and then to see just how far this differs from clinical circumstances in general and evaluations of interventions in psychiatry in particular.

A perfect trial

The perfect conditions for a trial would involve a disorder (D) which could be diagnosed with absolute precision at minimal cost and whose course was such that it did not matter when it was diagnosed or treatment started. We would then need a putative treatment (X) which had a compelling scientific basis for its use but whose efficacy was in doubt so that a trial was ethically acceptable. By preference there would be no other active treatment for D so that an inert placebo could be used as a comparator, and X should have no properties by which it could be distinguished from the placebo (e.g. taste, side effects, perception of effect) either by patient or doctor. D should also be sufficiently common and serious for it to be a good candidate for a clinical trial and full funding should be available.

For ascertaining outcome, we should have a perfect knowledge of the natural history of D and it should consistently lead to an unequivocal outcome, such as a disease-specific death, within a given time (say, one year on average). We should then be able to recruit a group of affected people who were absolutely representative of all people with D. These would be randomly allocated on a 1:1 basis to receive a course of X or placebo. We would then follow up all participants in both groups and measure after one year the death rate in the intervention and the control groups, comparing the two to ascertain the efficacy of X. The findings would be absolutely unequivocal. Just to make things perfect, X should be a compound which is not under drug company license and which is very cheap and very simple to manufacture and distribute so that the whole world can benefit from this work.

Preferably several independent research groups would have carried out separate similar trials at the same time, and they would all be published together. The role of X in the treatment of D would be systematically reviewed showing a consistent and powerful treatment effect in the individual studies and after meta-analysis. The fairy story would end with there being no political or clinical resistance to the introduction of the treatment and the health care delivery systems being universally available to make X available to all without prejudice. And we would all live happily ever after.

Clearly this is to argue by absurdity but it is important to make the point that the real world is a messy place full of uncertainly and complexity. Diagnosis or case ascertainment may be imprecise and difficult, and it may be modified by help-seeking behaviour which has an influence on outcome. There may be co-morbidity with other conditions and the patient may be taking other medication. Recruitment and obtaining informed consent may be difficult. There may be competing treatments and established practice may mean that placebos are not ethically justifiable. Treatments have side effects which may be unpleasant or serious, affecting both compliance and blinding to treatment group. Outcome may be difficult to measure accurately and loss to follow-up may compromise the validity of the study. When translating outcomes from RCTs into clinical practice, issues of cost and practicality invariably need to be taken into account.

'Scientific' vs. 'practical' studies—efficacy and effectiveness

One of the major fault lines in the design of trials is the dynamic between purity and generalizability. Generalizability is the degree to which findings of a study can be extrapolated from the study population to other populations of interest: most often to a much broader range of patients and services in general clinical settings. 'Scientific' (also known as efficacy, speculative or explanatory) studies take the view that it is important to investigate the effect of the intervention in ideal circumstances; while 'practical' (also known as effectiveness, pragmatic or management) studies seek to investigate whether the intervention works in real clinical settings. In practice the main differences between the two sorts of RCT lie in the participants selected for entry and the nature of the intervention. Issues which principally separate 'scientific' and 'practical' trials are the nature of the studied population (particularly regarding exclusion criteria) and way in which the intervention is delivered (Box 10.3).

It is worth considering some of the arguments put forward for each approach and the reasons why they might be articulated. As mentioned above, the arguments tend to revolve around the relative merits of maximizing either scientific purity or clinical generalizability. 'Scientific' studies produce data on the efficacy of an intervention: that is, the extent to which a specific intervention produces an effect in ideal conditions; while 'practical' trials produce data on the effectiveness of an intervention: that is the extent to which a specific intervention produces an effect under more normal clinical circumstances in terms of patients and services. Efficacy is of course necessary for effectiveness, but it is not always sufficient. The terms 'scientific' and 'practical' are problematic since 'practical' trails may be far better science than 'scientific' trials and occasionally 'scientific' trials may be of practical use. Therefore in the rest of this paper the terms efficacy and effectiveness will be used to describe the two types of study.

Box 10.3 **Scientific and practical studies**

	Scientific studies	Practical studies
Alternative terms	'Speculative', 'Explanatory'	'Pragmatic', 'Management'
What is measured	Efficacy	Effectiveness
	The effect of an intervention in ideal circumstances	The likely effect of an intervention in the settings where it will be applied
	'Does it work?'	'What is its likely impact?'
Exclusion criteria applied	Generally numerous	As few as possible
Effect size	Maximal	'Realistic'
Adverse events	Minimized	'Realistic'
Generalizability	Frequently limited	Maximal

Efficacy trials are designed to produce the maximum effect size and so are often smaller that an equivalent effectiveness study, but may take time to recruit participants due to multiple exclusion criteria. Part of their attraction to drug companies and researchers alike lies in this maximization of effect. Efficacy trials are more likely to come up with a positive finding, which is good for marketing a drug and good for the researcher's publication record. In contrast effectiveness studies generally have to be larger in order to measure smaller effect sizes. They also tend to be more complex to analyse and interpret because more 'typical' groups of participants may be less likely to want to participate in a trial, and more likely to be lost to follow-up. They may also be more likely to have incidental adverse events, such as death, since they are not selected on the basis of being unusually healthy as in many efficacy trials.

Incidental adverse events are worth dwelling on since they are another reason why drug companies may prefer efficacy trials. Severe adverse events are very problematic in a Phase III trial (see below for a description of the drug trial phases) and may occur entirely by chance. However, they are unlikely to be sufficiently common to assort equally across the intervention and control groups. They can get a drug a bad name (giving rival companies ammunition to attack the new drug) and even halt trials, whether or not they have occurred by chance. It is therefore often held that it is more sensible to exclude those with a greater likelihood of such events (e.g. the ill, the disabled, those with co-morbid physical disorder, those who are on other medication) from trials entirely rather than run the risk of losing the investment.

In reality there is a continuum with the gap between efficacy and effectiveness depending on the disorder being studied and the simplicity of the intervention. In our example of the perfect trial, efficacy is the same as effectiveness. However in many studies the gap between research findings and clinical applicability may be huge. An example of this is provided by a study of donepezil, a treatment for Alzheimer's disease (Rogers and Friedhoff 1996) whose exclusion criteria are listed in Box 10.4. No mention is made in this paper of exclusions on the grounds of concurrent medication, but this is also likely given that in follow-up trials (Rogers *et al.* 1998*a,b*) patients on anticholinergics, anticonvulsants, antidepressants, and antipsychotics were also excluded as well as potentially those taking other drugs with CNS activity. As a clinical old age psychiatrist these exclusions seem to result in a study population about as far away from those I am called to assess as possible, so bringing into question the applicability of the findings to clinical practice. This is not to say that such drugs are not of use, they may well be, but the evidence that we are often presented with means that real clinical practice is informed by an extrapolation of trial data rather then by its direct application.

Another striking example has been described by Yastrubetskaya *et al.* (1997). In a Phase III trial of a new antidepressant, 188 patients were screened

Box 10.4 **Exclusion criteria for one trial of dementia treatment**

(Rogers and Friedhoff 1996)

- age over 85, unable to walk freely or with a cane or walker;
- vision and/or hearing impairment interfering with testing;
- psychiatric or neurological disorder;
- previous or current active gastrointestinal, renal, hepatic, endocrine or cardiovascular disease;
- any form of diabetes;
- obstructive pulmonary disease, hematological or oncological disorders of onset within the last two years;
- B_{12} or folate deficiency;
- alcohol or drug abuse.

and 171 (91%) of them met the inclusion criteria of having sufficiently severe depression for the trial. However, when the multiple exclusion criteria were applied to this real-world sample of people with depression, only 8 (4.7%) of those eligible for inclusion could be recruited into the trial. Furthermore, at least 70% of the original sample required antidepressant treatment and were provided with it. Perhaps the way thorough these conundrums is to acknowledge that each study type has its place and it may be that at times a single study can provide efficacy data which are so clearly generalizable to clinical populations that they are in effect close to effectiveness data. However clinicians and purchasers need to know whether an intervention works in the real world. It may be that licensing organizations such as the MCA and FDA can suggest that such data are desirable and base their decisions more directly upon its availability. Alternatively where there are efficacy data but no data on clinical effectiveness, it may be necessary to commission effectiveness studies, either before or after licensing. This raises questions of who could and should fund such work. Should funding for effectiveness trials be levied from drug companies as a necessary part of the licensing procedure? Or should governmental and private agencies involved in purchasing health care fund such work? In either case there is a strong case for such trials being independent of those who stand to gain by the sale of the intervention and also those who stand to pay by purchasing the intervention.

Elements of a randomized controlled trial

In this section we will deal sequentially with some of the major practical elements of the design and conduct of RCTs. These cannot be dealt with in detail here due to constraints of space and the reader is referred to comprehensive texts such as Pocock's *Clinical trials: a practical approach* (1983) for further details and Last's *A dictionary of epidemiology* (1995) for succinct explanations of terms.

Review the literature

Before embarking on a trial there is a need to investigate systematically the existing evidence to ascertain the current state of the therapeutics of the disorder being studied and of the intervention being proposed. If there is already compelling evidence in the public domain then it may not be necessary, and therefore ethical, to carry out a trial. Techniques for the conduct of systematic reviews are increasingly well developed and the methods and outputs of the Cochrane Collaboration (see Chapter 11) should be consulted and used.

Clear formulation of a single primary hypothesis to be tested

The trial needs to have a single primary hypothesis which is to be tested by means of the RCT. There may then be secondary hypotheses but these should be limited to avoid multiple significance testing and 'data dredging'. At this point the level for statistical significance for the primary (e.g. $p < 0.05$) and secondary hypotheses should be set (e.g. $p < 0.01$).

Specify the objectives of the trial

The hypothesis should be stated clearly and simply, for example, 'the objective of the study is to test if Treatment B is more effective than Treatment A in Disease X'. However this means that you need to have decided what constitutes 'more effective'. If we know that A gets 30% of people with X better how much more effective does B need to be? These are complex questions when A is an acceptable, economic, and widely available treatment with known side effects. We may say that we are only interested in B if it gets another 20% of people with X better, but to an extent these figures will always be arbitrary. They are however vital to the study design since the effect size being sought will determine the size of the study, with larger studies required to detect smaller differences.

It is at this point that the pre-study power calculations need to be completed. At the very least these will require:

◆ an estimation of the treatment effect of your comparison group (i.e. the percentage of people with X who respond to known Treatment A, or in the case of a placebo-controlled trial the spontaneous recovery rate from X);

◆ an estimate of the minimum effect size of your new Treatment B for it to be considered useful;

◆ the level of statistical significance required for there to be accepted that there is indeed a true difference between the two groups. This is generally set at 0.05, that is, a random 'false positive' result (type 1 error) is acceptable on one in twenty occasions;

◆ the 'power' of the study to detect effect. This is generally set at 80–90%, that is, 'false negative' results (type 2 error) are acceptable on between one in five and one in ten occasions.

Power calculations are not generally complex but specialised statistical help is advisable. Lower acceptable rates of types I and II error and smaller potential differences in effect require larger numbers of participants. Recruitment targets also need to be inflated to allow for those who will withdraw from the study and those who are lost to follow-up.

The statement of the study objectives should form the start of a detailed study protocol which sets out why the study is being carried out and exactly how the study will be conducted and analysed. This will form the basis for the ethical approval which is necessary for all trials.

Define the reference population

Define the population to which you wish to generalise. In the case of the donepezil trial discussed above, this might have been 'extraordinarily fit and well people with Alzheimer's Disease'.

Select study population

It is not generally feasible to create a list of all people in a reference population and randomly select cases for inclusion in the study, unless the disorder is very rare and there are very careful records. It is more common that the work will be focussed in a single or a few sites for ease of administration and to control quality. These centres should ideally be representative of centres as a whole and their patients representative of the reference population. Reliance upon research-friendly 'centres of excellence' may compromise this. Even in the most inclusive of effectiveness studies there will be entry criteria to be applied to potential participants, these may be simple (e.g. age) or complex (e.g. stage of disorder). One should be careful not to select a study population which automatically and irrevocably limits the applicability of any findings obtained.

Participant identification and recruitment

In this phase participants are recruited by the plan set out in detail in the protocol. Since the RCT may be being carried out simultaneously at multiple sites, it is important that the same processes are adhered to in all study centres so that any selection bias can be minimized. Comprehensive and up-to-date lists of possible cases will need to drawn up and used as a sampling frame from which to randomly sample cases for assessment. Those participants who meet the pre-determined inclusion and exclusion criteria are eligible for entry into the study. A fairly solid rule is that the more exclusions there are, the more compromised is the generalizability of the study. An increasing number of scientific journals now require the CONSORT guidelines to be followed before they will publish a trial (Begg et al. 1996). These include a flow diagram summarising the effect of all inclusion and exclusion criteria and loss to follow-up through the study (see Fig. 10.1). The presentation of such data is an invaluable aid to assessing generalisabilty and therefore the clinical robustness of a study. Those studies presented without such data should be appraised with care.

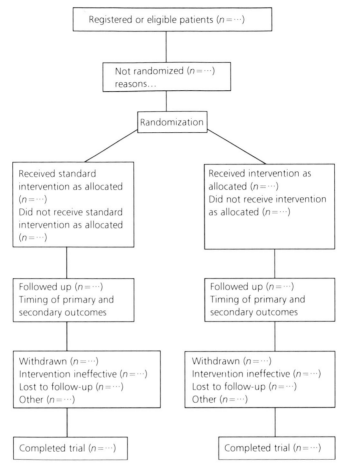

Fig. 10.1 Flow diagram summarizing progress of participants through both arms of a randomized controlled trial (Begg *et al.* 1996).

Informed consent

There is insufficient space here for a detailed consideration of ethical issues in RCTs, and major issues are well summarized by Edwards *et al.* (1998). If there is no doubt of the efficacy of an intervention then there is no ethical reason for withholding, and such withholding is implicit in a trial. If there is insufficient evidence of the potential for efficacy then there may be poor ethical grounds for conducting a trail and such evidence should be collected using other methodology. If a trial has insufficient statistical power to demonstrate the required difference between intervention and control groups then again it is unethical since it cannot provide useful data. Equally, poorly designed trials where any observed difference may be a function of bias or confounding are also unethical on the same grounds.

If the RCT design is satisfactory there remains the problem of recruiting participants into the study and the dilemma of how to obtained truly informed consent. In this chapter, I will leave to one side the issue of capacity to consent, which is of importance in mental health research, not only for people with dementia and learning disabilities, but also for people with psychotic and other disorders. Obtaining informed consent may involve a tension between the requirement to provide full information and the objectives for the trial itself. Comprehensive details of every conceivable risk may reduce participation, potentially compromising recruitment, generalizability, and the possibility of important therapeutic advances. Participants will need to receive written and verbal information on the trial and have the chance to discuss any questions they might have, they might need time to consider and consult with family, all of which is time-consuming and difficult for research teams. Consent will almost always need to be written and witnessed with stipulations of being able to withdraw at any time without giving any reason and without such withdrawal compromising their medical care in any way. These documents need to be submitted to and approved by appropriate research ethics committee.

Silverman and Chalmers (2001) have summarized elegantly some of these ethical issues and the value of random allocation of treatment: '... when there is uncertainty about the relative merits of the double edged swords we wield in medicine today, we are wise to employ this ancient technique of decision making. It is a fair way of distributing the hoped for benefits and the unknown risks of inadequately evaluated treatments'. There is a tension where recruiting physicians stand to gain from recruiting individuals into trials. This gain may be direct such as a financial payments from the pharmaceutical industry per participant recruited, or indirect mediated by the scientific kudos of completing a trial or being seen as successful by peers and seniors. In this context it is of great concern that reports from physicians recruiting patients into trials indicate that a half to three-quarters thought that few of the patients they had recruited understood that trial even though they had given written consent (Spaight *et al.* 1984; Blum *et al.* 1987; Taylor and Kelner 1987). In the circumstances that apply in a trial how good are doctors in protecting their patients' rights?

Baseline measurements

The literature review will have pointed to important possible confounding variables. These need to be measured with accuracy so that their potential effect on the outcome can be measured and controlled for in the analysis.

At this stage social, demographic, and other variables of interest (e.g. financial state, service use) which might change as part of the study need to be recorded. In mental health studies we seldom have hard outcomes such as unequivocal disease-related death. 'Change' scores are probably the most frequently used alternative. The measurement of the presence and/or severity of the disorder at recruitment is therefore a vital consideration. This must be achieved accurately and dispassionately, without conscious or unconscious bias, and without any knowledge of which treatment group the individual will be randomized to.

Randomization

Randomization is the single most powerful element of the RCT design. Its purpose is to ensure that all variables which might have an effect on outcome (known and unknown) other than the intervention(s) being studied are distributed as equally as possible between the intervention and the control group so that the effect of the intervention can be accurately estimated.

The application of randomization has developed over the course of the twentieth century. Its roots however are deeper, as early as 1662 a chemist named van Helmont advocated the drawing of lots to compare the effectiveness of competing contemporary treatments (Armitage 1982). His excellent concise protocol suggested: 'Let us take out of the hospitals... 200, or 500 poor People that have Fevers, Pleurises, etc. Let us divide them into half, let us cast lots, that one half may fall to my share, and the other to yours... We shall see how many funerals both of us shall have'. Another early proposal for the random allocation of treatments in human health referred to studies of cholera and typhoid in the first decade of the twentieth century (Greenwood and Yule 1915; Pocock 1983). While first actually applied in agricultural research in 1926 (Box 1980), stratified randomization of matched groups was used in a 1931 by Amberson *et al.* (1931) to investigate the efficacy of a gold compound in pulmonary tuberculosis (TB). However the first trial to be reported which used full randomization, using in this case sealed envelopes, was the Medical Research Council's (MRC) careful and methodologically advanced trial of streptomycin in TB in the late 1940s (MRC 1948). It is interesting to note that this trial was only ethically possible because the 'small amount of streptomycin available made it ethically permissible for the control participants to be untreated by the drug...' (D'Arcy Hart 1999).

Randomization uses individual-level unpredictability to achieve group-level predictability. So if randomization is on a 1:1 basis, we have no idea whether the individual in front of us will be randomized to the intervention or the control group. The result is that there will be a predictably equal distribution between the two groups of known *and unknown* potential confounders.

In small trials there is the possibility that variables of interest will not assort equally across the intervention and control groups. This may be controlled by the use of stratification at baseline (although this also imposes complexity) or by adjusting the analysis for baseline variables (Roberts and Torgerson 1999).

It is vital that the process of randomization is removed entirely from recruiting researchers since any knowing or unknowing compromise of the chance element to group allocation will undermine the whole basis of the study (Schulz 1995; Altman and Schulz 2001). This will usually require the involvement of a third party who can assure that strict randomization is implemented (e.g. telephoning with the name/study number and only then being assigned a randomization code). The method of assignment and concealment of allocation are important components. If there is an open list of random numbers (or if date of birth or hospital numbers are used) then the process of recruitment is open to influence. For example, if we were interviewing someone and felt that they might have a poor response to the treatment we were testing, and we had worked out that, because she had an even numbered birthday (or hospital number we had glimpsed on an appointment card), she would be allocated to the intervention group we might knowingly or unknowingly, in the process of gaining informed consent, discourage her from participation. Equally if we knew she would be in the control group then we might knowingly or unknowingly encourage her to participate.

Altman and Schulz (2001) suggest that there are two main requirements for adequate concealment of allocation. First, the person generating the allocation sequence must not be the same person determining whether a participant is eligible and enters the trial. Second, the method for treatment allocation should not include anyone involved in the trial. Where the second is not possible they conclude that that the only other plausible method is the use of serially numbered, opaque sealed envelopes although this may still be open to external influence (Schulz 1995; Torgerson and Roberts 1999). In practice, given the expense and complexity of trial design and the vital role that randomization and concealment of allocation plays in a trial it should be a priority to set up an external incorruptible system.

In an useful systematic review Kunz and Oxman (1998) demonstrated that studies which failed to use adequately concealed random allocation generated distorted effect size estimates with the majority overestimating effect. The effects of not using such concealed allocation were often of comparable size to those of the interventions. Another study by Schulz *et al.* (1995) suggested that RCTs without adequately concealed randomization produce effect size estimates that are 40% higher than trials with good quality randomization. They concluded that while the main effect was to produce a poorer response in the control group, there were also occasions where effects of interventions were obscured or reversed in direction. These data provide strong support for the use of robust and concealed methods for randomization and the need to be very sceptical about data from trials not using, or not declaring that they used, such methodology.

In this chapter the focus has been on simple individual intervention and randomization. However the unit of randomization need not be the individual. In a trial of a general practitioner (GP) psychoeducational package the unit might be the GP or a group of GPs in an individual practice, even though its efficacy is assessed by measurement of their patients. Equally where the intervention is population wide, as in trials of water fluoridation to prevent dental caries, the unit of randomization will be the entire catchment area of a reservoir system. Statistical power in such cluster randomization, depends more on the number of clusters (i.e. the number of units of randomization) than the numbers within the clusters, as well as the intra-cluster correlation of outcome (Kerry and Bland 1998).

Intervention, control groups, and blinding

At its most simple, participants are randomized into an intervention or a control group. The intervention group receives the novel treatment and the control group a placebo if there is no established treatment—or the best established treatment if there is one. If the study design is sound and the randomization robust then the control group should differ from the intervention group only in the treatment allocated to it.

The problems start when either the participant, the clinical staff or the researchers can work out which group they are in. There are fewest problems with drug trials. Placebos, or active control treatments can be formulated to look like the novel treatment. Inert placebos may however be discernable from active interventions if they differ in side effects (e.g. anti-cholinergic side-effects) which may alert a patient or clinician to the intervention status. The use of placebos which contain side-effect mimicking compounds may partially address this difficulty. Problems are far greater when the intervention cannot be concealed, for example, in a trial of psychotherapy. It is salutary to bear in mind Bradford Hill's (1963) defense of not subjecting control patients in the MRC Tuberculosis Trial to the four months of four times daily intramuscular injections which the streptomycin intervention group received, that there was 'no need in the search for precision to throw common sense out of the window'.

Blinding is different from concealment of random allocation, and concerns the degree to which participants and/or researchers are unaware of intervention groups after these have been allocated. This is an important tool in minimizing potential bias but may not always be possible depending on the nature of the intervention. *Single blind* studies usually describe a situation where the participant does not know their group but the researcher does. In a *double blind* study both the participant and the investigators are unaware of group membership. In a *triple blind* study the participants, the researchers, and the statisticians analysing the data are unaware of group membership. In an *open trial* everybody knows what is going on and making solid inferences can therefore be difficult. Blinding is not only important in RCTs: for example, the performance of diagnostic tests may be overestimated when the test result is known (Lijmer *et al.* 1999).

A particular issue for RCTs in mental health is the complexity of the intervention. Procedures which we wish to evaluate are often multifaceted and multidisciplinary rather than confined to different tablets (Banerjee and Dickenson 1997). This compromises blinding and may make intervention seem less precise. Certainly it can be difficult to pinpoint what element of intervention may be of help. These are issues across the whole of health care and the UK Medical Research Council (MRC) has published a framework for the design and evaluation of complex interventions to improve health (Campbell *et al.* 2000). In this the authors deal with interventions that are 'made up of various interconnecting parts' citing examples including the evaluation of specialist stroke units and group psychotherapies. They identify a lack of development and definition of the intervention as a frequent difficulty, and propose a five stage iterative process of trial development (Box 10.5).

Box 10.5 **Trial development for complex interventions**

(a) Theoretical phase—identifying evidence for the intervention.

(b) Phase I—defining components of the intervention using descriptive studies, and using modeling and qualitative methodologies to understand the components of the intervention and their interaction.

(c) Phase II—defining trial and intervention design including assessment of feasibility, acceptability, what should happen in the control group and even estimating potential effect sizes by carrying out a small scale exploratory trial where outcome measurement can also be tested.

(d) Phase III—the main trial with a detailed protocol development maximising generalizability. Concurrent qualitative work can help to understand why things are happening or not happening.

(e) Phase IV—promoting effective implementation putting evidence into practice.

Follow-up and reassessment

Given the obstacles to be overcome in getting this far, it is unlikely that assiduous attempts will not be made to follow up all participants in both groups. However the longer the study the more likely there are to be drop outs due to defaulters, and people moving or dying. It is important to attempt as complete a follow-up as possible and to get as much information on those lost to follow-up as possible since incompleteness introduces bias. Assessment of outcome may occur continuously during the trial (e.g. mortality in a cancer chemotherapy trial), intermittently at multiple predetermined timepoints or simply at the end of the defined period of the trial.

A cardinal rule is that assessment of outcome should be completed by a researcher who is blind to randomization group membership. This requires that personnel for the recruitment and the follow-up stages do not assess the same people if they have any knowledge of randomization group. Also any information which might unblind the assessor should be either collected in a different way or left to the end so as not to influence the assessment of outcome in any conscious or unconsciousness way.

Outcome measures should preferably be understandable if they are to be influential in changing clinical practice. Most drug trials rely on rating scales which generate continuous scores (e.g. of depression or cognitive impairment) where these have been widely used and are held to be sensitive to differential change with treatment. However it may be difficult to assess, for example, what a two point change on the Hamilton Depression Rating Scale or the ADAS-Cog actually means in a clinical situation. Clinically relevant outcomes such as recovery from depression need to be used more widely. There is also an increasing role for measures which take a more holistic view of the participant and the impact of the experimental intervention, such as health related quality of life (Guyatt *et al.* 1998).

Major trials will generally have a monitoring committee set up to inspect the data that emerge from the trial before completion. Their remit is to decide whether the trial needs to be stopped early. This may be because accumulating evidence for a strong benefit from the experimental intervention, or evidence that it appears to be harmful. Trials may also be stopped if they appear to be futile: that is where interim analyses show that there is no treatment benefit and that the remaining trial would not allow for a benefit to become manifest. An important considerations in setting up such committees is the need for confidentiality, regular review and pre-agreed criteria for discontinuation (Pocock 1992; Flemming *et al.* 1993).

'Intention to treat' analysis

The strategy for statistical analysis should be specified prior to the commencement of the study. The primary and secondary hypotheses are tested by comparing the outcomes of the intervention and the control groups. This will usually involve a multivariate analysis to control for the effects of any unevenly distributed confounders and to attempt to delineate the size of the treatment effect. Where continuous measures are used statistical methods such as analysis of covariance (ANCOVA) may be appropriate (Vickers and Altman 2001). As with cohort studies a major concern in RCTs is the completeness of follow up. It is often hard to persuade participants to stay in the trial, and if they drop out of treatment, it is usual for studies to collect no further information on them. This causes problems, especially if there is differential drop out between the treatment and control groups. If, for example, an antidepressant was highly effective in those who could tolerate it, but caused such unpleasant side effects that over half of participants dropped out of treatment, an analysis which compared outcome on just those who completed treatment and the placebo group (in whom only 10% dropped out of treatment), would tend greatly to exaggerate the effectiveness of the treatment. This would, in effect, be a form of selection bias.

Ideally, follow-up information should be collected on as many participants as are randomized. Follow-up information should be collected even if the participant has dropped out of treatment, because the outcome of those who are unable to tolerate treatment, or drop out because it is ineffective, is just as important as that of 'completers'. This process can be greatly enhanced if the outcome is a simple one (e.g. mortality), but in psychiatric RCTs there is a tendency to measure outcome on complex symptom inventories. The approach where data on all randomized participants are analysed irrespective of how much of the treatment they have received, is referred to as 'intention to treat analysis'. Using this form of analysis it is irrelevant whether an individual complied with treatment since it is the *offer* of the treatment which is being evaluated. As Last (1995) states 'failure to follow this step defeats the main purpose of random allocation and can invalidate the results'.

Inevitably, there are situations where it is impossible to gain full information on participants, and researchers have to account for such incomplete data. Probably the best approach is to present as much information as can be gathered from the data collected, and to then perform sensitivity analyses which account for missing data. One of the most common is to perform a 'last observation carried forward' analysis, where endpoint data a substituted with previous results. This is usually a conservative approach, but in situations where there is differential drop out, for example, in a psychotherapy trial comparing an active treatment, with treatment as usual, it is common for there to be more drop outs in the 'treatment as usual group'. Using 'last observation carried forward' in this situation would tend to lead to the treatment group appearing to have improved more. Another approach is to impute missing values using regression techniques. Using multi-level modelling is another suitable approach, which is particularly useful for handling missing data. However, no statistical approach is a substitute for good study design and conduct which minimize drop outs.

Interpretation of data

Following analysis, the data need to be presented in a way that can be understood. This is helped by the use of clinically relevant outcome measures, but the paraphernalia of statistical inference can be difficult to penetrate. The presentation of the *number needed to treat* may aid comprehensibility. This is the number of patients from your study population who need to be given the new intervention for the study period in order to achieve the desired outcome (e.g. recovery), or to prevent an undesired one (e.g. death). It is calculated as the reciprocal of the risk difference between treatment group and control (Sackett *et al.* 1991). If, for example, the outcome is recovery from depression, and the risk of recovery at 6 weeks in the treatment group is 0.7, whereas the risk of recovery in the control is 0.5, the risk difference is 0.2, and the NNT 5. To illustrate the meaning of this, one could imagine 10 patients receiving the control condition and five of them getting better. If the same number was given the new treatment, seven would get better. Therefore in 2 out of 10 the treatment would have been responsible for recovery (assuming that the results of the trial were valid), in other words, one would need to treat 5 patients with the treatment, to bring about one recovery attributable to the treatment. The NNT has the unusual characteristic of having a null value of infinity (i.e. one would need to treat an infinite number of patients to bring about a recovery, if the treatment was no better than control), and therefore where a non significant finding is being reported the 95% confidence intervals will span infinity (e.g. NNT = 40, 95% CI 25, ∞, −50). A negative value on the NNT suggests that the treatment is doing harm.

Publication, communication, and dissemination

Once a trial has been completed its findings need to be communicated. This usually requires the preparation of a scientific paper or series of papers and their submission to peer reviewed journals. This is a quality control measure, designed to assess the robustness and scientific strength of the study and its conclusions. Unfortunately publication bias can lead to a tendency for editors and authors to prepare and publish new and significant data rather than replications or negative findings. This can distort an estimation of the true effect of findings and the techniques of systematic review and meta-analysis have developed to attempt to locate unpublished data and to incorporate it into aggregate estimates of effect size. Publication should be seen as the start of a communication strategy for novel findings as it is by drug companies. McCormack and Greenhalgh (2000) have argued powerfully, using data from the UK prospective diabetes study, that there can be a problem with interpretation bias at this stage of a trial with widely disseminated conclusions being unsupported by the actual data presented in the papers. They identified powerful motivations for researchers, authors, editors, and presumably other stakeholders such as the drug industry and the voluntary sector to impart positive spin to trial data. The interpretive biases included the following:

- 'We've shown something here' bias—researcher enthusiasm for a positive result;
- 'The result we've all been waiting for' bias—prior expectations moulding interpretation;
- 'Just keep taking the tablets' bias—overestimating the benefits of drugs;
- 'What the hell can we tell the public' bias—political need for high impact breakthroughs;
- 'If enough people say it, it becomes true' bias—a bandwagon of positivity preceding publication.

That said, there is a need to ensure that important findings are made available, in a way that is accessible to them, for those who formulate policy and purchase services and also those who use them. Andrews (1999) has argued that mental health services may be particularly resistant to changing practice on the basis of empirical evidence, citing the persistence of psychoanalytic psychotherapy and the lack of implementation of family interventions for people with schizophrenia as examples.

Additional information on randomized controlled trials

In this section we will consider some of the more common supplementary questions raised by RCTs.

The phases of pharmaceutical trials

The meanings of and distinctions between the various phases of new drug development can seem opaque. They are best viewed as the necessary processes which need to be completed so that the drug company can satisfy regulatory authorities such as the United States Food and Drug Administration (FDA) or the United Kingdom's Medicines Control Agency (MCA). These phases explicitly refer only to experiments on human participants, there will have been a substantial programme of *in vitro* and animal experiments which will have been completed before the Phase I trials begin, which are beyond the scope of this chapter.

Phase I: Clinical pharmacology and toxicology. This represents the first time a drug is given to humans—usually healthy volunteers in the first place followed by patients with the disorder. The purpose is to identify acceptable dosages, their scheduling and side effects. These are most often carried out in a single centre, requiring 20–80 patients.

Phase II: Initial evaluation of efficacy. These are to determine whether the compound has any beneficial activity. They continue the process of safety monitoring and require close observation, they may be used to decide which of a number of competing compounds go through to Phase III trials. They may be single or multi-centre, and generally require 100–200 patients.

Phase III: Evaluation of treatment effect. This is a competitive phase where the new drug is tested against standard therapy or placebo. There may also be a further element of optimal dose finding. The format for this evaluation is that of an RCT. This phase usually requires large numbers (100s–1000s) and therefore a multi-centre design.

Phase IV: Post-marketing surveillance. Once a drug has been put on the market, there is a need to continue monitoring for rare and common adverse effects including mortality and morbidity. These may only become evident when the drug is used in large numbers in real clinical populations.

Other types of trial

Crossover trials: In a crossover trial the intention is that each patient acts as their own control. Randomization is to receipt of the intervention or the control followed by a wash out period then the treatment not received in the first phase.

Factorial trials: Interventions may be given alone or together so that their individual and joint effects can be evaluated.

Community trials: As discussed above, sometimes the unit of randomisation (i.e. the entity to which the treatment is given) is not an individual but is a community. A good example of this is water fluoridation for dental disease which can only be achieved on a population basis, so that the reservoir and the population it serves becomes the unit of randomization. The number within each community is of secondary importance and may add little to the statistical power of the study. With such interventions there are clear possibilities of problems with compliance (e.g. choosing to drink bottled water only); contamination (travel to fluoridated communities) and blinding (it may be politically unacceptable to prevent the community from knowing what is being done to them).

Other intervention designs

Comparison with historical controls

In this design a group of people are treated with a novel intervention and their progress is compared with a group that has been studied in the past with a different or no treatment and whose outcome is known. A major problem with this approach lies in the other changes which may have occurred as well as the intervention (e.g. lifestyle, diet, healthcare delivery, and other risk and prognostic factors). It may be difficult or impossible to adjust for these factors if they have been incompletely recorded or measured in a different way.

Simultaneous comparison of differently treated groups

This design strategy is subject to bias since there is seldom any element of randomization. The groups for treatment are usually selected either by the treating physicians or by the patients themselves and so are very unlikely to be representative of all individuals with the disorder. It may be impossible to adjust for the effects of variables other than the treatment being studied such as other healthcare provided, illness severity, and concomitant disorders. Inferences concerning the relative efficacy of the interventions may therefore be limited substantially. The same problems are associated with 'waiting list control' evaluations where there is the possibility of any discretion on the part of patients or treating physicians.

Patient preference trials

In trials of this sort the patient takes a more or less active role in deciding which of the treatment arms he or she will complete. This clearly compromises the power of randomization and blindness. However such approaches may be necessary where the belief systems of a study population mean that a standard RCT is not possible. In these trials patients with strong views as to treatment are given the intervention they want and those without preferences (and those with preferences who still agree) are randomized in the normal way. The data from such studies are often difficult to interpret and they will usually need to be very large to enable adequate statistical power for between group comparisons.

Practical

1. Discuss the following with respect to their implications for a randomized controlled trial:

(a) Extent of exclusion criteria—can you identify a true 'effectiveness' study in your field of research? Is this important?

(b) Randomization—how can this be achieved in service-level research?

(c) Blinding—is this feasible in Psychiatry?

(d) Sample size—can a study ever be too large?

(e) Intention to treat analysis—what outcomes should be assigned to people who are immediately lost to follow-up?

2. Pick a controversial treatment in a chosen area of practice—ideally an intervention which has proven efficacy but which is not yet fully accepted by clinicians and/or 'established' as cost-effective. Divide the students into three groups. One group are to represent patients or their advocates, one group are to represent prescribing doctors (or those who will deliver the treatment), and one group are to represent policy makers (e.g. advisors to a health minister) who have to consider the possible costs of the treatment (and assume that what is spent on this will have to be taken away from other aspects of care). Allow the groups about 30 min to prepare a brief presentation and let the fight commence! (*Note*: the choice of the 'treatment will depend on the nature of the class and current wider debate'. Previously successful examples have included atypical antipsychotic agents, anticholinesterase treatments for Alzheimer's disease and novel pharmacological interventions for smoking cessation. The purpose of the exercise is to emphasize that proof of efficacy is only the beginning…)

References

Altman, D.G. and Bland, J.M. (1999) Treatment allocation in controlled trials: why randomise? *British Medical Journal*, 318, 1209.

Altman, D.G. and Schulz, K.F. (2001) Concealing treatment allocation in randomised trials. *British Medical Journal*, 323, 446–7.

Amberson, J.B., McMahon, B.T., and Pinner, M. (1931) A clinical trial of sanocrysin in pulmonary tuberculosis. *American Review of Tuberculosis*, 24, 401–35.

Andrews, G. (1999) Randomised controlled trials in psychiatry: important but poorly accepted. *British Medical Journal*, 319, 562–4.

Armitage, P. (1982) The role of randomisation in clinical trials. *Statistics in Medicine*, i, 345–52.

Banerjee, S. and Dickenson, E. (1997) Evidence based health care in old age psychiatry. *Psychiatry in Medicine*, 27, 283–92.

Begg, C., Cho, M., Eastwood, S., *et al.* (1996) Improving the quality of reporting of randomized controlled trials: the CONSORT statement. *Journal of the American Medical Association*, 276, 637–9.

Benson, K. and Hartz, A.J. (2000) A comparison of observational studies and randomised controlled trials. *New England Journal of Medicine*, 342, 1878–86.

Blum, A.L., Chalmers, T.C., Deutch, E., Koch-Weser, J., Rosen, A., Tygstrup, N., *et al.* (1987) The Lugano statement on controlled clinical trials. *Journal of International Medical Research*, 15, 2–22.

Box (1980) RA Fisher and the design of experiments, 1922–1926. *American Statistics*, 34, 1–7.

Bull, J.P. (1959) The historical development of clinical therapeutic trials. *Journal of Chronic Disease*, 10, 218–48.

Campbell, M., Fitzpatrick, R., Haines, A., Kinmouth, L., Sandercock, P., Spiegelhalter, D., and Tyrer, P. (2000) Framework for design and evaluation of complex interventions to improve health. *British Medical Journal*, 321, 694–6.

Concato, J., Shah, N., and Horwitz, R.I. (2000) Randomised controlled trials, observational studies and the hierarchy of research designs. *New England Journal of Medicine*, 342, 1887–92.

D'Arcy Hart, P. (1999) A change in scientific approach: from alternation to randomised allocation in clinical trials in the 1940s. *British Medical Journal*, 319, 572–3.

Edwards, S.J.L., Lilford, R.J., and Hewison, J. (1998) The ethics of randomised controlled trials from the perspective of patients, the public, and healthcare professionals. *British Medical Journal*, 317, 1209–12.

Evans, S. and Pocock, S. (2001) Societal responsibilities of clinical trial sponsors. *British Medical Journal*, 322, 569–70.

Flemming, T.R. and De Mets, D.L. (1993) Monitoring of clinical trials: issues and recommendations. *Controlled Clinical Trials*, 14, 183–97.

Greenwood, M. and Yule, G.U. (1915) The statistics of anti-typhoid and anti-cholera inoculations and the interpretations of such statistics in general. *Proceedings of the Royal Society of Medicine, Sect Epidemiol State Med*, 8, 113–94.

Guyatt, G.H., Juniper, E.F., Walter, S.D., Griffith, L.E., and Goldstein, R.S. (1998) Interpreting treatment effects in randomised trials. *British Medical Journal*, 316, 690–3.

Hill, A.B. (1963) Medical ethics and controlled trials. *British Medical Journal*, i, 1943.

Ioannidis, J.P.A., Haidich, A.-B., and Lau, J. (2001) Any casualties in the clash of randomised and observational evidence? *British Medical Journal*, 322, 879–80.

Kerry, S.M. and Bland, M. (1998) The intracluster correlation coefficient in cluster randomisation. *British Medical Journal*, 316, 1455–60.

Kunz, R. and Oxman, A.D. (1998) The unpredictability paradox: review of empirical comparisons of randomised and non-randomised clinical trials. *British Medical Journal*, 317, 1185–90.

Last (1995). *A dictionary of epidemiology*. Oxford University Press, Oxford.

Lievre, M., Menard, J., Bruckert, E., Cogneau, J., Delahaye, F., and Giral, P., *et al.* (2001) Premature discontinuation of clinical trial for reasons not related to efficacy, safety, or feasibility. *British Medical Journal*, 322, 603–6.

Lijmer, J.G., Mol, B.W., Heisterkamp, S., Bonsel, G.J., Prins, M.H., van der Meulen, J.H., *et al.* (1999) Empirical evidence of design-related bias in studies of diagnostic test. *Journal of the American Medical Association*, 282, 1061–6.

Lilienfield, A.M. (1982) Ceteris paribus: the evolution of the clinical trial. *Bull History Medicine*, 56, 1–56.

Lind, J. (1753) *A Treatise of the scurvy*. Edinburgh: Sands, Murray & Cochran.

McCormack, J. and Greenhalgh, T. (2000) Seeing what you want to see in randomised controlled trials: versions and perversions of the UKPDS data. *British Medical Journal*, 320, 1720–3.

Medical Research Council (1948) Streptomycin treatment of pulmonary tuberculosis. *British Medical Journal*, ii, 769–82.

Pocock, S.J. (1983) *Clinical trials: a practical approach.* Wiley, Chichester.

Pocock, S.J. (1992) When to stop a clinical trial. *British Medical Journal*, 305, 235–40.

Roberts, C. and Torgerson, D.J. (1999) Baseline imbalance in randomised controlled trials. *British Medical Journal*, 319, 185.

Rogers, S.L. and Friedhoff, L.T. (1996) The efficacy and safety of donepezil in patients with Alzheimer's Disease: results of a US multicentre, randomised, double-blind, placebo-controlled trial. *Dementia*, 7, 293–303.

Rogers, S.L., Farlow, M.R., Doody, R.S., *et al.* (1998*a*) A 24-week, double-blind, placebo-controlled trial of donepezil in patients with Alzheimer's Disease. *Neurology*, 50, 136–45.

Rogers, S.L., Doody, R.S., Mohs, R.C., *et al.* (1998*b*) Donepezil improves cognition and global function in Alzheimer's Disease. *Archives of Internal Medicine*, 158, 1021–31.

Sackett, D.L., Haynes, R.B., Gutatt, G.H., *et al.* (1991) *Clinical epidemiology: a basis science for clinical medicine.* Little Brown, Boston.

Sacks, H., Chalmers, T.C., Smith, H. (1982) Randomized versus historical controls for clinical trials. *American Journal of Medicine*, 72, 233–40.

Schultz, K.F. (1995) Subverting randomisation in controlled trails. *Journal of the American Medical Association*, 274, 1456–8.

Schultz, K.F., Chalmers, I., Hayes, R.J., and Altman, D.G. (1995) Empirical evidence of bias. Dimensions of methodological quality associated with estimates of treatment effects in controlled trails. *Journal of the American Medical Association*, 273, 408–12.

Silverman, W.A. and Chalmers, I. (2001) Casting and drawing lots: a time honoured way of dealing with uncertainty and ensuring fairness. *British Medical Journal*, 323, 1467–8.

Spaight, S.J., Nash, S., Finison, L.J., and Patterson, W.B. (1984) Medical oncologists' participation in cancer clinical trials. *Progress in Clinical Biological and Research*, 156, 49–61.

Taylor, K.M. and Kelner, M. (1987) Interpreting physician participation in randomized clinical trials – are patients really informed? *Journal Health and Social Behaviour*, 28, 389–400.

Torgerson, D.J., and Roberts, C. (1999) Randomisation methods: concealment. *British Medical Journal*, 319, 375–6.

Vickers, A.J. and Altman, D.G. (2001) Analysing controlled trials with baseline and follow up measurements. *British Medical Journal*, 323, 1123–4.

Yastrubetskaya, O., Chiu, E., and O'Connell, S. (1997) Is good clinical research practice for clinical trials good clinical practice? *International Journal of Geriatric Psychiatry*, 12, 227–31.

Chapter 11

Research synthesis: systematic reviews and meta-analysis

Joanna Moncrieff

Introduction

The process of synthesizing data from different studies is known as meta-analysis. The techniques were developed in the social sciences and only recently applied to medical research. There has been intense debate about the validity of the process and its potential contribution to research. In medicine the widest application of research synthesis techniques has been with intervention studies. In particular the Cochrane Collaboration[1] has promoted the use of systematic reviews and meta-analysis to evaluate medical treatments. Recently there has been increasing attention paid to meta-analysis with other types of study (Altman 2001). This overview will focus on intervention studies, and, after describing the uses and limitations of research synthesis and the particular issues arising for psychiatric researchers, will illustrate the stages in conducting a systematic review or meta-analysis.

Definitions

For the purposes of this chapter systematic reviews will be taken as referring to reviews which aim to achieve comprehensive coverage of the relevant literature and meta-analysis refers to the statistical process of combining quantitative data from different studies.

The need for research synthesis

(1) The exponential increase in medical research over recent decades makes it impossible for doctors to have a comprehensive knowledge of research in every area relevant to their practice.

(2) By virtue of bringing a fresh perspective to an area, systematic reviews may be able to reach a more objective view of the evidence.

---

[1] For further information contact the UK Cochrane Centre, Summertown Pavillion, Middle Way, Oxford, OX2 7LG.

(3) Health economists and policy makers need an overview of research and a reliable estimate of efficacy to facilitate the process of resource allocation.

(4) Collation of research in different settings is valuable in order to obtain a picture of the range of action of a particular intervention.

(5) Many studies are not large enough to detect small effects that may be clinically useful. Combining data enhances the power of the analysis to detect such effects.

(6) Systematic collation of evidence indicates which areas require more research.

Disadvantages of research synthesis (Box 11.1)

There is a perception that a well-conducted meta-analysis provides a definitive answer about the hypothesis in question. However, the results of meta-analysis are just as susceptible to bias as primary research, and may, in fact, be more so. The results of meta-analysis may differ from the results of supposedly definitive 'mega' trials and different meta-analyses in the same area may reach different conclusions. The problems involved have led some commentators to argue that the results of meta-analysis are frequently misleading (Eysenck 1994).

The following issues pose specific problems for meta-analysis.

Publication bias

Negative studies are less likely to be published than positive ones (Egger and Smith 1995). This poses a serious threat to the ability of syntheses of published research to reach unbiased conclusions, although thorough searching may help locate some unpublished material.

Magnification of study bias

Results of individual studies will reflect a variable amount of bias, which usually tends in the direction of overestimating the effect of an intervention. Combining data from different studies adds together these positive biases.

Box 11.1 **Disadvantages of research synthesis**

Disadvantages of research synthesis

- Publication bias
- Magnification of study bias
- Heterogeneity
- Subjectivity

Thus meta-analysis should be regarded conservatively and potential sources of bias should not be overlooked.

Heterogeneity

Individual studies in any field are likely to vary according to the characteristics of the participants, the intervention and many aspects of the design and conduct of the study. It is not meaningful to summarize information from very different situations. In addition, interventions may operate differently under different conditions and combining results of studies with different characteristics may obscure these effects.

Subjectivity

Meta-analysis involves various processes of selection and estimation, which are inevitably based on subjective decisions made by the reviewer. Examples are, the selection of studies for inclusion in the analysis and the choice of outcome measures, measurement points and analytical procedures for use in the combined analysis. Where inadequate data is supplied, estimation of parameters, such as standard deviations, may be undertaken.

Planning rationale for selection and estimation prior to the beginning of the study aids the transparency of the process but it may not be possible to anticipate all the necessary decisions. Usually investigators replicate data extraction and quality rating using a second rater allowing inter-rater reliability to be measured.

The arithmetic nature of meta-analysis may obscure these subjective elements and the inherent uncertainty of the process. Thus the technique should not be used indiscriminately and should be interpreted cautiously. It may be preferable to collate studies, examine their individual characteristics, discuss sources of bias and conclude that statistical combination is inappropriate rather than proceed with a quantitative analysis that may be misleading.

Systematic reviews in psychiatry

Principles of research syntheses in psychiatry are essentially no different from elsewhere. However, there are aspects of psychiatric research, which arguably make the process of meta-analysis more fraught than in other areas of medicine. Psychiatric conditions are difficult to define and diagnose reliably, thus patient groups may vary considerably across studies despite the use of standardized diagnostic criteria, making heterogeneity a particular problem.

The subjective nature of most outcomes in psychiatry means that there is always a debate about the most appropriate measures to use. In addition, again because of the subjective nature of outcomes and because of the power of suggestion in some psychiatric conditions, studies in psychiatry may be more susceptible to subtle sources of bias than research in other areas of medicine. There is therefore a particular danger that small amounts of bias present in individual studies may be magnified in the process of combining study results.

Stages of a systematic review and meta-analysis

It is as important to draw up a protocol for a systematic review as it is for a primary research project. The following stages should be considered (Box 11.2).

Frame objectives

Just as for primary research, it is important to frame the research question as precisely as possible, defining the nature of the intervention as well as the control or comparison group and the context from which the question arises.

Define inclusion criteria

Specify in advance what sort of studies will be included in the review. The inclusion criteria should flow from the objectives. The nature of the interventions should be described and the types of participants that will be included. For example, what age group will be included, and are any participants to be excluded on medical or other grounds? Specify the design of studies, such as randomized trials or perhaps only double blind trials. In areas where it is

---

Box 11.2 **Stages of a systematic review and meta-analysis**

Stages of a systematic review and meta-analysis
- Frame objectives
- Define inclusion criteria
- Finding studies
- Quality assessment
- Data extraction and computation of effect sizes
- Dealing with heterogeneity
- Combining outcomes
- Subgroup analysis
- Consideration of publication bias

suspected that there are few randomized trials, or where randomization is inherently difficult, it may be necessary to include all controlled trials.

Finding trials

A thorough search is important to avoid obtaining a biased selection of trials. As well as electronic databases, such as PSYCHLIT, MEDLINE, and EMBASE, systematic reviews of interventions can also use the Cochrane Collaboration registers of randomized controlled trials. Investigators should consider the existence of unpublished studies and how to locate them.

Quality assessment

Quality assessment is important because there is evidence that quality affects the outcome of studies. In particular, lack of rigorous procedures to control bias, such as random allocation and double blinding produces inflated estimates (Shultz *et al.* 1995).

There are numerous different ways to assess the quality of studies and there is no single agreed best method to use. There are quality scales available such as the scale devised by Jadad *et al.* (1996), which has proved popular, is simple to use, but may not discriminate well between trials in psychiatry (Bollini *et al.* 1999). A more detailed assessment instrument has been devised and tested with trials of interventions for depression and neurosis (Moncrieff *et al.* 2001). This provides a more comprehensive assessment of all aspects of study quality but is more complex and hence the overall score is more difficult to interpret. Although reasonable inter-rater reliability has been demonstrated for some of these scales (Jadad *et al.* 1996; Moncrieff *et al.* 2001), there is an irreducible element of subjectivity in quality assessment. For this reason it is important that criteria are made explicit and that detailed results are presented or at least available.

Researchers may exclude certain studies from the combined analysis on the basis of specific methodological criteria, such as all studies that were not conducted double blind. This aims to reduce bias by ensuring the meta-analysis is based only on trials employing rigorous methods. It is also possible to use some key quality variables as co-variates in a meta-regression analysis (see below), although it is generally not recommended that the overall score obtained from a quality rating scale be used in this way because of the difficulty of interpreting the meaning of such a score (Juni *et al.* 2001).

Data extraction and computation of effect sizes

Ideally a meta-analysis would be based on the outcome measure with the greatest validity for the question under consideration. However, it is sometimes difficult to specify in advance which outcomes will be used most frequently and in practice, meta-analysis is often limited to the outcome measures for which adequate statistical details are available. Authors need to consider whether categorical or continuous measures best address the research question. This will probably reflect what has generally been used in the primary research, although it is possible to convert categorical into continuous data and vice versa.

Where studies use a variety of different measures, a standardized mean difference, also known as an effect size, can be computed using continuous measures. This allows comparisons across different studies and outcome measures, and can be calculated using the formula in Box 11.3. There is some debate as to whether to use the pooled standard deviation, recommended by Hedges and Olkin (1985), or whether to use the standard deviation of the control group, which is the method suggested by Glass *et al.* (1981). Standardized mean differences can now be calculated and combined if appropriate by the Cochrane software package REVMAN (Review Manager is available to people who wish to conduct systematic reviews with the Cochrane Collabaroration).

Heterogeneity

It is important to try to anticipate sources of heterogeneity and plan how to manage them in advance. For example, an intervention may theoretically

---

Box 11.3 **Calculation of the standardized mean difference or effect size**

$$\text{Standardized mean difference} = \frac{\text{mean of experimental group-mean of control group}}{\text{pooled standard deviation}}$$

The formula for pooled standard deviation is $= \dfrac{s_1{}^2(n_1-1)+s_2{}^2(n_2-1)}{(n_1-1)+(n_2-1)}$

where n_1 and s_1 are the number of subjects and the standard deviation of the mean, respectively, in the first group and n_2 and s_2 are the same parameters for the second group.

The approximate variance of a standardized mean difference
$$= (n_1 + n_2)/n_1 n_2$$

and confidence interval is therefore:

$$d - 1.96^* \left[(n_1 + n_2)/n_1 n_2\right]^{1/2} \text{ to } d + 1.96^* \left[(n_1 + n_2)/n_1 n_2\right]^{1/2}$$

work differently in patients with severe compared with more minor complaints. Data obtained from different groups of patients could then be used to perform a subgroup analysis.

Once studies have been collected the results should be inspected graphically to look for heterogeneity, which might reveal patterns such as a single outlying trial or distinct groupings of trials. Explanations for these patterns can then be sought. Computer packages that calculate combined statistics produce a 'heterogeneity statistic', the significance of which can be ascertained using χ^2 tables. The degrees of freedom are the number of trials used in the combined analysis minus one. However, these tests lack power and a non-significant heterogeneity statistic does not necessarily indicate sufficient homogeneity among the trials used. The test should not replace the process of anticipation of sources of heterogeneity and inspection of results.

Researchers should seek explanation rather than combining trials with widely discrepant results (Abramson 1990/1991; Thompson 1994). However, some reviews employ statistical models called random effects models (in contrast to the fixed effects models which are employed with homogenous groups of trials) to perform meta-analysis where there is a high degree of unexplained heterogeneity.

Heterogeneity may also be investigated by sensitivity analysis, when meta-analysis is repeated with different combinations of trials. The effect of omitting certain trials, or groups of trials, on the results of the combined analysis may indicate sources of heterogeneity, which can be followed up by re-examination of the trials involved.

Meta-regression analysis using variables thought to explain heterogeneity as covariates can also be conducted. Covariates such as aspects of study design or quality, characteristics of the patient population and characteristics of the intervention can be investigated, but should not be performed with small numbers of trials because of the danger of spurious positive results.

Combining outcomes

If trials seem reasonably homogenous, their outcomes can be combined to produce a pooled measure of effect, which is a weighted average of the outcomes of different trials. Although various methods of weighting exist, weighting by the inverse variance is usually the preferred method. This is the variance of the statistic used, such as the odds ratio, mean difference or standardized mean difference. The variance of an odds ratio and the calculation of the pooled effect are given by the formulae in Box 11.4. The variance of a mean difference is the square of the pooled standard deviation of the two groups. The variance of the standardized mean difference is given above

Box 11.4 **Combining outcomes**

$$\text{Pooled effect} = \Sigma(\text{mean, OR or SMD*weight})/\Sigma\text{weights}$$

where the weight = 1/variance

$$\text{Variance of an odds ratio} = 1/a + 1/b + 1/c + 1/d$$

where

a = number of subjects with the outcome in the exposed group

b = number of subjects with the outcome in the unexposed group

c = number of subjects without the outcome in the exposed group

d = number of subjects without the outcome in the unexposed group

Variance of a mean difference = (pooled standard deviation)^2

$$\text{where pooled standard deviation} = \frac{s_1^2(n_1-1)+s_2^2(n_2-1)}{(n_1-1)+(n_2-1)}$$

(n_1 and s_1 are the number of subjects and the standard deviation of the mean, respectively, in the first group and n_2 and s_2 are the same parameters for the second group.)

$$\text{Variance of a standardized mean difference} = (n_1 + n_2)/n_1 n_2$$

Table 11.1 Illustration of the computation of pooled effect

Trial	Outcome statistic (e.g. mean difference, odds ratio or effect size)	1/ variance (weight)	Statistic*weight
Smith *et al.* 1990	11.7	0.06	0.7
Turner *et al.* 1986	8.2	0.69	5.7
Morris *et al.* 1993	6.0	0.21	1.2
Total		0.96	7.6

(see Box 11.3). Occasionally weighting by the number of participants has been used where there is inadequate information to calculate the variance.

Table 11.1 provides an example using hypothetical trials and data. In this case the pooled effect is 7.6/0.96 = 7.9. The units are the units of the outcome statistic used.

EXAMPLE | 211

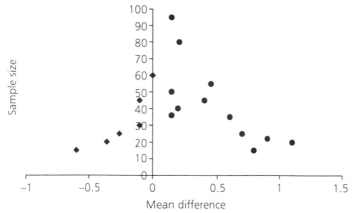

Fig. 11.1 Funnel plots: ♦ indicates small negative studies which if omitted may indicate publication bias combine with small positive and larger studies represented by ● to give a symmetrical funnel plot.

Publication bias

Publication bias can be assessed by constructing a 'funnel plot', which consists of the effect size on the *x*-axis against some measure of study size on the *y*-axis. The resulting plot should be symmetrical about the true effect since small studies, assuming they are conducted under the same conditions as larger ones, should give a wider scatter of results around the true effect with larger studies being closer to the true effect. The resulting graph thus has a shape that resembles an inverted funnel as illustrated in Fig. 11.1. If some small negative studies are not published the plot is asymmetrical.

However readers should note that funnel plots might also be asymmetrical if smaller studies are biased due to poorer quality. There may also be instances where small studies show a genuinely larger effect if, for example, they are conducted on a subset of patients with whom the intervention is truly more effective (Sterne *et al.* 2001).

Example

Meta-analysis of trials of drugs acting on the serotonin system for the prevention of relapse in people with alcohol problems.

Protocol

Objectives

This review aims to evaluate the efficacy of drugs acting on the serotonin system compared with placebo in the treatment of alcohol misuse. These drugs have been employed to reduce the amount of alcohol consumed. A secondary objective will be to determine the effects of these drugs in a subgroup of patients who are alcohol dependent. We hypothesize that drug treatment may not be superior to placebo in this group of people with more severe problems.

Inclusion criteria

Interventions: Studies will be included in the review if they concern a drug that acts on the serotonin system in a way that theoretically enhances the activity of the system.

Participants: The subjects must be people regarded as having alcohol problems using any reasonable definition and be over 16 years of age. A subgroup analysis will use studies which have data for patients diagnosed as having alcohol dependence syndrome using a recognised diagnostic system.

Methodology: Only studies using random allocation to groups will be considered.

Quality assessment

The quality of the trials will be assessed on the following parameters: principle outcomes were specified *a priori*, assessment was conducted blind, all subjects were included in the analysis (an intention to treat analysis) and relevant differences between groups were adjusted for in the analysis. In addition a quality rating scale designed for alcohol treatment studies will be used to obtain a quantitative overview of the quality of each study (Moncrieff and Drummond 1998). All trials meeting inclusion criteria will be included in the meta-analysis regardless of other aspects of quality.

Data extraction

We anticipate that trials will use a variety of measures of drinking to assess outcome. An analysis based on the mean difference of the number of drinks per day at the end of the study will be used if enough studies use this measure. A secondary outcome of interest will be the proportion of people relapsing or remaining abstinent. If studies have no single outcome measure in common, a standardized mean difference will be calculated for each study using the principle continuous outcome at the end of the study.

Heterogeneity

Sources of heterogeneity include the initial severity of the alcohol problems of participants and the action of the drug used and we have planned subgroup analyses accordingly. We will conduct subgroup analyses for trials using different classes of drugs where there are more than two trials. In addition, effect

EXAMPLE | 213

sizes from all individual trials will be displayed graphically to look for hetero-geneity and any patterns associated with it.

Calculation of pooled effect

If inspection of trial results indicates reasonable homogeneity, selected out-comes will be combined to produce a pooled statistic, which will be a weighted average of individual study outcomes. We will use REVMAN computer pack-age to provide heterogeneity statistics.

Subgroup analysis

A subgroup analysis will be performed using only data concerning patients with alcohol dependence syndrome. Further subgroup analyses may be per-formed by grouping trials according to the mode of action of the drug used. Post hoc subgroup analyses may also be conducted if the investigation of heterogeneity reveals any other plausible characteristics that might predict the results of studies.

Publication bias

This will be investigated using funnel plots.

Results

Extensive searching lead to the identification of four trials that fulfilled inclu-sion criteria (see Table 11.2).

Table 11.2 suggests that the trials differ considerably with respect to the drug used, the sorts of participants and the level of severity of their alcohol problems, methods of recruitment, duration of treatment and follow up after treatment, outcome measures used and the proportion of subjects included in the analysis. In addition, it was difficult to determine how many subjects were used in the analysis and how this analysis was done. Thus it is unlikely that one would proceed to combine outcomes numerically, however, this has been done in Table 11.3 to provide an example using the mean difference of number of drinks per day. The overall weighted mean difference can be calculated as sum of the last column divided by the sum of the penultimate column as follows:

$$0.89/0.614 = 1.45$$

The overall mean difference between subjects taking a drug and those taking placebo calculated on the basis of the four trials is 1.45 alcoholic drinks per day.

Note the weights of the different studies depend on the variances, which are very different in these studies. Studies with the smallest variances have the largest weights. In general these will tend to be the largest studies, but as can be seen from this group of trials this is not necessarily the case.

Table 11.2 Characteristics of trials selected for inclusion in the meta-analysis of drugs acting on the serotonin system in relapse prevention for alcohol problems

Trial	Subjects	Total number of subjects randomized	Treatments	Length of treatment and follow up	Main drinking related outcome measures	Proportion of subjects included in analysis
Kranzler et al. 1995 (fluoxetine)	People with alcohol dependence (DSM-III-R) recruited from advertisements	101	Fluoxetine (mean dose 47 mg/day) vs. placebo	12 weeks treatment +6 months follow up	Drinking days, drinks per day, drinks per drinking day	95/101 = 94%
Kranzler et al. 1994 (buspirone)	People with alcohol dependence (DSM-III-R) recruited from advertisements	61	Buspirone mean maximum daily dose 52.5 mg/day	12 weeks treatment +6 months follow up	Weeks to first drinking and heavy drinking day, drinking days, drinks per day, drinks per drinking day	100%
Naranjo et al. 1995 (citalopram)	Heavy social drinkers recruited from advertisements drinking >28 drinks per week	99	Citalopram 40 mg/day + brief psychosocial intervention	12 weeks treatment + 8 week FU	Mean daily drinks, days abstinent, drinks per drinking day, alcohol dependence (ADS) and alcohol problems (MAST)	62/99 = 63%
Naranjo et al. 1995 (ritanserin)	Heavy social drinkers recruited from advertisements drinking >28 drinks per week	42	Ritanserin 5 mg and 10 mg/day	2 weeks treatment	Mean daily drinks, days abstinent, drinks per drinking day	39/42 = 93%

Table 11.3 Calculation of a composite mean difference in the meta-analysis of drugs acting on the serotonin system relapse prevention in alcohol problems

Trial	n analysed for drinks per day drug/placebo	Period of last measurement	Mean difference for drinks per day (placebo-drug)	Pooled s	Weight (1/s²)	Mean difference/ variance
Kranzler et al. 1995 (fluoxetine)	40/45	Last 6 months of follow up	$2.4 - 1.6 = 0.8$	3.87	$1/14.96 = 0.067$	0.05
Kranzler et al. 1994 (buspirone)	31/30	Last 6 months of follow up	$4.8 - 0.9 = 3.9$	1.85	$1/3.42 = 0.29$	1.14
Naranjo et al. 1995 (citalopram)	31/31	Last 4 weeks of follow up	$2.6 - 3.6 = -1$	2.23	$1/4.95 = 0.20$	-0.20
Naranjo et al. 1995 (ritanserin)	14/25	2 weeks of treatment	$5.73 - 7.53 = -1.8$	4.25	$1/18.13 = 0.055$	-0.10
Total					0.614	0.89

A more sensible way to proceed in this case would be to give a qualitative summary of the studies and a discussion of the need for further research.

Practical

A. Critically assess the following meta-analysis by answering the questions below:

Hazell, P., *et al.* (1995) Efficacy of tricyclic drugs in treating child depression: a meta-analysis. *British Medical Journal*, **310**, 897–901.

(1) Comment on the search strategy used.

(2) What were the inclusion criteria and were these appropriate to the objectives?

(3) Discuss the way the quality of included trials was assessed.

(4) How was the process of the selection of outcome measures for use in the meta-analysis justified?

(5) Discuss the way in which heterogeneity was managed. Do you think this was adequate?

(6) What statistical methods were used to combine results?

(7) What could have been done to assess the possibility of publication bias?

B. Answer the following questions on

Bech, *et al.* (2000) Meta-analysis of randomised controlled trials of fluoxetine vs. placebo and tricylic antidepressants in the short term treatment of major depression. *British Journal of Psychiatry*, **176**, 421–8.

(1) Comment on the inclusion and exclusion criteria. How representative of the research were the trials selected in this way?

(2) Identify three different ways in which heterogeneity was managed. Discuss how further assessment of heterogeneity could have been made.

(3) What other sources of heterogeneity could have been investigated?

(4) Was there any consideration of trial quality? What else could have been done to assess this?

(5) Was there any consideration of publication bias or any protection against it?

Suggested reading

Egger, M., Smith, G.D., and Altman, D.G. (eds) (2001) *Systematic reviews in health care: Meta-analysis in context.* BMJ Books, London.

Abramson, J.H. (1990–1991) Meta-analysis: a review of pros and cons. *Public Health Reviews*, **18**, 1–47.

Glass, G.V., McGaw, B., and Smith, M.L. (1981) *Meta-analysis in social research.* Sage Publications, Beverly Hills, CA. Chapters 5 and 6.

Knipschild, P. (1994) Systematic reviews. Some examples. *British Medical Journal,* 309, 719–21.

Mulrow, C.D. (1994) Rationale for systematic reviews. *British Medical Journal,* 309, 597–9.

Thompson, S.G. (1994) Why sources of heterogeneity in meta-analysis should be investigated. *British Medical Journal,* 309, 1351–5.

Eysenck, H.J. (1994) Meta-analysis and its problems. *British Medical Journal,* 309, 789–92.

References

Abramson, J.H. (1990–1991) Meta-analysis: a review of pros and cons. *Public Health Reviews,* 18, 1–47.

Altman, D.G. (2001) Systematic reviews of evaluations of prognostic variables. *British Medical Journal,* 323, 224–8.

Bollini, P., Pampallona, S., Tibaldi, G., Kupelnick, B., and Munizza, C. (1999) Effectiveness of antidepressants. Meta-analysis of dose-effect relationships in randomised clinical trials. *British Journal of Psychiatry,* 174, 297–303.

Egger, M. and Smith, G.D. (1995) Misleading meta-analysis. *British Medical Journal,* 311, 753–4.

Eysenck, H.J. (1994) Meta-analysis and its problems. *British Medical Journal,* 309, 789–92.

Glass, G.V., McGaw, B., and Smith, M.L. (1981) *Meta-analysis in social research.* Sage Publications, Beverly Hills, CA.

Hedges, L.V. and Olkin, I. (1985) *Statistical methods for meta-analysis.* Academic Press, Inc. San Diego.

Jadad, A.R., Moore, R.A., Carroll, D., *et al.* (1996) Assessing the quality of reports of randomised clinical trials: is blinding necessary? *Controlled Clinical Trials,* 17, 1–12.

Juni, P., Altman, D.G., and Egger, M. (2001) Assessing the quality of controlled clinical trials. *British Medical Journal,* 323, 42–6.

Kranzler, H.R., Burleson, J.A., Del Boca, F.K., *et al.* (1994) Buspirone treatment of anxious alcoholics. *Archives of General Psychiatry,* 51, 720–31.

Kranzler, H.R., Burleson, J.A., Korner, P., *et al.* (1995) Placebo-controlled trial of fluoxetine as an adjunct to relapse prevention in alcoholics. *American Journal of Psychiatry,* 152, 391–7.

Moncrieff, J., Churchill, R., Drummond, D.C., and McGuire, H. (2001) Development of a quality assessment instrument for trials of treatments of depression and neurosis. *International Journal of Methods in Psychiatric Research,* 10, 126–33.

Moncrieff, J. and Drummond, D.C. (1998) The quality of alcohol treatment research: an examination of influential controlled trials and development of a quality rating system. *Addiction,* 93, 811–23.

Naranjo, C.A., Bremner, K.E., and Lanctot, K.L. (1995) Effects of citalopram and a brief psycho-social intervention on alcohol intake, dependence and problems. *Addiction,* 90, 87–99.

Naranjo, C.A., Poulos, C.X., Lanctot, K.L., Bremner, K.E., Kwok, M., and Umana, M. (1995) Ritanserin, a central 5-HT$_2$ antagonist, in heavy social drinkers: desire to drink, alcohol intake and related effects. *Addiction,* 90, 893–905.

Schultz, K.F., Chalmers, I., Hayes, R.J., and Altman, D.G. (1995) Empirical evidence of bias: dimensions of methodological quality associated with estimates of treatment effects in controlled trials. *Journal of the American Medical Association*, **273**, 408–12.

Sterne, J.A.C., Egger, M., and Smith, G.D. (2001) Investigating and dealing with publication and other biases in meta-analysis. *British Medical Journal*, **323**, 101–5.

Thompson, S.G. (1994) Why sources of heterogeneity in meta-analysis should be investigated. *British Medical Journal*, **309**, 1351–5.

Section 3

Interpretation

Chapter 12

Inference 1: chance, bias, and confounding

Robert Stewart

Inference is the process of passing from observations to generalizations. As such, it is a key activity in all research. An observed association between two factors does not mean that one definitely caused the other. In Epidemiology, before any other consideration of cause and effect can be entered into, the role of chance, bias, and confounding need to be assessed and then the direction of causality considered. If an association is observed, might it have occurred by chance? Might it have arisen because of error intrinsic to the study design (bias)? Might the association have arisen because of other factors (confounding)? Has an association between factors A and B arisen because A has caused B or because B has caused A (direction of causation)? (Box 12.1).

Chance and bias represent relatively simple concepts to evaluate and should be the first considerations in study design and critical appraisal. These address the 'translation' of inference from the sample to the population. For example, 'here is an association between two factors in a sample. But can I assume that this is true for the source population?' Confounding and direction of causation are conventionally included as similar considerations. However they address potentially more complex issues: 'here is an association which I believe to be present in the source population (having considered the roles of chance and bias). But what does this tell me about how this disease or event is caused?' Confounding will be considered with chance and bias out of convention, but the issue of inferring cause and effect will be then be taken up in more detail in the following chapter.

Chance

The role of chance in explaining an observed association is assessed in the statistical analysis of results. Statistical inference involves generalizing from sample data to the wider population from which the sample was drawn. Inferences are made by calculating the range around an observed property of

Box 12.1 **Inference**

Chance	What is the likely value in the population (95% confidence intervals)?
	What is the probability of chance (*p*-value)?
Bias	Through sampling/participation/follow-up (selection bias)
	Through measurements applied/information obtained (information bias)
	From participants/from observers
	Differential/non-differential
Confounding	'An alternative explanation'
	Addressed in the study design (by restriction/matching/randomization)
	Addressed in the analysis (by stratified/multivariate analysis)
Further considerations	Relationship between prevalence, incidence, and survival
	Relationship between the ecological- and individual-level
	Direction of causation
	Mediating factors
	Effect modification
	Background literature
	Implications for research/clinical practice/Public Health

the sample within which the 'true' property of the population is likely to lie (confidence intervals) or, less commonly now, the probability that chance alone might have accounted for a given observation (the *p*-value).

Sampling error and sampling distributions

Chance operates through sampling error. If we wanted to estimate the mean alcohol intake in people aged 16 and over in the United Kingdom, we would not go to the trouble of interviewing the whole nation. We would instead draw a representative sample, possibly from a population register. Non-random selection might give rise to unrepresentative samples—this situation is considered under 'bias' below. For the moment, a random and entirely representative sample is assumed. If, say, 100 people were interviewed we would have a mean alcohol intake for that sample. Assuming a symmetrical 'normal' distribution for alcohol intake, 95% of people in the sample will have intakes within approximately two (nearer 1.96) standard deviations either side of this mean (because this is a property of the normal distribution). If however we were to interview another random sample of 100 people, the mean intake would not be exactly the same. Which one should we believe? If we were to repeat the study over and over again we would end up with a distribution of mean intakes. This hypothetical distribution is referred to as the *sampling distribution*. The observed means from repeated sampling will be normally distributed. This tends to be true even if the trait itself is not normally distributed in the population (the proof is referred to as the *central limit theorem*). The mean of the sampling distribution will be the population mean; sample estimates for the mean which deviate considerably from the true population mean will be observed much less commonly, and appear in the tails of the distribution. Note that if the size of the samples were to be increased (i.e. above 100 in this example), then the variance (i.e. spread) of these means would decrease. This is because larger samples give more precise estimates.

Standard errors and confidence intervals

The standard deviation for the sampling distribution is known as the standard error of the mean—so 95% of *sample means* obtained by repeated sampling will lie within approximately two standard errors either side of the population mean (because of this property of the normal distribution). This information can therefore be used to estimate limits of uncertainty around an observed *sample* mean, giving the range of likely values for the *population* mean. These limits of uncertainty are referred to as *95% confidence intervals*. They represent the range in which 95% of mean values would lie if sampling was repeated under identical conditions.

Confidence intervals for other types of observations in a sample are calculated in a similar way (by estimating the standard error), for example, proportions (e.g. the prevalence of depression), mean differences (e.g. gender differences in alcohol intake), odds ratios (e.g. for associations between gender and major depression), or rate ratios (e.g. for male/female incidence rates of depression). The calculation of standard errors is relatively simple for many situations and some formulae are given in Box 12.2. For small sample sizes, other formulae may have to be used and these are described in most generic Statistics guides (e.g. excellently in Kirkwood 1988). A pocket calculator is sufficient but computers generally 'take the strain'. Useful algorithms may also be downloaded from the website of the 'Medical Algorithms Project', Chapter 39 at *http://www.medal.org/index.html*. Slightly more complicated equations

Box 12.2 Formulae for calculating standard errors and confidence intervals

Situation 1: A single proportion 'p' in a sample of size 'n'

$$SE = \sqrt{\{p\,(1-p)\}/n} \quad 95\% \text{ CI} = p \pm 1.96 \times SE$$

(suitable when np and $n\text{-}np$ are 10 or more).

Situation 2: A mean for a sample of size 'n' and standard deviation 's'

$$SE = s/\sqrt{n} \quad 95\% \text{ CI} = \text{mean} \pm 1.96 \times SE$$

(suitable for sample sizes above 20).

Situation 3: The difference between two proportions 'p_1' and 'p_2' in samples with sizes 'n_1' and 'n_2' respectively

$$SE = \sqrt{\{p_1(1-p_1)/n_1\}+\{p_2(1-p_2)/n_2\}}$$
$$95\% \text{ CI} = \text{difference} \pm 1.96 \times SE$$

(suitable when both samples fulfil criteria for (1) above).

Situation 4: The difference between two means in samples with sizes of n_1 and n_2 and a standard deviations of s_1 and s_2 respectively

$$SE = \sqrt{(s_1/n_1 + s_2/n_2)} \quad 95\% \text{ CI} = \text{difference} \pm 1.96 \times SE$$

(suitable when both samples fulfil criteria for (2) above).

are used for generating standard errors and confidence intervals for odds and rate ratios. These are outlined in Chapters 8 and 9 respectively. The principle is still that 'out there' in the whole source population (e.g. UK adults) is a true proportion, mean difference, odds ratio, rate ratio, etc. This cannot be directly measured without recruiting the whole population but, for a representative sample, 95% confidence intervals give a range of values within which the true value will lie on 95% of occasions. The choice of '95%' for defining confidence intervals is entirely arbitrary, but there is generally little reason to stray beyond convention.

Statistical tests and *p*-values

Statistical procedures are used to test whether a hypothesis about the distribution of one or more variables should be accepted or rejected. In the case of a hypothesized association between a risk factor and a disease, we can estimate the probability of an association of at least a given size being observed if the *null hypothesis* were true (i.e. that there is no real association and the observed association merely arose through chance). Conventionally, the threshold for statistical significance is taken to be 0.05 (i.e. findings are accepted as present if the probability that they occurred by chance is 5% or less). As with confidence intervals, it is important to remember that there is nothing magical about the $p = 0.05$ threshold. It represents nothing more than a generally agreed acceptable level of risk of making what is known as a *Type I error*, that is falsely rejecting a null hypothesis when it is true (a 'false-positive' finding). This is generally based on the assumption that a two-tailed statistical test will be used (see note on p-values below). The probability of rejecting the null hypothesis when it is indeed false (i.e. detecting a true association) is the study's *statistical power*. The converse scenario, accepting a null hypothesis when it should have been rejected (i.e. failing to detect a true association) is referred to as a *Type II error* (1-power).

For differences in proportions and mean values between two groups, estimating the p-value for a given observation is, like confidence intervals, relatively simple since it just involves calculating the number of standard errors the observed difference is away from the null value. For these estimations, the null hypothesis is that there is no difference between group A and group B (e.g. men and women) with respect to a mean value or a proportion (e.g. mean alcohol consumption or prevalence of depression). For example, you might observe that men drank 4 units of alcohol per week more than women (assuming, for the sake of argument, a normal distribution for alcohol intake). You might then calculate that the standard error for that difference was 1 unit/week. The observed difference is therefore four standard errors away from the null. This is called a 'z-score'. We know already that 1.96 standard errors away from the null give 95% confidence intervals—and are therefore equivalent to a p-value of 0.05 (for a two-tailed test—see note on p-values below). So the p-value for a difference of four standard errors is considerably less than 0.05—therefore 'highly significant'. We really knew this anyway because 95% confidence intervals for the mean difference would have been approximately 2–6 units/week (i.e. nowhere near the null value of zero). The equivalent z-score for a p-value of 0.01 is 2.58, for 0.001 is 3.29 and for 0.0001 is 3.89. So for our analysis, the p-value is less than 0.0001. Tables linking z-scores more precisely to p-values are given in most statistics textbooks. In general, a computer will come up with a needlessly precise estimate. The calculation of p-values for other situations (e.g. odds ratios) are slightly more complex, although with similar underlying principles, and are described in other texts (e.g. Kirkwood 1988).

The relationship between *p*-values and confidence intervals

There are therefore two ways in which the role of chance can be estimated for a given association. One is to give the probability that the association might have arisen through chance (the *p*-value). The other is to estimate that range of values within which the true strength of association is likely to lie (confidence intervals). The problem with *p*-values is that they only give a single probability (related to whether the null hypothesis is true or not). The size of the *p*-value gives little indication of the strength of association (a weak association of little clinical significance may be detected with a 'highly significant' *p*-value if the sample is very large). Confidence intervals on the other hand describe both the likely magnitude of an association as well as giving an idea of whether it is present or not (i.e. for a significance cut-off of 0.05, whether 95% intervals overlap the 'null' value—which would be 1.0 for an odds ratio, or 0.0 for a difference in means). They are therefore preferred and there are now a decreasing number of circumstances where calculation of a *p*-value is considered helpful or necessary.

A note on hypotheses

It is important to bear in mind that two different sorts of hypothesis are referred to in Research Methods literature. In papers and funding applications, one or more 'positive' hypotheses are generally required, that is, that X and Y will be associated, or that X will occur at a greater frequency in group Y than group Z. A requirement for the paper or funding application is to demonstrate that the design and sample size are sufficient to test these according to refutationist principles (discussed in Chapter 13). In order to carry this out in statistical analysis, the starting point is always from the opposite point of view, that is, that there is no association between X and Y (the 'null hypothesis'). The task is then to establish whether this can be disproved and with what degree of certainty.

A note on *p*-values

It is customary practice to apply what are known as *two-tailed* statistical tests for significance. These test whether an observation is *different* from the null rather than specifically whether it is either *greater* or *less*, that is, it concerns *both* tails of the normal distribution. A common mis-interpretation of the two-sided *p*-value is that it represents the probability that the point estimate is as far or further from the null value as was observed. For large samples, this probability is approximately the square of the *p*-value (i.e. considerably lower). This problem with interpreting two-sided *p*-values is another reason to focus on confidence intervals instead.

A note on confidence intervals

In the absence of bias, 95% confidence intervals will, over unlimited repetitions of the study with a given sample size, include the true parameter on at least 95% of occasions. A common misinterpretation of confidence intervals is that there is a 95% probability or 'likelihood' that they contain the true parameter. This situation only applies to confidence intervals derived using Bayesian analysis, and cannot be assumed for those calculated using standard procedures.

Bias

Bias refers to systematic error arising from the design or execution of a study. It is an entirely undesirable feature, which, unlike confounding (see below) cannot be 'adjusted for' once data has been gathered. The only hope is to limit the scope for bias in the way in which the study has been designed. Then, where the potential for bias still exists, care must be exercised in drawing inferences. Bias can be mainly categorized into that which arises from deriving the sample or comparison groups from the 'base' population (selection bias) and that which arises from the measurements made on study participants (information bias). Particular study designs are more or less prone to particular sources of bias. Therefore readers are also referred to the chapters on ecological studies (Chapter 6), cross-sectional surveys (Chapter 7), case–control studies (Chapter 8), cohort studies (Chapter 9), randomized controlled trials (Chapter 10) and systematic reviews and meta-analyses (Chapter 11) for a more detailed account of the role of bias in these study designs.

Information bias

Information bias arises from systematic error in measurements applied to participants. All measurements are potentially subject to error, whether they are an assay for cholesterol levels, a genetic test, a questionnaire assessment of personality traits, or a structured clinical interview diagnosis of major depression. Error in categorical measures such as diagnoses is conventionally referred to as misclassification. The effect of the bias depends upon whether the error is *differential* or *non-differential*. In *differential misclassification*, the misclassification depends on the values of other variables; thus where the proportion of participants misclassified on exposure depends on outcome status, or the proportion of participants misclassified on outcome status depends on exposure status. For example, in a prospective cohort study misclassification of outcome (incident depression) may depend upon whether or not they were exposed at baseline (to a recent stressful life-event). In a case–control study misclassification of exposure (to a head injury) may depend upon whether they are a case or a control (dementia present or absent). Where *differential misclassification* has occurred, *bias might operate in either direction*, that is, the 'true' strength of the association (between head injury and dementia) may be over- or underestimated. If misclassification is *non-differential* (i.e. occurring to the same extent and in the same direction in cases and controls or among those exposed and unexposed), then results will be *biased towards the null*. This means that the 'true' strength of association will be underestimated.

Participant-derived information bias (recall bias)

In a case–control study bias occurs if cases are systematically more or less likely to recall and/or relate information on exposure than controls. For example, people with multiple episodes of major depression as an adult (cases) may be more likely to recall and report childhood abuse (the exposure of interest) than people with no history of mental health problems (controls). This will give rise to a spuriously strong association between abuse and depression unless measures are taken to prevent this bias (not always simple or even possible). The experience of disease encourages an 'effort after meaning' whereby the participant has already gone over their life history in an attempt to understand why they have become ill.

Investigator-derived information bias (observer bias)

In a case–control study, an investigator who believes that child abuse causes major depression in adulthood, might put extra effort into obtaining disclosure of abuse from major depression cases than from controls (giving rise to a spuriously strong positive association between exposure and outcome).

Information bias is a particular problem for case–control studies and cross-sectional surveys, since exposure and outcome have already occurred by the time that each is ascertained and hence there is always the potential for assessment of the one to be influenced by the participant's status with regard to the other. In prospective cohort studies, assessment of the exposure cannot in principle be affected by knowledge of the outcome, which has not occurred and cannot be predicted reliably either by participant or investigator. However, assessment of the outcome can be affected by knowledge of the exposure. For example, in randomized controlled trials, which are really a special type of cohort study, if participants either know or can guess their treatment allocation they may be more or less likely to report an outcome of interest (whether this is clinical improvement or side-effects). Attempts are made to conceal allocation from participants (to reduce recall bias) in 'single-blind' trials, and from both participants and investigators (to reduce observer bias) in 'double-blind' trials (see Chapter 10). Note that blinding also has a place in case–control studies as a tactic to reduce information bias. Participants may be blinded to the hypothesis under study, and investigators may be blinded to a participant's case status, and to the study hypothesis. Clearly neither of these procedures is universally feasible.

Selection bias

Selection bias is again a particular problem in case–control studies. Cases selected for the study should be representative of all cases from the base population and controls should be representative of all controls. Selection bias may occur where selection as a case or control is to some extent dependent upon an exposure under study as a hypothesized risk factor. For example, a case–control study of risk factors for Alzheimer's disease finds that arthritis (an exposure) is more common in controls than cases, hence is inversely associated with the outcome. However cases were recruited from specialist outpatient clinics whereas controls were recruited from people attending primary care clinics. Arthritis is a common reason for primary care consultation and therefore the odds of this exposure may have been spuriously higher in controls; the association had arisen purely from the selection procedures, and may not have reflected a true protective effect of arthritis in the pathogenesis of Alzheimer's Disease. For a case–control study, cases and controls should be drawn from the same base population (one useful check is to ask yourself the question 'if this control had developed the disease would he have been included in the case group?'). Inclusion and exclusion criteria need to be examined carefully. In principle they should be the same for case and control groups.

In an observational cohort study, selection of the baseline sample is unlikely to have differential effects upon outcome for the exposed and unexposed groups (or vice versa), particularly if there is a lengthy follow-up period. Loss to follow-up (i.e. selection through 'survival') could potentially lead to bias as it is often associated with the outcome and also with exposure status. If loss to follow-up is differential with respect to both exposure and outcome, bias will occur. However for cohort studies generalizability is the more important consideration. For example, a major piece of evidence that smoking might cause lung cancer came from following up a 'convenience' sample of British physicians. Would the findings also apply to women, or to the general population? Similar considerations apply to randomized controlled trials (see Chapter 10).

Other 'bias'

Two other situations are commonly described as sources of bias, namely 'prevalence bias' and 'ecological bias'. However limitations in inference relate to fundamental properties of the individual study designs rather than arising from a source of error in their application.

Prevalence bias

This refers to the fact that prevalence (the proportion of people having a disease at a particular time) is a product both of the rate at which new cases arise (the incidence) and the rate at which cases cease to have the condition (e.g. through recovery or death). Factors which are identified in a cross-sectional study as positively associated with a disease will include those which are associated with increased incidence, and those associated with increased duration (or 'maintenance') of illness. For most aetiological studies, associations with incidence are of principal interest. It is therefore usual to move from cross-sectional to prospective research to distinguish influences on incidence from those on duration. For disorders with little variation in duration, the two may be equated. Schizophrenia approximates to this condition since the diagnosis reflects lifelong vulnerability rather than a transient state (so symptom resolution is referred to as 'remission' rather than 'recovery'). Mortality will, however, still influence prevalence. Prevalence 'bias' is a particular issue with more fluctuating 'state' diagnoses such as depression where prevalence is more strongly influenced by state-duration. One approach, used particularly in case–control studies is to restrict 'case' participants to those with a recent onset and hence limited duration. This procedure does require some means of dating the 'onset' of the condition (to estimate duration), a procedure with dubious validity for many psychiatric disorders.

Ecological bias

Issues concerning ecological studies are described in Chapter 6. A fundamental limitation is that it cannot be inferred that associations observed at a group level also apply at an individual level. This is referred to, somewhat confusingly and apparently interchangeably in many texts, as 'ecological bias', 'ecological confounding', and the 'ecological fallacy'. The second two terms are more appropriate than the first. Confounding is an important issue in ecological studies, and individual-level generalizations from ecological data are better described as 'fallacy' than bias since they represent a failure to draw appropriate inferences rather than an error in the methodology of the study itself.

Bias, inference, and critical appraisal

Sometimes a study may have a major flaw in its design or execution, which precludes any inference being drawn. For example, in a cohort study with

30% follow-up rates, it may be impossible to conclude anything about exposure–outcome relationships in the remaining participants. Thankfully, however, critical appraisal is rarely so clear-cut for the large proportion of published research. The task in critical appraisal is therefore not only to identify potential sources of bias, but also to decide whether these might have influenced results and, if so, to what extent and in what direction. It is demoralizing and of little purpose merely to criticise and 'bring down' a paper without considering how methodological obstacles might have been overcome. For many areas of psychiatric research this is a formidable task and some degree of bias is inevitable.

Confounding

The term confounding derives from the Latin *confundere*, meaning to mix up. Confounding describes a situation in which the measured effect of an exposure is distorted because of the association of that exposure with other factors that influence the disease or outcome under study. A confounding variable might cause or prevent the outcome of interest, is not an intermediate variable, and is independently associated with the exposure under investigation. As discussed earlier, consideration of confounding factors represents an intermediate step between relatively simple questions of whether an association is true or not and the nature of the causal pathways which it represents.

An illustration of confounding would be an observed association between grey hair and increased mortality. This observation might have arisen from a rigorously designed study with a representative sample, perfect outcome ascertainment and with statistical tests indicating a strong association with narrow confidence intervals. The association in the sample therefore appears to be entirely valid: that is, true for the source population as well as the sample. However it quite obviously does not imply that grey hair *causes* mortality. The limitation in the inferences which can be drawn is that age is a likely confounding factor which has not been taken into account. Increased age is associated with grey hair and is more likely to be a cause of mortality. It therefore represents an *alternative explanation* for the observed association. *A factor providing an alternative explanation for an association* is probably the simplest way to understand a confounder. Confounding may be addressed either in the design of a study or, more usually, in the statistical analysis of results. It is important to remember that confounding, like bias, may lead to true associations being missed as well as false associations being identified. It may even lead to an association being reversed in its direction. For example, driving a fast car might be found to be associated with lower mortality. However people who drive fast cars are also likely to have higher incomes and socioeconomic status. If the association was adjusted for income, driving a fast car might instead be associated with higher mortality.

Addressing confounding through study design

Strategies in the study design to limit confounding operate by removing variation in confounding factors between comparison groups of interest. A potential confounding factor cannot influence an observed association if it is evenly distributed between groups compared. An extreme method is sample *restriction*, that is, the sample is limited so that the confounding factor does not vary at all. For example, if gender was believed to be an important confounder, a study might be carried out only in men or only in women. This has the obvious limitation of reduced generalizability (results in women could not be assumed to be the same as results in men). A second approach for case–control studies is matching. In this method, control participants are specifically chosen to be as similar as possible to cases with respect to a given confounding factor. In the example above, for each person with grey hair, another person without grey hair might be recruited who was of the same age (one to one matching) or within a similar age-range (restriction matching). Matched designs have limitations and, with increasingly accessible statistical procedures, have few advantages except in small case–control studies. There are obvious logistical difficulties with matching on more than one or two factors and there is a danger of 'over-matching' (i.e. creating groups which are so similar that they are partially matched on the exposure of interest). Specific statistical procedures have to be used for the analysis of matched samples.

Ultimately the best method for removing confounding effects is through *randomization*. If an intervention is randomly assigned then all other factors should be evenly distributed between intervention and control groups (given reasonable sample sizes). Any difference in outcome between comparison groups can therefore be reasonably attributed to the intervention. An important advantage is that randomization controls for both measured *and unmeasured* confounding factors. In observational studies on the other hand, researchers can only do their best to measure and take into account everything they can think of and hope that there are no other major factors 'out there' that have been missed. However, randomization is limited ethically to interventions which might be beneficial but where no strong evidence exists one way or another. In observational studies, the most common method for dealing with confounding is through statistical 'adjustment'. The obvious implication for study design is that potential confounding factors need to have been identified and measured as accurately as possible.

Addressing confounding through statistical analysis

The simplest and most appropriate 'first stage' for investigating confounding is the *stratified analysis*. For the grey hair–mortality example, if we had a sufficiently large sample, and were to subdivide the sample into 5-year age bands, we would probably find that the association between grey hair and mortality was no longer present (or at least substantially reduced) within each of these bands. Relatively simple statistical equations (e.g. for odds ratios, the Mantel–Haenszel procedure) allow stratum-specific estimates to be 'combined' for the whole sample to produce an 'adjusted' estimate (in this case, an age-adjusted association between grey hair and mortality). The limitation is that only one, or at the most two, confounding factors can be considered before strata become too small. More advanced forms of statistical analysis, collectively referred to as *multivariable analyses* (and discussed in more detail in Chapters 15), have been developed which can adjust simultaneously for the effects of several potential confounding variables. The choice of analysis depends on the nature of the outcome (or 'dependent') variable. Linear regression and analysis of variance (ANOVA) are used for continuously distributed outcomes (e.g. level of alcohol intake), logistic regression for binary outcomes (e.g. presence or absence of depression), and Cox proportional hazards models where the outcome is a rate or 'survival' (e.g. onset of depression, mortality). Multivariable analyses need to be used with caution and careful forethought. Most importantly, effect modification may be missed if stratified analyses are not first carried out (discussed in Chapter 13), and there is a danger that confounding and mediating factors may not be distinguished (discussed below).

Confounding, inference, and critical appraisal

The example of grey hair and mortality is a simple one with a clear single confounding factor. 'Real world' situations are inevitably more complicated, possibly particularly so in psychiatric research (as will be discussed in the following and final chapters). An important first step for evaluating the role of a potential confounding factor is interpreting 'adjusted' values. There is no 'test' for confounding and the judgement is a subjective one on the part of the researcher and of each person reading their report. The point of focus should be on the estimate of the strength of an association. This might be an odds ratio, or a mean difference, or a correlation coefficient. The extent to which this estimate changes following adjustment, gives the best idea of the extent to which the association was explained by a confounding factor. For example, the rate ratio for mortality associated with the presence of grey hair might be 7.0 (i.e. the mortality rate is seven times higher in people with grey hair than those without). If after adjustment for age this ratio was reduced to 1.0 (i.e. implying equal rates), it would imply that all of the association was potentially 'explained' by age as a confounder. If the age-adjusted rate was reduced to 2.0, the situation would be less clear and would raise the possibility of another confounder accounting for the remainder of the association (e.g. mental or physical stress causing premature physiological ageing and also mortality).

The concept of *residual confounding* is an important consideration at this stage of appraisal. Any measurement error in a confounding factor will reduce the effect of adjustment on the association of interest. In the grey hair–mortality example, adjustment for age would have less effect on the rate ratio of interest if age was measured (and entered into the multivariate analysis) in decades rather than one-year units. However some degree of measurement error or misclassification is inevitable for most potential confounding factors. Furthermore, even in the most rigorous study, it is likely that there is a cluster of minor unmeasured confounding factors which have not been taken into account. The combination of unmeasured factors and error in measured factors is known as 'residual confounding', and there is no means of addressing it through any procedures apart from randomization in intervention studies as discussed earlier. Statistical adjustments therefore should always be assumed to *underestimate* confounding. The decision about residual confounding is entirely subjective in critical appraisal and again depends on the difference between the adjusted and unadjusted strengths of association. If an association is little changed (e.g. an odds ratio changes from 5.0 to 4.8) following adjustment for all conceivable major confounding factors (and if these have been measured satisfactorily), it is unlikely that residual confounding will explain a substantial further proportion. If an association is markedly reduced in strength (e.g. an odds ratio changes from 5.0 to 1.5) following adjustment, residual confounding is more of a concern even if the adjusted association remains 'significant'.

A frequently confusing issue in critical appraisal is whether the role of chance should be considered before or after confounding. If a 'significant' association is 'no longer significant' after adjustment, what should be concluded? This again appears to be subjective, since there is no consensus on the matter. As mentioned above, if an association remains statistically significant but substantially reduced following adjustments, there is the concern of residual confounding. If on the other hand an odds ratio and 95% confidence intervals were to change from 3.3 (1.4–7.8) to 3.2 (0.9–10.8) following adjustment for all major potential confounding factors, it might be reasonable to assume a true association which was not substantially explained by confounding. The widening of the confidence intervals are most likely to be explained by the large number of other variables in the regression models, although the reader would need to examine the report carefully to ensure that there were no missing data for confounding factors. Most regression procedures will exclude cases with missing data on any entered variable so that the sample at the end of the analysis may be different from that at the beginning. In general the problem with this aspect of appraisal is imparting too great an importance to the arbitrary 5% significance cut-off. For the adjusted odds ratio above, 90% confidence intervals might well have excluded the null value. Would inferences have been any different?

Confounding factors, causal pathways, and planning a statistical analysis

In considering confounding factors, and particularly in planning the statistical analysis of a study, it is important to develop first an idea of potential causal pathways. This is discussed in more detail towards the end of Chapter 13. The principal danger is to confuse confounding and *mediating factors*—since the results of statistical 'adjustment' appear the same. For example, lower social class is generally found to be associated with increased depression. Part of that association may be because people with lower status are more likely to suffer traumatic life-events. The association between social class and depression might therefore be reduced after adjustment for recent life-events. However life-events are not a confounding factor because they probably lie on the causal pathway *between* the exposure and outcome of interest. Life-events are not an *alternative* explanation for the association of interest. Instead, they provide *additional* information on why risk of depression is higher in people with lower status. If the association between social class and depression were to 'disappear' (i.e. return to the null value—e.g. a rate ratio of 1.0) after adjustment for life events, this would not imply that there was no causal link between the two. It would instead imply that any causal link was *mediated* by life-events, that is, that the effect of social class on life events entirely explained the effect of social class on depression. If the association remained present but reduced after adjustment, the residual association would be that which was not mediated by life-events (i.e. operating along other causal pathways—e.g. reduced access to healthcare, family tensions, substandard accommodation, occupational strain). Causal pathways are potentially complex in psychiatric research. For example, particular life events might conceivably cause a downward social drift as well as later depression (and therefore be confounding rather than a mediating factors). For both cross-sectional and prospective research, there are often difficulties in inferring the direction of causation because of the nature of the disorders which we study. These issues will be discussed in Chapter 13.

Summary

A fundamental process in interpreting one's own or another's research is to consider what the observations 'mean', that is, what can be *inferred* from them. This involves a series of questions and considerations (Fig. 12.1). The first step theoretically is to decide whether observations can be believed in the first place. It is the duty of the guarantor for any submitted research paper to ensure that the data and results derived from analyses are valid—and to

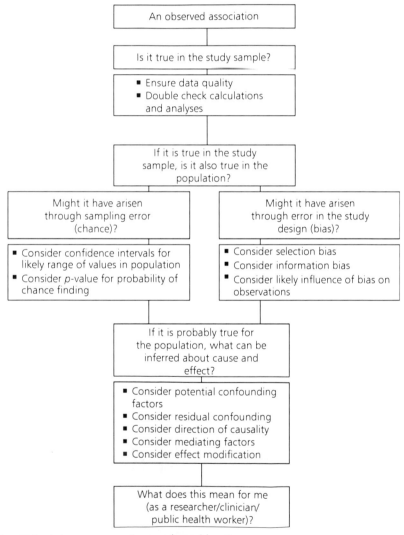

Fig. 12.1 Inference—questions and considerations.

withdraw a submission promptly if there are any concerns over this. Readers have no choice but to assume the integrity of the raw data. The first formal stage of appraisal is to decide to what extent the observations in the *sample* are likely to apply to the source *population*. The principal considerations here are chance and bias. If the reader is happy that a population-level association is likely, the next stage is to consider what can be inferred concerning cause and effect. This begins with considering whether the association between proposed exposure and outcome is a direct one and not confounded by other factors. After this point, there are a series of more complex decisions regarding causal pathways, which may not always be inferred from a single study but may require a more broad knowledge of the background literature. These are discussed in Chapter 13 and include the direction of causality (whether an association between A and B is because A causes B or vice versa), mediating factors (does A cause C because A causes B which in turn causes C, or are there other pathways by which A and C are related?), and effect modification (does A cause B to a uniform extent across the population or does the strength of association depend on other factors being present?). Finally, the implications of these inferences need to be considered with respect to developing new hypotheses and investigations, as well as for clinical practice and Public Health.

Exercise

An understanding of chance, bias, and confounding is vital for interpreting most forms of research. This is best assessed through the critical appraisal of a research paper. Students should be able to define confidence intervals, *p*-values, selection and information bias, the relationship between prevalence, incidence and duration, and confounding factors. They should also be able to define the meaning of these concepts in relation to a given research paper. The paper under discussion should be of reasonable quality so that students can discuss the strengths as well as the weaknesses of the study. They should also be encouraged to discuss ways in which weaknesses might be addressed in a future study (how they would do things differently) and the 'real-world' logistical issues involved in setting up such a 'perfect' study. In an extension to the critical appraisal exercise, a literature search might be carried out to investigate how different study designs (with their strengths and weaknesses) have been used to address the research question of interest.

Reference

Kirkwood, B.R. (1988) *Essentials of medical statistics.* Oxford, Blackwell Science.

Chapter 13

Inference 2: causation

Robert Stewart

The study of cause and effect forms the basis for most human interaction. The repetitive investigation of actions and their consequences can be readily seen in children's behaviour. Adult behaviour may be more complex but essentially involves identical principles. When we speak to someone for the first time, an initial impression is formed. If the conversation proceeds, the impression (hypothesis) is tested and refined through evaluating actions (what we say) and their consequences (the reaction or reply this provokes). If an unknown factor is present (e.g. the other person is preoccupied with something else), the relationship between cause and effect may be misinterpreted resulting in a false impression (e.g. that they are rude or unfriendly). The process can be seen as a repeated series of experiments, albeit unconscious. All of us are therefore involved in active cause–effect research for most of our waking lives. However the inferences (whether true or false) derived from these day-to-day experiments apply only to ourselves. Science and philosophy on the other hand seek to uncover truths that are generalizable beyond the individual. Because of this, their experiments require greater scrutiny.

Research may be divided into that which is observational (describing what is there) and that which is analytic (explaining why it is there). Deducing cause and effect relationships is central to analytic research. The 'result' of any given experiment is indisputable. What is open to interpretation is what caused that result. As discussed in Chapter 12, a series of questions have to be asked. What is the likelihood of it having occurred by chance? Was it caused by problems in the design of the study (bias), by the influence of a different factor to that hypothesised (confounding), or by a cause–effect relationship in the opposite direction to that anticipated ('reverse' causality)? If the anticipated cause–effect relationship is supported, what precise cause and effect were being measured in the study under consideration and how might other factors contribute to this? And what are the implications of the findings? The focus for critiquing a research report (apart from allegations of deliberate falsification) strictly speaking should not be the reported 'Results' but the 'Discussion and Conclusions'—the inferences (particularly regarding cause and effect) which can be drawn from the results and therefore the generalisability of findings beyond the experimental situation.

Determinism and the boundaries of cause–effect research

Is it possible that one day we will be able to explain the causes of all diseases in all people? This is surely the ultimate objective of all risk factor research. However it is fair to say that, for many of the more common non-infectious disorders, analytic research is beginning to 'run dry'—that is, the major risk factors have already been identified and what is left may take considerably more effort to clarify. Possible new directions for epidemiological research will be discussed in Chapter 21 and it is likely that there are important risk factors still 'out there' and unidentified. There will also be large numbers of risk factors (such as specific gene polymorphisms) accounting for much more minor degrees of variation and undoubtedly complex risk factor interactions which will keep researchers busy for a long time to come. However, what is the final target? How much of the variation for a given disorder might ultimately be explained by identifiable causes and their interactions? The determinist viewpoint is that all variation can ultimately be explained. In Epidemiology this attitude became prominent with the original focus on infectious diseases. Smallpox is caused by a single identifiable 'cause' and vaccination (effectively removal of the cause) has resulted in the complete eradication of this disease, a situation which would have been viewed as nothing short of miraculous two centuries ago. For many other infectious diseases, the principal obstacles to eradication are logistical rather than fundamental.

Many disorders were once viewed as essentially random occurrences with only limited modification by external influences. Optimism arising from infectious disease research was carried over to other disorders and supported by early findings for clear risk factor-outcome associations (e.g. smoking and lung cancer). Science will undoubtedly continue to uncover important causal processes, even if newly identified risk factors are steadily weaker in their influence and interactions more complex. However it cannot be assumed that outcomes will ever be predicted with 100% accuracy. Do diseases ever occur by chance? A sceptic might point to many examples in the natural world (for instance in weather systems) where early optimism about ultimate predictability has been challenged, because even the slightest uncertainty about initial conditions leads to vast uncertainty about outcomes. What amount to random events may therefore substantially limit the extent to which 'causation' can be investigated.

In psychiatry, a deterministic view has been particularly prevalent, possibly because disorders affecting a person's thoughts and behaviour are intuitively felt to be 'explainable'. The tradition of the psychiatric formulation, for example, has required generations of psychiatrists to provide sufficient reasons why *this* person developed *this* disease at *this* time. However, even if a disorder is readily attributable to a discrete cause, the cause itself (e.g. an adverse life-event) may have considerably less predictable origins. This is important from a preventative point of view—how do you stop people having adverse life-events? Determinism is understandably popular in research because it implies that further discoveries are 'out there'. However there may be a danger in over-optimism and a lack of awareness of science's limitations. Where discoveries within a field prove elusive, demoralization can result in important areas of research (and, for those suffering the disorder in question, potentially important opportunities for prevention/treatment) becoming sidelined in favour of 'easier targets'.

Principles underlying cause–effect research

Inductivism

Assuming that analytic investigation still has life left in it and important findings are 'around the corner', how should cause and effect be investigated? Inductivism describes a conceptual framework going back to Francis Bacon's writings in the early seventeenth century, a time when science and philosophy were closely and openly inter-related. From a scientific viewpoint, an often quoted example of induction concerns Jenner's observation that smallpox occurred less frequently than expected in milkmaids. From this observation, Jenner surmised that cowpox (to which milkmaids had a high exposure) might confer immunity to smallpox. From an observed relationship between two factors, an interpretation is therefore made concerning cause and effect. Taking another example, if a light comes on after a switch is flicked, an interpretation is made, particularly after repeated trials, that the switch controls the light. However there are obvious unsatisfactory elements to this approach. The observation that two events occur together in temporal succession does not necessarily imply cause and effect. If dawn is always preceded by a rooster crowing, does this imply that the rooster causes the sun to rise?

Refutationism

Dissatisfaction with inductivism, raised initially by David Hume in the eighteenth century, led to the alternative theoretical framework of Refutationism, refined and supported in the twentieth century by Karl Popper. A central tenet is that cause and effect can never be proved but only refuted. For example, the rooster is silenced and the sun still rises; water heated at high altitude or under pressure shows that its boiling point is not always 100 °C; Newtonian principles are superceded by those of relativity. Popper suggested instead that good science advances through conjecture and refutation. Through this process, a hypothesis should always lead to predictions which can be tested through an appropriate experiment. The hypothesis may be supported but never proved absolutely. On the other hand it may be refuted by inconsistent observations and replaced by another hypothesis which explains these more satisfactorily.

Hypothesis generation

Refutationism at its extreme is disparaging of inductivism, pointing out that it consists of little more than assumption and circular argument. However an important deficiency in refutationist theory is that assumes that a hypothesis is already there to be tested. Where should hypotheses come from in the first place? A rather optimistic viewpoint is that they arise *de novo* from a good scientist's intuition—that is through 'brainwaves'. However any worthwhile intuition is likely to be grounded in experience and observation, that is, inductivism. From a clinical perspective, the case series is a good example of inductivism, and it is important to bear in mind that most modern medical knowledge has its origins in careful observation and induction—and also that important treatments (for disorders from psychoses to male erectile dysfunction) have arisen out of chance observations during trials of agents for entirely different disorders. Inductivism is therefore fundamental to hypothesis generation. However causal inferences are limited and refutationism provides the most appropriate framework for testing and refining hypotheses. Depending on the nature of the experiment, a certain amount of induction may also be involved in interpreting the results and considering ways to refine the hypothesis. This is particularly important in epidemiology as will be discussed below. The process of hypothesis formulation and testing is therefore a cyclical process involving both inductivist and refutationist principles as described in Fig. 13.1.

Limitations for refutationist epidemiology

A hypothesis concerning the causal relationship between two factors, according to refutationist theory, should lead to predictions which can be tested through an appropriate experiment. Epidemiological research faces two difficulties in this respect. The first is that there is no 'clean' experimental environment. Epidemiology is carried out in the natural world with all its uncertainty and unknown variation. A hypothesis may be formulated, predictions clearly delineated and a study properly conducted to test this. If the observations support

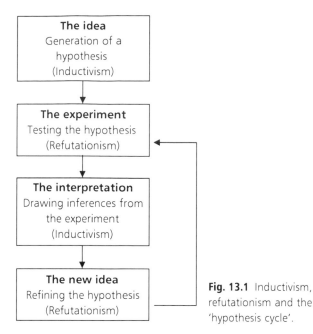

Fig. 13.1 Inductivism, refutationism and the 'hypothesis cycle'.

the hypothesis, all well and good but, as discussed above, hypotheses can never be proved absolutely. If observations are inconsistent with the study hypothesis, it may be more difficult to refute this in epidemiology than other scientific disciplines. If a different population had been sampled, would a different association have been observed? There are therefore obvious difficulties in determining cause and effect relationships if a hypothesis can neither be proved or disproved absolutely. A second, but related difficulty is that epidemiology is largely an observational science. Interventional research is substantially limited by ethical considerations. People cannot be randomly exposed to a hypothesised risk factor and, once there is a suspicion that something may be a risk factor it becomes steadily less ethical to observe the 'natural' course of events.

Epidemiological research, as it is currently conceptualized in papers and funding applications, is also more fundamentally inconsistent with refutationism. A researcher may hypothesize that risk factor A is associated with outcome B. According to refutationist principals, he or she must then set up an experiment which allows the hypothesis to be supported or refuted—and Popperian principles are that only refutation can be definite. However statistical analyses only allow the *null hypothesis* (i.e. that A and B are *not* associated) to be refuted (to a given degree of probability). It is impossible to prove that an association is absent, only that it is unlikely to be present beyond a given strength (e.g. outside 95% confidence intervals). 'Positive' hypotheses (as are expected in protocols for funding applications) cannot therefore be refuted, only supported (having refuted their absence to a given degree of certainty).

Causal criteria

If hypotheses cannot be proved or disproved absolutely and research findings are principally derived from observation rather than experiment, causal inference in epidemiology comes perilously close to pure inductivism with all of its associated shortcomings. One attempt to remedy this situation has been the use of 'causal criteria', particularly those drawn up by Bradford Hill (the origins of which lie in the work of Hume) although Hill referred to these as 'standards' rather than 'criteria'. The intention was to provide a framework for judging causality with respect to an observed association. A prior assumption is that competing explanations for the association such as chance, bias, and confounding have already been considered. Limitations of individual criteria are outlined in Table 13.1 and an excellent and more comprehensive critique is given by Rothman and Greenland (1998). An over-riding difficulty is that these standards do not move very far beyond inductivism since they rely heavily on the subjective judgement of the reviewer. The criterion of temporality could be reasonably claimed to be the most important—hence the weight given to evidence from prospective research. However, as described in Table 13.1, it should not be taken to indicate that cause and effect are always in one direction. A particularly dangerous criterion is that of biological plausibility. A degree of speculation as to biological mechanisms underlying observations has become acceptable and possibly even expected in epidemiological research reports. However, with a vast and expanding biomedical literature and sophisticated search engines, it is not difficult to find evidence from basic science which backs up any association found (in whatever direction it happens to be) conferring a spurious respectability.

Bayesianism

Epidemiology is therefore caught between the ideal of pure refutationist science and the real world of chaotic natural processes, observational research with sampling error, and conclusions which are derived to a large part through inductivist principles. Like many areas of science, it is also saddled with a regular flow of seemingly important findings which attract interest but which cannot subsequently be replicated. Inductivism and refutationism alone may be an insufficient framework for clarifying causation. A third approach, Bayesianism, again rooted in eighteenth century philosophy, has been used to address some of these difficulties. There is insufficient space in this chapter to discuss this theoretical framework in detail but essentially it espouses a more transparent acceptance of

Table 13.1 Criteria for causation (Hill 1965)

Criterion	Description	Limitations
1. Strength	A strong effect size for an association	This reduces the chance of minor unmeasured confounding, but assumes that major confounding factors have been accounted for. Weak associations may also be causal.
2. Consistency	Repeated observations of an association in different populations/circumstances	This assumes that all necessary causal factors are evenly distributed between populations. If a risk factor-outcome association were present only in men, would this imply non-causality?
3. Specificity	A risk factor leads to a single outcome	There is no reason why a risk factor should be associated with a single disorder (e.g. multiple disorders associated with alcohol misuse).
4. Temporality	The cause should precede the effect	A study should ideally demonstrate this. However the fact that one event follows another does not rule out the opposite direction of causation in other circumstances. For example, depression may cause physical ill-health but the opposite may also occur.
5. Biological gradient	A 'dose–response' relationship	This assumes that the 'ceiling' of risk has not been reached. A single life-event may be sufficient to cause depression with no influence of further events. Of little use for cross-sectional associations since a 'dose–response' pattern of association would be predicted with either direction of causation.
6. Plausibility	That the hypothesis is biologically plausible	Frequently a highly subjective judgement, given the volume of the biological literature. There are many historical examples of important findings rejected on the ground of implausibility at the time (e.g. Darwin's theory of the Origin of Species).
7. Coherence	That the interpretation does not conflict with the know biology of the disease	This depends heavily on the quality of the ancilliary information. It also is not entirely consistent with the principle of hypothesis refutation.
8. Experimental evidence	Evidence from interventional research	Interventional research may not be ethical and/or feasible for many cause effect investigations. The intervention may not be discrete enough to infer causation.
9. Analogy	Similar associations in other fields	A highly subjective judgement.

probability rather than certainty both in observations from a study and in the assumptions which underlie those observations. A more detailed discussion of Bayesian theory in epidemiology can be found in the textbook of clinical epidemiology by Sackett *et al.* (1991). This approach has been helpful in relieving scientists from a perceived responsibility to provide absolute proof/disproof.

Consensus

Perhaps the most important force underlying causal inference in epidemiology is that of consensus. In the broader field of science, the concept of truths held and evaluated by the academic community is most strongly associated with the writings of Thomas Kuhn. This issue is particularly pertinent in epidemiology because of the difficulties with conducting 'pure' refutationist research. Ideally, observations from a single study are not viewed in isolation but in the context of other epidemiological findings and broader opinion. An important example of the development of consensus has been in the expansion of research synthesis which in turn has led to recommendations regarding evidence-based clinical practice. To date these have principally focused on interventional research. However guidelines have now been published for meta-analyses of aetiological investigations (Stroup *et al.* 2000), suggesting that the process of more formalized consensus will continue to expand its area of influence. An advantage of consensus is that the interpretation of causation becomes less dependent on an individual's subjective judgement. Also, heterogeneity in epidemiological findings can be taken into account, or even (ideally) investigated in its own right as a clue to other causal process. Disadvantages, as with all consolidation, are that anomalous findings which challenge a prevailing hypothesis may be ignored as 'outliers', and originality in research design may be stifled. A narrow focus on the quality of the evidence may also distract attention from the restricted populations from whom the evidence base is derived.

The *a priori* hypothesis

Consensus therefore acts to limit speculative interpretation of research findings. On a more individual level, the approach to the research project is also important. If observations are 'explored' without clear forethought, it is much more likely that inferences will be biased and causation misrepresented. 'Negative' findings, which might have been important refutationist contributions to a particular field of interest, may be glossed over and a large number of between-variable correlations filtered for those which are positive and 'significant'. Having drawn inferences (and this process may be as easy for a finding in one direction as another) it is not difficult, as discussed above, to search for other data to back up a finding that may well have arisen through chance. The more interesting the finding, the more demoralizing the consequences for other research teams who are unable to replicate the result. Causal inferences in this situation are derived entirely through induction, although the sample size and meticulous study design may mask the fact that no hypothesis was being tested when the data came to be analysed. A much more satisfactory approach is to formulate the hypothesis (through insight, intuition, observation, background reading, etc.) before the study is designed, or at the very least before the data are analysed. A certain amount of subjectivity may still be involved in the process of drawing conclusions. However this is likely to result in a substantially more reliable interpretation. A useful and popular procedure is to draw up and label 'dummy' tables for results before commencing data analysis. Minor revisions may still be needed but most of the thought and work will have been done and the quality of the resulting paper will have been improved.

Box 13.1 **Principles underlying cause and effect research**

Underlying principles

- Inductivism—from an observed co-occurrence of two factors, a cause and effect relationship is inferred.
- Refutationism—a hypothesis is generated. Predictions are made which are tested in an experimental situation.

Limitations in epidemiology

- No 'clean' experimental environment. Difficult to test hypotheses with absolute certainty.
- Principally an observational science. Interventional research limited substantially through ethical considerations.
- Therefore inductivism strongly involved in interpreting cause and effect relationships.

Solutions

- Causal criteria—but these still require a considerable degree of subjective judgement.
- Bayesianism—allows cause and effect relationships to be considered in terms of probabilities rather than absolutes.
- Consensus—synthesizing research findings to reduce subjectivity.
- The *a priori* hypothesis—limiting *post hoc* subjective inference.

The role of exploratory studies

Are all 'exploratory' studies invalid? The objectives of epidemiology are to describe as well as to explain the distributions of health states. Where a disorder is being investigated in a new population which differs substantially from other samples, it may not always be appropriate to approach with pre-formed hypotheses. For example, the distribution and determinants of affective disorder may differ substantially between different cultures. In investigating these issues in a new setting where there has been little previous research, pre-formed hypotheses about cause and effect relationships may even be counter-productive since they will narrow the focus of the investigation and ignore potentially important influences. In these cases it may be preferable to begin with a 'clean slate', and describe relationships in order to generate rather than test hypotheses. However, it is important that this approach remains transparent in any research report and that caution is exercised in drawing causal inferences until hypotheses have been tested.

A second example of exploratory analysis is where potential causes are too numerous to investigate individually. This issue is particularly important for genetic epidemiology. Obviously with enormous numbers of potential 'causes' and increasingly sophisticated techniques to identify them, there is a high risk of false positive findings and post hoc inference. Specific techniques for approaching this type of data will be discussed in a later chapter. One important step in the reporting of gene-disorder associations has been for the highest impact journals to restrict eligibility to studies where replication has already been achieved in an independent sample.

A structure for cause–effect relationships

Induction and latent periods

The assumption behind causation is that there are factors which contribute towards the probability of an 'outcome' such as a disease. The outcome therefore requires a sufficient number or combination of these factors to have exerted their influence. (For non-determinists this position remains tenable if random occurrences are allowed to contribute to this process.) The period during which causal factors operate is referred to as the *induction period*. Once the final factor has exerted its influence, the outcome becomes inevitable. The ensuing period from this point until the clinical manifestation of the disease is the *latent period*.

This framework has been useful for describing causal processes in many areas of epidemiology. Induction and latency are clearly important considerations in cancer, and infectious disease research. However the focus on disease 'onset' has obvious limitations for psychiatric epidemiology. For psychiatric disorders manifesting in early adulthood, distinctions with abnormal mental states in adolescence or childhood may be difficult to draw because of changing symptom patterns (such as in schizophrenia) or a longstanding fluctuating 'subclinical' course (such as in affective disorder). When then do these disorders have their onset (i.e. become inevitable)? For Alzheimer's disease, where underlying pathological processes are at least more clearly defined, an induction/latency model has been proposed as a framework for discussing causation (Mayeux and Small 2000). The 'onset' in this case was defined as the first appearance of characteristic pathological changes. This is believed to occur a decade or more before clinical manifestations and hence a long latent period is proposed. However it can be argued that the distinction between these periods cannot even be applied to Alzheimer's disease since most people with Alzheimer pathology do not develop symptoms of dementia. Onset is not therefore inevitable at early pathological stages and other 'causal' factors must continue to operate. Survival is also an important issue. A factor may act to reduce the probability of dementia occurring by postponing its onset to a later date. By this time a person may have died from another disorder and dementia can be said to have been prevented. Whatever caused the earlier mortality is also in theory preventative in this respect. If dementia is not inevitable until the onset of symptoms, it has no latent period.

The time-course of causation

An induction/latency distinction may be of little use for outcomes (i.e. most, if not all psychiatric disorders) which are defined in terms of clinical symptoms since causal influences will always operate up to the time of manifestation. Contributing causes are sometimes subdivided into 'predisposing' and 'precipitating' factors on the basis of the believed proximity between their influence and the outcome event, although distinctions may not always be clear, for example, when does an adverse life-event become a precipitating rather than predisposing factor for depression? However some idea of the time course over which causes exert their influence is important in drawing inferences from observed relationships between two or more potentially causal factors. In Fig. 13.2, four examples are given with respect to two hypothetical risk factors (A and B) and an outcome (C). The associations shown in the results tables illustrate the importance of thinking through potential causal pathways (and developing hypotheses) before analysing the data. For scenarios 2, 3 and 4, identical results might have been obtained if the association between B and C had been 'adjusted' for A in a regression analysis (i.e. the association between B and C would be reduced in strength after adjustment). Conducting a stratified analysis is sufficient to illustrate *effect modification* (scenario 4) but will not

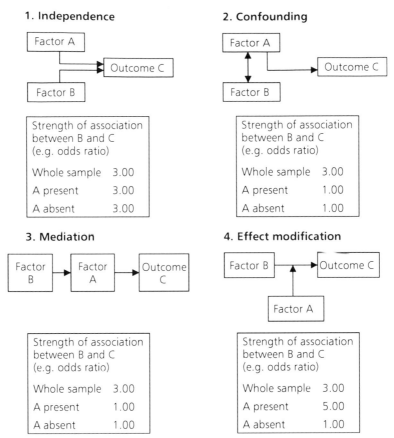

Fig. 13.2 Illustrating different ways in which causal factors may combine.

distinguish between confounding and mediation, even in prospective studies. Statistical procedures such as lag time analyses may be of assistance but require large sample sizes and multiple examination points. For most studies the distinction can only be made through considering what is known about A and B—in particular the relationship between them and the likely times of their influence on C. As emphasized in the previous chapter, these questions are far better considered before approaching the data, rather than in a *post hoc* discussion of puzzling findings.

Interactions between causal factors and effect modification

Taking the scenarios in Fig. 13.2, a hypothetical situation can be imagined where A and B are only two possible causes for outcome C. The simplest situation is that each cause exerts its influence independently (scenario 1). This implies that A and B are both in themselves sufficient to cause outcome C. Assuming no random occurrences were involved, everyone with *either* A *or* B would develop C. An example of this situation might be certain conditions with a very strong genetic influence, such as Huntingdon's chorea or early-onset Alzheimer's disease, where the presence of particular mutations are in themselves sufficient to make the disease inevitable and where the occurrence of the disease is stereotyped with respect to age of onset (i.e. nothing short of early mortality will prevent its occurrence). However these examples, although devastating for those at risk, are fortunately rare. An alternative scenario is that causes combine in their influence on the outcome. Therefore C depends on both A and B being present. This is illustrated by scenario 4 (effect modification). B is therefore only associated with C if A is also present. The results of the analysis in the table would be the same if the association between A and C was stratified by B. The importance of effect modification is inherently acknowledged in the diagnostic formulation for psychiatry and other medical specialties. In particular the division of identified potential causes into predisposing and precipitating factors acknowledges that single causes are usually insufficient to bring about the outcome and that 'precipitants' may require a 'predisposition' in order to exert their effects (and *vice versa*). However, despite this, statistical analyses for the majority of studies appear to be carried out entirely to distinguish between independence and confounding, with no consideration of the possibility that causes might interact.

Multivariate analyses which assume that significant independent variables are either independent causes or confounding factors, may fail to identify effect modification. Another important issue arising from the example discussed above is that the nature of causation may be misinterpreted if one of the factors has a high prevalence. This is illustrated in more detail in Fig. 13.3. As described above, the hypothetical situation is that outcome C depends on both causes A and B being present. However if A is already present in most members of a particular population, someone's risk of C will principally depend on whether they have B. For a population with a high prevalence of B, the risk of C will depend on A. An often quoted example of this principle is Rose's comment that if everyone smoked, lung cancer would appear to be a genetic disease (Rose 1985). Where epidemiological samples are drawn from homogeneous populations, there is a danger that important risk factors for a particular disorder may be missed because there is insufficient variation between individuals. This issue will be discussed again in Chapter 21.

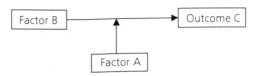

Situation	Observed relationship	Causal inference
A is common B is rare	Frequency of C will depend on B	B causes C
A is rare B is common	Frequency of C will depend on A	A causes C

Fig. 13.3 Effect modification and assumed causation.

Exercises

1. Why are hypotheses important? Discuss.

2. How can we get beyond guesswork in interpreting cause and effect? Discuss with respect to epidemiology in general and then specifically with respect to psychiatric research.

3. Choose a cause–effect relationship of interest in psychiatric research and apply Bradford Hill's criteria. Discuss their implications with respect to research design.

4. Take an example of two causes and an outcome. Think of as many ways as possible in which these causes might plausibly interact in their influence (with reference to Figs 13.2 and 13.3). This should be done without considering evidence for any particular combination. For many areas of psychiatry confounding, mediation and effect modification can be considered with the causal factors arranged any way around. Possible examples might be diabetes and depression as risk factors for dementia; family strain and socioeconomic deprivation as risk factors for schizophrenia; poor health and social isolation as risk factors for depression.

5. For the above example, try swapping around the 'outcome' with one of the causes (e.g. diabetes and dementia as risk factors for depression; schizophrenia and family strain as risk factors for socioeconomic deprivation; depression and poor health as risk factors for social isolation). Repeat the exercise. This illustrates the importance of considering 2-way directions of causation and complex interplay between risk factors in psychiatric research.

6. For the above example(s) discuss implications for prevention/treatment which arise out of each combination. Are there any differences? Does causation matter?

7. How might a research project disentangle some of these difficulties? Discuss.

References

Hill, A.B. (1965) The environment and disease: association or causation? *Proceedings of the Royal Society of Medicine*, **58**, 295–300.

Mayeux, R. and Small, S.A. (2000) Finding the beginning or predicting the future? *Archives of Neurology*, **57**, 783–4.

Rose, G. (1985) Sick individuals and sick populations. *International Journal of Epidemiology*, **14**, 32–38.

Rothman, K.J. and Greenland, S. (1998) Causation and causal inference. In *Modern epidemiology* (ed. K.J. Rothman and S. Greenland), pp. 7–28. Lippincott Williams & Wilkins, Philadelphia, PA.

Sackett, D.L., Haynes, R.B., and Tugwell, P. (1991) *Clinical epidemiology. A basic science for clinical medicine*. Little, Brown & Co, Boston.

Stroup, D.F., Berlin, J.A., Morton, S.C., *et al.* (2000) Meta-analysis of observational studies in epidemiology. A proposal for reporting. *Journal of the American Medical Association*, **283**, 2008–12.

Chapter 14

Statistical methods in psychiatric epidemiology 1: a statistician's perspective

Michael E. Dewey

Introduction

In this chapter we shall look at methods of statistical analysis used in psychiatric epidemiology. We shall focus on the issues which arise in trying to make sense of a small real dataset. We assume that readers are already familiar with the concepts of confidence interval, means, correlations, and odds ratios.

What makes statistical analysis in psychiatric epidemiology different?

We have given more space to methods dealing with measures than would be usual in a general text on epidemiology. This is quite deliberate. What makes psychiatric epidemiology different is the emphasis on measurement. By contrast most outcomes in medical statistics were historically binary (usually dead vs. alive). This is beginning to change (note for instance the increased interest in measuring quality of life almost everywhere). Of course psychiatry as a branch of medicine has used the concept of diagnosis freely, and so naturally we also include methods for handling such binary outcomes.

We start by discussing methods for predicting an outcome, whether a measurement or a binary outcome. We then discuss a group of methods used for exploring the relationship between groups of variables where there is no single outcome.

Prediction

Some first steps

For our first few examples we shall consider 115 cases selected from the ALPHA study (Saunders *et al.* 1993). This was a population sample studied for the incidence of dementia. Initially we shall analyse *variables* from the first wave of interviews, but later we shall also incorporate the second wave from two years later. The original sample was age and sex stratified so that there were approximately 500 people in each five year band (starting at 65) for each sex. The upper band (age 90 and over) for men falls short of this as there were not enough men in Liverpool to achieve 500. At each wave everyone was interviewed in phase one, and a selected sub-sample was re-interviewed approximately three months later by a psychiatrist in phase two. The sample selected for our example consists of all those who were seen on all four occasions (both phases in both waves).

We have available on these 115 cases:

- sex—coded 1 for women and 2 for men;
- age—in years at initial interview;
- Mtot1—Mini-mental state examination (MMSE) score at initial interview;
- Mtot2—MMSE at follow-up approximately three months after the initial interview;
- Mtot3—MMSE at two year follow-up;
- Mtot4—MMSE approximately three months after Mtot3;
- Dem—whether diagnosed by the psychiatrist as having dementia at the time of collection of Mtot2, coded 0 for not having dementia, 1 for having it;
- rater—a code for the rater who collected the original Mtot1.

To start with we just consider the variables collected at the first wave. We might ask whether sex and age influence Mtot2 (the second MMSE score). If we knew nothing about multivariate methods what might we do?

We might make some plots and we might calculate some simple summary statistics. Perhaps not surprisingly we find that age is related to Mtot2, $r = -0.36$ (95% CI -0.51 to -0.19) and perhaps slightly more surprisingly men have higher scores, the means being 22.5 and 26.5 mean difference -4.01 (95% CI -6.56 to -1.46).

So far so good. But the sceptical reader may well want to point out that in the older population, older women outnumber older men and so we may not have discovered two separate things, but the same thing under two different guises. We would really like to have an estimate of

- the difference between the sexes holding age constant;
- the effect of age holding sex constant.

In fact because of the rather complicated way in which this sample arose the women are not much older on average than the men, 78.2 as opposed to 77.3 years, mean difference [95% CI -1.98 to 3.85] but that might account for some of the effect.

Multiple regression is useful
- To form a prediction system
- To adjust variables which are interesting for the effects of others less interesting
- To construct hypothesis-led exploration of the effects of different variables

Fig. 14.1 Why use regression?

Table 14.1 Fitting the simple model Mtot2 as a function of sex and age

	Coefficient	se
Age	−0.31	0.077
Sex	3.72	1.21
Constant	43.3	6.40

The answer is to fit a regression model (Fig. 14.1) where we try to predict Mtot2 using both sex and age simultaneously. At this point we need to introduce some mathematical notation. Apart from the brevity which the correct notation introduces there is the practical point that readers who want to go beyond the level of the present text will need at least a reading knowledge of the formulae used.

The *linear model* which we have been using is usually written

$$y_{ij} = \sum \beta_j x_j + \epsilon_i \tag{1}$$

where i indexes the subject and j indexes the X variables. The ϵ_i term is the *residual*. We assume the ϵ_is are independent and identically distributed with mean 0. If we want to form confidence intervals we need to further assume that they are normally distributed with standard error σ. We might write this as $\epsilon \sim N(0, \sigma)$ where $\sim$ can be read 'is distributed as' and N represents the normal distribution. The reader who has seen these models before will be wondering where the *constant* or *intercept* has gone. We incorporate that by including an X variable whose value is always 1. Its coefficient is the intercept.

Table 14.1 shows the results. We shall see a number of these models so some effort studying the various components of the fit is worthwhile. Each term in the model has a *coefficient* and a standard error for that coefficient. The coefficient for age implies that for each additional year of age the MMSE score drops by 0.31 and the coefficient for sex implies that men have a higher score than for women by 3.71. Note that this is smaller than the mean difference which we saw earlier and this is because the value here is the difference adjusting for age. If we wanted to predict the score for a given person we would just substitute in the formula

$$Mtot2 = 3.72 * sex - 0.31 * age + 43.3 \qquad (2)$$

where sex is 1 or 2 depending on whether it is a woman or a man and age is measured in years.

We might also want to see how well the model fits overall and for this we might examine the value of r^2 the proportion of the variability in Mtot2 which can be predicted from a knowledge of sex and age. For this model $r^2 = 0.20$. This implies that 20% of the variability in Mtot2 can be predicted if we know the values of age and sex. The residuals (the ϵ_is in Eq. (1)) have standard deviation of 6.47. So the predictions have quite a wide range of error.

The fitting method used for the regression is known as *least squares* fitting. It estimates the value for the βs which minimizes the sum of squared residuals $\sum \epsilon_i$. We should as part of our *model criticism* look at the residuals from the fit but we shall defer that for the moment and look at some more models first.

Change

Are we really interested in predicting the value of Mtot2 or are we really interested in change? This is of course a scientific not statistical question but the analysis we have given so far only looks at predicting final value. What if we were to try to take the initial value, Mtot1, into our model? As one might expect Mtot1 is correlated with Mtot2 ($r = 0.78$, [95% CI 0.70–0.84]) and Fig. 14.2 shows the relationship between age and Mtot1 and Mtot2. There is a certain amount of overprinting in these graphs but we can see the correlations quite clearly. A slightly worrying feature is the small number of points which seem to have one low value of MMSE and one high one so standing out from the rest of the points.

We could take several different approaches here:

◆ model Mtot2 as a function of Mtot1 + sex + age;
◆ form the difference Mtot2 − Mtot1 and model that as a function of sex + age;
◆ form the difference and model it as a function of Mtot1 + sex + age.

It does make a difference which we choose, as we shall see, and so we shall take them in turn. If we model Mtot2 as a function of sex, age and Mtot1 we get the results summarised in Table 14.2. The model fits much better as evidenced by

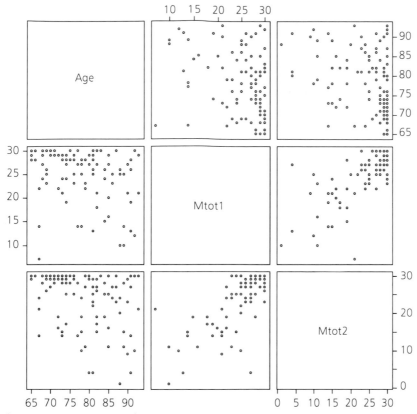

Fig. 14.2 Age vs Mtot1 and Mtot2.

Table 14.2 Incorporating Mtot1 into the model

	Coefficient	se
Age	−0.15	0.054
Sex	0.31	0.870
Mtot1	0.97	0.084
Constant	11.1	5.156
r^2	0.64	
Resid se	4.38	

the larger value for r^2. We are getting an improved prediction by taking account of the original individual variability in MMSE score.

Table 14.3 shows what happens when we model change between time 1 and time 2. The model does not fit at all well. This is not too surprising that we get

Table 14.3 Modelling change without Mtot1

	Coefficient	se
Age	−0.15	0.052
Sex	0.21	0.815
Constant	10.2	4.319
r^2	0.07	
Resid se	4.36	

Table 14.4 Modelling change with Mtot1

	Coefficient	se
Age	−0.15	0.054
Sex	0.31	0.870
Mtot1	−0.03	0.084
Constant	11.1	5.156
r^2	0.07	
Resid se	4.38	

a different picture here as we are trying to do something quite different. On the one hand we are trying to predict final value, on the other to predict how much people change from time 1 to time 2. It might very well be that age predicts final value, but not the amount of change.

Table 14.4 shows what happens if we repeat the analysis of change but incorporate Mtot1 into the model.

Some software and some authors describe the models in a compact format due to Wilkinson and Rogers. For simple models like those we have seen so far there is an obvious form.

Table 14.5 Some terms used and some synonyms for them

Outcome (variable)	Dependent variable, Y variable
Predictor (variables)	Independent variables, X variables, covariates
Factor	Categorical variable
Variate	Covariate
Residual	Deviation, error

	Outcome	Predictors	See Table
A	Mtot2	~ Sex + Age	1
B	Mtot2	~ Sex + Age + Mtot1	2
C	Mtot2 − Mtot1	~ Sex + Age	3
D	Mtot2 − Mtot1	~ Sex + Age + Mtot1	4

Note that this makes it clear that models B and C are closely related. C is just B with the coefficient of Mtot1 forced to be −1. Models B and D are effectively the same. The difference is that the coefficient of Mtot1 in model D is always 1 less than in Model B. Model A is distinct.

Some terminology

Table 14.5 shows some of the terms used in this chapter, and some synonyms used by others. As can be seen there is far from uniformity in the use of terms.

Model criticism

We should check the residuals from our model to see whether they do have the desired properties. Some plots may prove useful here.

The first plot in Fig. 14.3 shows the residuals plotted against the predicted value. This should show a band of points evenly distributed about the zero-axis (shown in the figure) and not increasing in variability to the right (or more rarely the left) end of the plot. In this case the picture does not look too bad except for one or two points with unusually large residuals (in magnitude). The most extreme of these have been numbered so that they can be traced back to the original dataset for checking.

The second plot attempts to portray normality graphically. The residuals are plotted against the expected values from a normal distribution. This is a Q–Q plot (short for quantile–quantile). The points should lie along a straight line from bottom left to top right. It is rather hard to see what is going on here because of the same three unusual points.

The third plot combines information about the residual and the influence of the points. This uses the *Cook's deleted residual statistic* (named after R. D. Cook, there is no culinary reference).

We have assumed that the relationship between the predictors (Age and Mtot1) and the outcome (Mtot2) is linear. We should check this. One way is to plot some more graphs of residuals. If we look at Fig. 14.4 we can see the residuals plotted against the predictors. The line shown is a locally smoothed line through the points. If the points (or the line) showed evidence of a U-shape (or something more complex) we might consider adding a quadratic term in

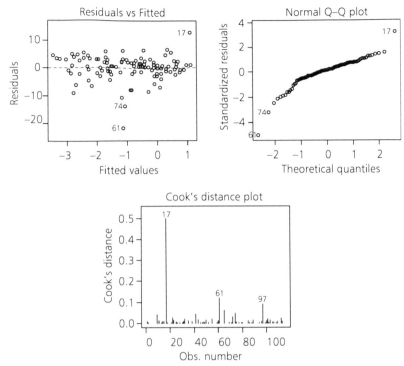

Fig. 14.3 Residuals plotted against the predicted values.

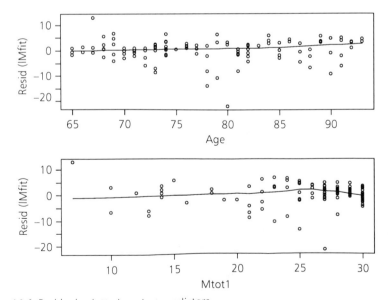

Fig. 14.4 Residuals plotted against predictors.

Table 14.6 Sex as a factor

	Coefficient	se
Age	−0.15	0.054
Sex		
Women	Ref	
Men	0.31	0.870
Mtot1	0.97	0.084
Constant	11.4	5.156
r^2	0.64	
Resid se	4.38	

age (or Mtot1). To do that we would just form a new variable which contains the square of age (or Mtot1) and add that to the model. The graphs do not suggest any profit in doing that.

We might also recode age so that it was a series of categories (perhaps five year agebands) and then add that to the model instead of the linear term in age. The usual thing would be to tell the model that the codes for age represented what are called *levels* on a *factor* and it would then model it appropriately. You need to know how your software does this. Most programs will set one of the levels as a *reference level* and express the other levels as differences from it. This is by no means universal. As an exercise we shall do this. At the same time we shall take the opportunity to code sex as a factor. For a binary factor like sex it does not really make a big difference in terms of modelling, but some programs need to know the information.

We might also consider adding *interaction terms*. Up until now we have assumed that the slope for age was the same for men and for women. Suppose it was different? We shall fit the model with separate slopes first.

Going back to one of our earlier models (shown in Table 14.2) we repeat it with sex as a factor (Table 14.6). The coefficients are the same except the constant has had 0.31 added to it (the coefficient for sex) as sex is now being treated as coded 0 and 1 rather than 1 and 2. We have added an extra line so that it is clearer that women are the reference category. The value of r^2 is unchanged as is the residual standard error.

Table 14.7 shows us what happens when we add the different slopes (the age–sex interaction). The value of r^2 rises but to such a small extent that to 2 decimal places it is the same. The residual standard error is slightly smaller. Evidently the effect of adding the interaction is minimal.

Table 14.7 Adding an interaction term

	Coefficient	se
Age	−0.15	0.054
Sex		
Women	Ref	
Men	−11.0	8.199
Mtot1	0.96	0.084
Age		
Men	0.15	0.11
Constant	16.7	6.395
r^2	0.64	
Resid se	4.36	

Many of the coefficients have changed quite dramatically and we need to explore why that is. The predicted value is 16.7 − 0.21Age + 0.96Mtot1 for a woman and 16.7 − 11.0 − 0.21Age + 0.96Mtot1 + 0.15 Age for a man. If we substitute zero for age and Mtot1 we see that the intercept is the predicted value for a woman aged 0 years scoring 0 on the MMSE and a man of that age and MMSE score is predicted to score 11 points lower (the coefficient for sex). The difficulty in interpretation is that the range of age is from 65 upwards so the coefficients are telling us what happens in a part of the data space which is of no interest. It would be better to transform age. The usual thing to do is to *centre* variables like this by subtracting the mean, or a convenient value near the mean. In this case we might also consider just subtracting 65 the lower limit of age.

Table 14.8 shows the result of using age-75 as the predictor. The coefficients now have more sensible interpretations. In particular the coefficient for sex now represents the difference at age-75 at a score of 0 on the MMSE. The value of r^2 and the residual standard error remain unchanged. We could also have centred Mtot1, but there seems less benefit in doing this as 0 is a value of the MMSE which does occur, and indeed does occur in the dataset as can be seen from Fig. 14.6.

Collinearity

One of the reasons for using these multivariate methods is to deal with predictors which are correlated. Problems can arise both in fitting and

Table 14.8 Centring age and adding an interaction term

	Coefficient	se
Age-75	−0.22	0.072
Sex		
Women	Ref	
Men	−0.06	0.906
Mtot1	0.96	0.084
Age		
Men	0.15	0.11
Constant	0.49	2.130
r^2	0.64	
Resid se	4.36	

interpretation if predictors are too closely related. This is often referred to as the problem of *collinearity*. Modern software should always give some sensible result without giving up, but it may refuse to use all the predictors if one is a linear or near linear combination of the others. One way in which this can arise is if the total scale score and the score on a number of subscales are all entered together.

If you have a pair of closely related variables like income this year and income last year you might consider replacing them by their average and difference. These are usually much less correlated. If you want to add quadratic terms (like age squared) you might well want to centre age first to remove some of the correlation between age and age squared.

Predicting binary outcomes

In the above we have been predicting a measured outcome (Mtot2). As well as the measures we have discussed above the example dataset also has available diagnosis made by the psychiatrist at the second phase which is a binary variable. We will try to predict this using the variables we already have used: age, sex, and MMSE score at the first phase. For various reasons it turns out to be better not to try to predict the 0/1 variable of dementia directly but instead to predict the probability of having dementia. Furthermore we do not predict probability itself directly because such a model is unattractive as:

- it can predict any value whereas we only want values between 0 and 1;
- probabilities have a natural scale which is not linear.

We shall solve this problem by predicting the *logit* (or *log odds*) of the probabilities instead

$$\text{odds} = \frac{p}{1-p} \tag{3}$$

And so using ln for the natural logarithm (logs to the base *e*).

$$\text{logit}(p) = \ln \frac{p}{1-p} \tag{4}$$

If you never came across *e* before you will have to take on trust that it is an important number whose value is approximately 2.71828. Figure 14.5 shows the relationship between *p* and its logit. The values plotted are 99 values of *p* equally spaced from 0.01 to 0.99. As can be seen the logit stretches out the values near 0 and 1. (In fact it stretches them to $-\infty$ and ∞ respectively.)

So what we do is to set up an equation for predicting the logit of the probability of having dementia (Fig. 14.5).

$$\ln \frac{p}{1-p} = b_0 + b_1\text{age} + b_2\text{sex} + b_3\text{Mtot1} + \epsilon$$

If we do this we end up with something like Table 14.9.

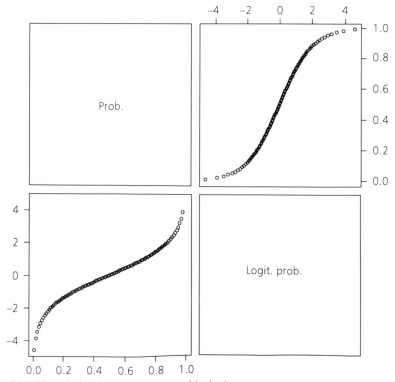

Fig. 14.5 The relationship between *p* and its logit.

Table 14.9 Logistic fit

	Coefficient	se
Age-75	0.17	0.052
Sex		
Women	Ref	
Men	−2.19	0.816
Mtot1	−0.32	0.077
Constant	6.32	1.832

Table 14.10 Logistic fit—odds ratios

	Odds ratio	95% CI
Age-75	1.19	1.07 to 1.31
Sex		
Women	Ref	
Men	0.11	0.02 to 0.55
Mtot1	0.73	0.62 to 0.84
Constant		

This is not as helpful as it might be as these coefficients do not mean much. What is preferable if to think in terms of odds ratios. We can convert the coefficients to odds ratios by exponentiating them (raising e to that power often written exp). So the odds ratio for age will be $\exp(0.17) = e^{0.17} = 1.19$.

Table 14.10 shows the results. Most software will give you the odds ratios as well as the coefficients. So we see that for each additional year older people had a 19% greater chance of having dementia. For each additional point on the MMSE at baseline they had 73% of the chance of having dementia, and if they were men their chances were about 11% of that of the women. Bear in mind, as we have already stressed, that this is a very unusual sample and generalizing to the population is difficult.

There is no generally accepted equivalent to r^2 for models except the linear one. The general goodness of fit of the model is expressed in terms of the *deviance* (which is distributed as a χ^2) and differences between models can be evaluated by differences in deviance.

There are of course methods for examining residuals for logistic models too.

More than one source of random variability

Up until now we have looked at models where the only source of random variation was between participants. Now we shall extend that to what are sometimes called multi-level and sometimes mixed models. There are two interesting ways in which we can use such models here.

♦ The way in which people took part in the study may mean that they are grouped in some way so that we suspect that people within groups may be more similar than between groups.

♦ The measurements may in fact represent repeated measurements on the same of participants.

Clusters of participants

Sometimes people may have entered the study in some sort of meaningful group. They may represent geographical groups like towns, administrative groups like electoral wards, or other groups like general practices. In the example dataset the participants were visited by one of a small number of raters. (In fact there were 20 in all.) The question might then arise as to whether the scores obtained by participants interviewed by one rater might differ from those obtained by those interviewed by another. So there might be random variability between raters, and random variability between participants. In the terminology of multi-level modelling this is therefore a two-level model.

Table 14.11 shows the number of participants seen by each rater. So there are 5 raters who each saw only 1 participant, 3 who saw 2 and so on up to 1 rater who saw 14.

The model we are going to fit is

$$\text{MMSE} = b_1\text{age-75} + b_2\text{sex} + \beta_j + \epsilon_i \tag{5}$$

where the β_j represents the effect of the jth rater and we assume that $\beta \sim n(0, \sigma)$.

We fitted the model without rater variability as a random effect earlier and the results are shown in Table 14.12 although there we used age rather than age-75. There the residual standard error was 4.38 (between participants), now we have two sources of residual variability that due to raters 0.358 and that between participants 4.367. The main difference is that as well as getting estimates of individual variability we also get rater variability.

We could also allow for a random coefficient for MMSE (Fig. 14.6). This would mean that the relationship between Mtot1 and Mtot2 would be allowed to be different between raters. For brevity we shall omit that. We can also

Table 14.11 Number of participants
seen by each rater

Number of participants	Number of raters
1	5
2	3
3	1
4	1
5	1
6	2
7	2
8	1
9	1
10	
11	2
12	
13	1
14	1

Table 14.12 Model with rater variability

	Coefficient	se
Age-75	−0.15	0.054
Sex		
Women	Ref	
Men	0.32	0.868
Mtot1	0.97	0.084
Constant	−0.23	2.178

calculate the *intra-class correlation coefficient* from the variabilities. This is sometimes known as the *intra-cluster correlation coefficient*

$$\text{icc} = 0.358/(0.358 + 4.367) \qquad (6)$$

giving a value of 0.0758.

Repeated measures

In many cases we follow people over time.

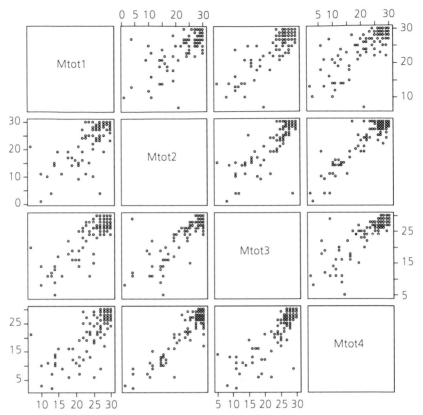

Fig. 14.6 Four administrations of the MMSE.

Figure 14.6 shows the plots of the four administrations of the MMSE.

One possibility would be to carry on using the same sort of prediction model and predict score on the fourth administration of the MMSE from age, sex and the three other administrations of the MMSE. This would not necessarily be a foolish thing to do.

Table 14.13 shows what happens when we do that. But is this really what we want to do with a longitudinal dataset like this? There does not seem to be any good reason why we are more interested in the last MMSE than any of the others. Are we not really more interested in seeing what happens to the profile of the MMSE scores over time? We would then have four repeated measures on MMSE for each person and we would have participants as a random factor.

It is perhaps easiest to look at a concrete example of the data layout. The top row of Table 14.14 shows the layout for the regression model in Table 14.13 The remaining rows show the same person's dataset laid out for the repeated

Table 14.13 Final MMSE

	Coefficient	se
Age-75	−0.05	0.034
Sex		
Women	Ref	
Men	0.24	0.529
Mtot1	0.09	0.090
Mtot2	0.65	0.066
Mtot3	0.30	0.092
Constant	−2.66	1.304

Table 14.14 Data layout for repeated measures

Participant	Time	Age-75	Sex	Mtot	Mtot1	Mtot2	Mtot3	Mtot4
1		11	1		25	27	28	24

Participant	Time	Age-75	Sex	Mtot
1	0	11	1	25
1	3	11	1	27
1	24	11	1	28
1	27	11	1	24

Table 14.15 Repeated measurements model

	Coefficient	se
Age-75	−0.26	0.64
Sex		
Women	Ref	
Men	3.73	0.999
Time1	−0.05	0.011
Constant		

measures analysis. We cannot just process it as it stands, but we have to ensure that the program is instructed that the first four rows belong together in a block, and that those blocks are a source of random variability.

Table 14.15 shows what happens. The new variable time suggests that the decline in MMSE score is about 0.05 per month. We could now go on to see whether this decline is predictable from the covariates. For instance did men have a different profile of change over time than women? For brevity we again omit that.

Software

Readers of a text on psychiatric epidemiology may be presumed to have at least some acquaintance with biology, and may be interested in looking at software choice from an evolutionary perspective. In the beginning people wrote their own, or used their colleagues' special purpose software. Then some of these programs grew and took on wider functions but usually within one area (SPSS was originally statistics package for the social sciences, and BMDP was biomedical data package, SAS was always bolder in its claims as statistical analysis system). Then they tried to expand to do more. At about this point we could consider that a researcher might learn one package which would do everything.

Then arose new hardware and new statistical techniques and so new packages arose which could take advantage of them (we can think of graphics, computer-intensive methods like bootstrapping). Then the old programs tried to incorporate the new methods but found it difficult, although not impossible. So new general purpose packages grew up which implement modern techniques as well as the older ones (we might think of STATA and the language S, implemented as the commercial product S-PLUS or the free open source R). Specialized packages also arise, EQS, LISREL for the structure of variance–covariance matrixes, STATXACT and LOGXACT for exact methods, MLWin for multi-level modelling. We should not forget that the handling of the database might well best be taken care of by specialized data base management software. At this point it becomes clear that no researcher can rely any more on doing everything within a single package. Life is too complicated for that.

What advice can one give?

- Pick a general purpose system used locally so you can ask a guru.
- Even though most systems let you use point and click interfaces make sure your system lets you save commands and learn to use them. If you do that you will have an audit trail of what you did.
- Expect to have to use several systems for your work so do not be too worried if your chosen general purpose system does not do everything.

The example analyses in this chapter were carried out using R.

Where next?

The next step is probably to look at a book which specializes in one area. More about linear models in Morrison (1976) which also introduces the linear algebra. Structural equation models (including factor analysis) is introduced in Dunn (2000).

References

Dunn, G. (2000) *Statistics in psychiatry*. Arnold, London.

Morrison, D. (1976) *Multivariate statistical methods*. McGraw-Hill, New York.

Saunders, P.A., Copeland, J.R.M., Dewey, M.E., Gilmore, C., Larkin, B.A., Phaterpekar, H., and Scott, A. (1993) The prevalence of dementia, depression and neurosis in later life: The Liverpool MRC-ALPHA study. *International Journal of Epidemiology*, **22** (5), 838–47.

Chapter 15

Statistical methods in psychiatric epidemiology 2: an epidemiologist's perspective

Martin Prince

Introduction

In Chapter 14 on 'statistical methods in psychiatric epidemiology' Michael Dewey has provided a practically oriented guide to the application of statistical methods to the study of the aetiology of mental disorders in populations. The focus is upon multivariable methods, in particular the use of different types of regression analysis to study the independent effects of variables upon a given mental health outcome. In this companion chapter we consider the specific application of these procedures to mental health research, together with some observations upon sound strategies for model building, and inferencing data output from these analyses.

   While the focus of this chapter is upon regression analyses, we would strongly recommend the use of classical stratified methods of statistical analysis (covered in Chapters 8 and 12) for initial exploration of confounding and interaction effects.

Types of regression

Linear regression

The previous chapter opens with a description of linear regression, used to model associations with a continuously distributed outcome. This is particularly appropriate given that many of our mental health outcomes take this form (see also Chapter 2 for further details), whether they be psychological morbidity scales (the General Health Questionnaire or the Clinical Interview Schedule), trait neuroticism (the Eysenck Personality Questionnaire), depression symptoms scales (the Centre for Epidemiological Studies Depression scale), or cognitive function in the elderly (the Mini-Mental State Examination; MMSE). Each of these scales may be dichotomized to identify those with a high probability of having a diagnosable disorder. However, to do so potentially involves throwing away useful information, and underestimating the association between a risk factor and the trait that underlies the propensity to develop and exhibit the disorder in question.

Use of linear regression to model continuous outcomes is in our experience relatively little taught in generic epidemiology, possibly reflecting the origins of the discipline in infectious disease and, later, cancer and cardiovascular epidemiology. The cardiovascular physiologist Pickering complained in relation to this tendency that 'it (essential hypertension) is difficult for doctors to understand because it is a departure from the ordinary process of binary thought to which they are brought up. Medicine in its present state can count up to two but not beyond' (Pickering 1968). Pickering had recognized that hypertension was not a disease that one had or did not have, but was a continuously distributed pathological trait with major implications for risk for heart disease and stroke. Interestingly, generic epidemiologists are now increasingly investigating continuously distributed 'intermediate phenotypes' essentially the proximal biological markers underlying a disease process, CD4 lymphocyte count for HIV/AIDS, arterial intimal thickness for atherosclerosis and heart disease, fasting glucose for type II diabetes. Arguably, many of the continuously distributed outcomes in psychiatric epidemiology have a similar relationship with our own standardized diagnostic outcomes.

A practical difficulty that we need to face is that many of our continuous measures have pronounced floor effects in the general population. Most people have no depression symptoms, no or very few cognitive deficits detectable by the MMSE and so on. The distribution of these variables therefore have a pronounced positive skew with a minority of impaired participants in an elongated tail of the distribution, while the central tendency as reflected by the median is close to zero. Non-parametric methods, which model the rank order of participants rather than the absolute value of their scale score are one appropriate method of dealing with this problem, at least for univariate analyses that seek to compare the distribution of the outcome for those who are and are not exposed to a risk factor. However, the standard multivariable methods for continuous outcomes (including linear regression) make parametric assumptions, in particular that the outcome measure is, more or less, normally distributed. Non-parametric regression methods have been developed, but are not generally available on standard statistical software packages (Fox 2000). The previous chapter covers some of the other approaches for dealing with this problem. Continuous scale scores may be transformed to make them more normally distributed, a logarithmic transformation for positively skewed outcomes, or a square root or cube root transformation for negatively skewed outcomes. Bootstrapping is increasingly advocated, a method in which robust standard errors for the mean difference are generated by analysing repeated random subsamples of the study sample. Specialist statistical advice is indicated. When dealing with extremely skewed outcome data (costs associated with service use are one example, with, frequently a few extreme positive outliers, and the bulk of the population having no service use and no associated cost) the only viable approach may be to ignore Pickering's dictum and dichotomise the continuous data distribution into, for example, the top 10% of service use cost vs. the bottom 90%, and then to use the logistic regression methods described below.

Logistic regression

Description of logistic regression, for dichotomous disease outcomes appropriately follows that of linear regression. The classical linear regression equation, with its coefficients and constants allowing prediction of a continuous outcome based upon knowledge of the levels of continuous or dichotomous independent predictor variables, is intuitively straightforward for most students. The equation for logistic regression is at first sight more demanding, but it is important not to be blinded by the mathematical notation, and to appreciate that the equation follows exactly the same form as that for linear regression. The only difference is that in the case of logistic regression one is modelling on (and predicting) the log of the odds of having a disorder (a dichotomous outcome) rather than the absolute value of a continuously distributed outcome. Thus, for example, the log of the odds of having major depression, rather than the CES-D depression symptom scale score. Having grasped this point, and having understood that the log of the odds can be antilogged to give the odds, and that the odds can be readily converted to probability (probability = odds/ 1 + odds), the logistic regression output is demystified. The logistic regression equation, with its coefficients and constant can thus be used to predict the probability that an individual with given predictor characteristics, has the disease outcome. The odds ratio gives a measure of effect, the predicted odds of developing the disease for an exposed participant compared with the predicted odds for an unexposed participant.

Cox's proportional hazards regression

One other form of regression, not covered in the chapter is probably worth a brief footnote. Cox's proportional hazards regression models on survival times, that is the time taken to develop the outcome of interest for those at risk. There are two parameters in this model:

(1) The outcome either (a) developing the outcome of interest or (b) being censored. Participants are censored when they are no longer at risk, either because they have completed the follow-up period without developing the outcome, or they have died or otherwise been lost to follow-up before the end of the follow-up period.

(2) The time in days, weeks, months or years to the outcome, either (a) or (b) above.

Instead of modelling on the log of the odds of developing the disease, as in logistic regression, one is modelling on the instantaneous hazard, the risk of developing the disease for an individual with particular characteristics at a particular juncture in the follow-up period. The hazard ratio has a similar interpretation to the odds ratio in logistic regression, the instantaneous hazard for an exposed participant compared with that for an unexposed participant. Cox's proportional hazards regression is widely and appropriately used in generic epidemiology to model the effects of aetiological factors upon discrete time limited health outcomes. This might be death, myocardial infarction or stroke. The problem in relation to psychiatric epidemiology is that it is very difficult precisely to date the onsets of many outcomes, which by their nature have an insidious onset. This is clearly the case, for example, for dementia, depression, and schizophrenia. For this reason, its use in psychiatric epidemiology is likely to remain relatively limited.

Multi-level modelling

Multi-level modelling, a relatively new technique, the mathematical basis for which is described in the previous chapter, has several possible applications in psychiatric epidemiology. As a historical footnote, the technique was first developed in the field of agricultural science, where it was recognized that certain ecological variables (e.g. farm, soil type or prevailing climate) impacted upon crop yields *at a different level* to the characteristics of individual seeds (crop strain, planting techniques, etc.). The analytical techniques developed to partition variance between these different levels of analysis were further developed by educationalists who were interested in the added value of particular school-based educational environments (characteristics of the school impacting on all pupils) having adjusted for the individual characteristics of the pupils attending that particular school. The popular MLn/MLWin multi-level modelling statistical software, now in widespread use in health sciences was developed by the Institute of Education in the United Kingdom.

The essence of the multi-level model is that one set of observations can be considered to *nested within* another, and that the observations can be attached to one or other of these levels. Thus seed types are nested within farms, pupils are nested within schools, and residents in a national population survey are nested within administrative districts. In the latter example, individual characteristics such as personal income, life events, and number of friends are attached to the individual, while supra-individual observations, for example, the Gini index of income inequality, the proportion of single resident households, or the level of social capital within the district are attached to the higher level of observation, that of the administrative district. These supra-individual observations are considered to be a property of the district rather than of individuals within the district, and through the use of multi-level modelling, in appropriately designed studies, one can test the hypothesis that they have an impact upon risk for a mental health outcome independent of the effect of individual characteristics.

The development of this statistical method has coincided with an increased interest in the role of supra-individual contextual variables upon health in general, and mental health. This is particularly the case for social capital and income inequality. Research questions that can only be answered adequately through the use of multi-level modelling include:

(1) Is there a discernable effect of local social capital (e.g. community trust, community activity, the extent to which people know each other and interact with each other) upon risk for mental health that is independent of the extent of individual's social networks and social support? That is, it is not your own level of social support that is critical but rather the social enmeshment of the community in which you live.

(2) Is there a discernable effect of income inequality at district, regional or national level upon risk for mental health that is independent of the income level or occupational status of the individual. That is, it is not your own socio-economic status that is critical but rather the degree of equity in this respect in the community in which you live.

To test these hypotheses, one needs an appropriate research design, and to date psychiatric epidemiologists, and generic epidemiologists, have been slow to adapt their research designs to the strengths and limitations of the multi-level modelling paradigm. First, this is a parametric approach, and at the higher of the two or more levels observations are assumed to be normally distributed between regions, school or farms. A practical implication is that multi-level modelling is only really worth attempting if there are at least 20 clusters within the higher level of observation. At the lower level of observation it is necessary to have sufficient individuals to realise an adequately precise estimate of the individual level parameters. An ideal multi-level design for the testing of the hypothesis that income inequality at district level had an independent effect upon GHQ scores would therefore include at least 20 districts selected on the basis that they exhibited reasonable degrees of variance in income inequality. However, in each of these districts one might need only one to two hundred randomly selected participants to realise adequate precision in estimates of GHQ score distributions and other important individual level covariates and confounders. Epidemiologists are used to conducting large scale surveys, often organized on a convenient locally circumscribed catchment area basis. Multi-level designs require more catchment areas with varying district level characteristics, but fewer individual participants in each second-level cluster.

In addition to testing specific multi-level type aetiological hypotheses, multi-level modelling may be appropriately used in traditional survey designs in which individuals can be considered to be nested within households and or districts. Individuals within households will tend to share habits, lifestyles, exposures and propensity to suffer from mental health disorders. They will be more like each other in these respects than others in the surrounding community. To an extent there will therefore be an *intra-cluster correlation* on these various observations that can be measured directly using the method indicated in the accompanying chapter. Where intra-cluster correlation exists it will have an impact upon sampling error and by extension upon the standard errors and confidence intervals for estimates of means, proportions, and effect sizes for associations. Generally these will have been underestimated. To take an extreme example, if there is an intra-cluster correlation of 1, that is, all residents of households share the same outcome characteristic, then the effective n of the study is the number of households, not the number of individuals studied. At the other extreme, if the intra-class correlation is 0, that is, individuals in households are no more likely to share the same outcome with co-residents than with anyone else in the survey, then the effective n is the number of individuals. In practice of course, the intra-class cluster tends to be somewhere in between zero and one, and usually closer to zero. Important degrees of clustering have been observed at household level, within families, and in marital pairs, but not generally within communities. Schools and classes within schools are another setting where intra-cluster correlation has been observed to be significant. In the accompanying chapter data are presented to the effect that intra-class correlation within interviewer (participants at the first level considered to be nested within interviewers at the second level) in a population survey is negligible, and can probably be discounted. This issue may also arise for group interventions where the response of participants to the intervention may be correlated within groups because of the particular favourable or unfavourable prevailing group dynamic or the charismatic qualities of the therapist. Multi-level approaches may therefore also be appropriate for analysis of data sets of this kind. In this instance, the impact of likely intra-cluster correlation needs to be built into the sample size calculation, as well as the subsequent analysis of the data. If substantial, then a sample size calculation carried out traditionally, based on the number of individual participants may fail to realise adequate statistical power. Again, using the extreme analogy cited above, if response is perfectly correlated within group, then the effective n for the trial will be the number of groups rather than the number of individual participants.

A final application for multi-level modelling is again mentioned in the accompanying chapter. Where continuous outcome measures are used in longitudinal mental health research, it is often the case that repeated measures are taken over time. The previous chapter covers several possible approaches for dealing with this situation. Others, with particular relevance to mental health outcomes are described in a separate section below. Multi-level modelling is appropriate where one is interested not so much in the change between two discrete measures over time, as in the effect of an exposure on the general levels of the outcome variable over the outcome period taking account of all of the repeated outcome measures. In the multi-level modelling paradigm, these repeated measures are considered to be *nested within* participants. Thus the repeated measures are at the lower level of observation and the individual participants at the second level. This neatly deals with the problem of *auto-correlation*, the tendency for repeated measures to be correlated within participants. In the same way that individuals within a household are more like each other than others in the community, then repeated measures within individuals are more similar to each other than to observations in other individuals. In, for example, antidepressant treatment trials, one often sees investigators reporting *t*-tests for differences in depression scale outcomes at 6 weeks, 3 and 6 months. This is technically incorrect. These outcomes will be auto-correlated and are not independent of each other. It is more correct to use multi-level modelling to test the hypothesis that in general, taking account of the phenomenon of auto-correlation, those randomized to anti-depressant have lower outcome symptom scores than do those on placebo over the entire follow-up period.

Strategies for model building in multivariable analysis

Whether using linear regression, logistic regression, Cox's proportional hazards regression or multi-level modelling, certain basic principles apply in the construction of multivariable predictive models.

The aims underlying the construction of such models are generally two-fold:

(1) to control for confounding, when testing the hypothesis that a particular exposure is independently associated with an outcome;

(2) to develop a parsimonious model, in an exploratory analysis.

In either case it is important to act judiciously, and to justify carefully the inclusion and exclusion of variables in the model.

Controlling for confounding

In the first case the aim in principle is to include in the model all potential confounding variables in order to establish whether or not there is an independent association, free of confounding. Potential confounding variables will be independently associated with both the exposure and the outcomes, so a useful first step is to carry out an exploratory univariate analysis to discover which of the variables assessed in the study meet these criteria. For example, in an imaginary example of a case control study testing the hypothesis that the experience of child sexual abuse (CSA) may be associated with major depression in young adulthood, you may detect the following pattern of associations

Potential confounder associated with exposure (CSA)	Potential confounder associated with outcome (major depression)
Female gender	Female gender
Leaving school early	Leaving school early
No qualifications	No qualifications
Lower parental social class	Lower parental social class
Parental divorce	Parental divorce
Alcohol dependency	Alcohol dependency
Deliberate self harm	Deliberate self harm
	Recent adverse life events
	Family history of major depression
Learning difficulties	
Remote rural residence	Urban residence

In this instance female gender, low education, lower parental social class, parental divorce, alcohol dependency, and deliberate self-harm are identified as potential confounders. However, caution must now be exercised.

(1) In establishing whether or not there is an association between potential confounder and both exposure and outcome you should focus more on the size of the effect for the association rather than the p-value or statistical significance. Remember that the latter will be dependent upon the statistical power for the comparison, which may be limited for uncommon exposures that may nevertheless be important confounders. If in doubt, include it in the final model.

(2) There may be a lot of missing values for certain potential confounding variables. The regression model will be derived from the subset of participants with *complete data for all variables included in the model*. Inclusion of such variables in the adjusted model will certainly lead to loss of power, and may also bias the estimate of the association under study.

(3) A confounder is *independently associated* with both exposure and outcome. Therefore the association with the outcome does not depend upon the association with the exposure and the 'confounder' is not *on the causal pathway* between exposure and outcome. Looking at the examples above, it seems highly likely that alcohol dependency, given our knowledge of likely mechanisms, is on the causal pathway, rather than a true confounder. The traumatic experience of CSA is likely to lead to alcohol dependency, which in turn increases the risk for major depression. It would be incorrect to adjust in the final model for such a causal pathway variable as it is likely to lead to an underestimate of the true association between CSA and major depression. Under these circumstances a successful intervention targeted at alcohol dependency would reduce the prevalence of major depression, while an intervention targeted at the prevention of CSA would reduce the incidence both of alcohol dependency (the mediating variable), and of major depression (the ultimate outcome of interest). Conversely remote rural/urban residence looks like a true potential confounding variable. It is likely to exert its effects on CSA and major depression via different pathways. Isolated rural families with few possibilities for same sex or different sex relationships may have a high prevalence of within family sexual abuse. People living in cities seem to have a higher risk for all forms of mental disorder, whether because vulnerable people drift in to cities, or because the pace of life and social anomie associated with city dwelling is directly causative. Under these circumstances, an intervention associated with moving vulnerable families from crowded cities to rural locations may increase risk for CSA and reduce risk for major depression. If the potential confounding effect of area of residence is not accounted for, then the true strength of the association between CSA and major depression may be underestimated.

(4) Some true potential confounders may be highly correlated with each other. The obvious example in the above list is 'leaving school early' and having 'no qualifications'. Most of those in the first category would also be in the second category and there would be very few individuals who have left school early and have qualifications. Under these circumstances the correct approach is to include one or other of the variables in the final model, but not both. They are effectively measuring the same thing, so nothing is lost through this strategy in terms of control of confounding. If both variables are included then there is a high risk of *collinearity* in the resulting model. This phenomenon is discussed in technical terms in the accompanying chapter. In practical terms, as a consequence of some cells in the model being empty or being represented by few participants, there is considerable imprecision in the estimation of the model coefficients. The results are likely to be capricious, with either both variables 'knocking themselves out' of the model or one being associated with a very large effect size but also a very large standard error.

Having finalized the list of potential confounders for which adjustment is to be made, inexperienced investigators are prone simply to enter the hypo-thesized exposure and all of the potential confounders simultaneously into the model in a single step. The correct approach is first to enter the hypothesized exposure, and then to enter, one by one, the potential confounding variables. At every stage, the effect of entering the new confounder upon the effect size for the main hypothesized exposure should be observed and recorded. In this way, the confounding effect of each and every variable can be elicited. To use the example above, with imaginary data, had all of the variables been entered simultaneously one might arrive at a model as below

CSA	1.0 (0.5–1.5)
Female gender	2.5 (1.6–3.7)
Leaving school early	2.1 (1.4–2.9)
Lower parental social class	1.4 (0.7–2.9)
Parental divorce	3.0 (0.8–9.9)

The inference is that there is no association between CSA and major depression having adjusted for the potential confounding effects of female gender, leaving school early, lower parental social class, and parental divorce. However, we are none the wiser as to which of these variables is responsible for the confounding effect.

Entering the variables sequentially one may observe the following results

	Step 1	Step 2	Step 3	Step 4	Step 5
CSA	2.4 (1.2–4.8)	1.3 (0.6–2.0)	1.3 (0.6–2.0)	1.2 (0.6–1.8)	1.0 (0.5–1.5)
Female gender		2.6 (1.7–3.6)	2.3 (1.4–3.2)	2.4 (1.5–3.5)	2.5 (1.6–3.4)
Leaving school early			1.9 (1.2–2.5)	1.9 (1.2–2.5)	2.1 (1.4–2.8)
Lower parental social class				1.6 (0.9–3.3)	1.4 (0.7–2.9)
Parental divorce					3.0 (0.8–9.9)

Step 1   CSA

Step 2   CSA + gender

Step 3   CSA + gender + leaving school early

Step 4   CSA + gender + leaving school early + parental social class

Step 5   CSA + gender + leaving school early + parental social class + parental divorce

From the above data it is immediately apparent that the univariate association between CSA and major depression (OR 2.4) is likely to be spurious, confounded by gender. Women are at increased risk for major depression, and independently are more vulnerable to CSA. This impression could be confirmed by repeating the sequential modelling process, entering first CSA, then leaving school early, parental social class, and parental divorce (likely to have a minimal effect upon the univariate association—OR 2.4), and then in a final step entering gender (likely to substantially reduce the OR for the association between CSA and major depression.

Building a parsimonious predictive model

The overriding objective here is to identify the best and most efficient prediction for the outcome measure, at the cost of the fewest degrees of freedom. This contrasts with the strategy for control of confounding where the aim is to saturate the model with inclusion of all plausible confounding variables, while concentrating upon the impact of these potential confounders upon the association with the single, hypothesis defined exposure of interest. The analysis is by definition *post hoc* and exploratory, rather than hypothesis driven, but the findings, on the apparent independent effects of multiple variables may be used to generate hypotheses for future study. Hence, in the case of the example of the case–control study described above, the parsimonious model might well include recent adverse life events and family history of depression, which were univariate risk factors for major depression, whilst not associated with CSA, as well as CSA, and the potential confounders listed above. The strategy for model-building should still be judicious. For example, likely mediating variables, on the pathway between CSA or other risk factors and major depression might still be excluded. For the generation of such parsimonious models, forward or backward stepwise regressions are popular. In forward stepwise regression the statistical software first enters the most strongly associated variable according to a variety of possible criteria, for example, the likelihood ratio, the reduction in likelihood (essentially the improvement of fit of the model) divided by the number of degrees of freedom consumed. Next it tests whether model fit can be improved significantly by adding in another variable and/or by removing the first variable. This process is continued until the fit of the model cannot be improved by entering or removing any more variables. Backwards stepwise regression uses essentially the reverse process. All variables are entered and then sequentially, variables are removed and/or re-entered until no further variables can be removed or re-entered without a significant deterioration in the fit of the model. These approaches are superficially attractive, but can under certain circumstances lead to capricious results. While they may be worth considering as an initial step to identify a subset of independent predictor variables of interest, it is always worth further exploring by building predictive models manually, to see if a more informative result can be achieved. There is no one correct approach. This is after all an exploratory technique, and the final results should be inferenced with due caution. As with the stepwise regressions, you can judge for yourself whether extension of an existing model to include an additional variable significantly improves upon the fit of the model, by carrying out a likelihood ratio test (in logistic regression) or an F-test (in multiple linear regression).

Some observations on the nature of mental health outcomes and attendant implications for statistical analysis

Dichotomous outcomes

As noted above, much generic epidemiology focuses upon discrete disorders, rather than continuously distributed underlying traits. Furthermore, in the classical disease incidence model, best represented by the example of cancer studies, individuals in cohort studies are exposed or not exposed to a risk factor but free of the disease at baseline. They then either do develop the disorder, in which case they are considered to be no longer at risk and censored, or do not develop the disorder over the period of follow-up. In contrast many mental health disorders, depression being a case in point, are classically remitting and relapsing in character. Over a period of follow-up an individual may experience none, one, two or more episodes of the disorder. If an individual is free of the disorder at baseline and has the disorder at follow-up, all we can say with certainty is that they have experienced an odd number of transitions between depression-free and depression status. They may have experienced one, or more episodes in between. If an individual is free of the disorder at baseline and free of the disorder at follow-up, all we can say with certainty is that they have experienced an even number of transitions between depression-free and depression status. They may have experienced none, one or more episodes in between. It follows that longitudinal studies require some kind of ongoing surveillance between the beginning and end of the follow-up period, either through repeated outcome assessments at even intervals, or, less satisfactorily through retrospective recollection by the participant of the intervening period. If repeated measures have been used, then some kind of special strategy is required to analyse them in an appropriate and statistically robust manner. The binomial theorem that underpins probabilistic statistical approaches for the estimation of risk for discrete events, assumes that each event is independent from others. Thus if you toss a coin 10 times and it comes up heads every time, then the probability of it coming up heads on the 11th throw is still 0.5, as for all the previous throws. Onsets of depression are likely to deviate from this basic assumption. They are more likely to follow the pattern observed for, for example, factory accidents, falls in the elderly or urinary tract infections in women, where one event indicates an underlying vulnerability and increases the risk of another episode occurring. Two episodes increases the risk of a third even further. Modelling numbers or rates of such discrete but non-independent events requires a different approach, and use of the reverse Poisson distribution has been advocated as providing a better fit to the data and hence as being more statistically robust under these circumstances (Glynn and Buring 1996). Expert statistical advice would be indicated. Alternative approaches for summarizing a relapsing and remitting recurring disorder of this kind would be to model on the time with, or time free of the disorder over the follow-up period. Other investigators have characterised the clinical course into several discrete typologies e.g. continuously well, continuously ill, prevalent case remitted, incident case remitted, incident case not remitted and variable course (Beekman *et al.* 1995). Risk factors for these different categorical outcomes, with reference to those who are continuously well, can then be studied.

Continuous outcomes

The use of multi-level modelling to deal with the problem of autocorrelation arising from repeated continuous outcome measures within participants has been advocated and described both in the previous chapter and earlier in this chapter. An equivalently robust technique, perhaps somewhat easier to apply, involves summarizing the repeated outcomes into a single observation that in some fashion captures the information contained in the repeated measures. The nature of the summary technique will depend on the general pattern of the repeated observations *within individuals*. This approach is covered in an excellent review article (Matthews *et al.* 1990).

Growth variables are a special case in which there is a trend for progress-ive increase or decrease in the levels of the observed outcome over time. Cognitive decline in older people is a good example. Test scores on measures of cognitive ability tend to deteriorate progressively over time. This pattern can be checked by 'eyeballing' the data in a graphical plot with lines linking observations within individuals. If the pattern seems to apply in general, while some individuals decline less than others, and some may even perversely improve over time, it may be appropriate to summarize the outcome with the gradient of the least squares regression line, estimating the decline in score per year within each participant. This then becomes the outcome variable for the analysis. This approach was used to study the impact of various risk factors for cognitive decline in a study nested within a hypertension treatment trial in older persons (Prince *et al.* 1996).

Change over time may be discontinuous rather than linear, for example, in the study referenced above, blood pressure levels typically declined precipit-ately over the first year of the study, and then remained relatively stable there-after. In this case the change in blood pressure level was summarized as the initial observation minus the mean of subsequent observations.

In the case of depression symptoms scores, as previously observed the natural history is for these to increase and decrease in a cyclical fashion, or to remain stable and high, or stable and low. These present a particular problem for summary in a single figure, but possible approaches include the mean of all measures (when evenly distributed in time), the area under the curve (when unevenly distributed in time) or possibly the variance of the measures for each participant where instability versus stability is the outcome of interest.

Conclusion

We hope that these two chapters, while providing students with greater confidence in approaching the analysis of their data sets, will also have raised as many questions as they have provided answers. It should by now be evident that there is no single, set, correct way to analyse a given data set; many will argue with some of the approaches advocated in these chapters. The import-ant thing is for students to be aware of the diversity of methods currently available, and to proceed judiciously in the analysis and inferencing of their data, constantly aware of the strengths and limitations of the techniques that they are using. Also, it is important to recognize that biostatistics is a constantly and rapidly evolving discipline. The introduction of logistic regression in the 1970s revolutionized modern epidemiology, influencing the design of our studies as well as the methods used to analyse them. The more recent development of multi-level modelling is likely to have a similarly profound effect upon the type of research questions that we formulate, as well as the designs that we use to test these new hypotheses. Statistical methods are therefore not just the tools that statisticians, working with epidemiologists use to analyse data. They also, as they develop drive the research agenda and influence all aspects of methodology. Ever increasing collaboration between biostatisticians, epidemiologists, and clinical researchers is therefore essential if the full creative potential of this momentum is to be realized.

References

Beekman, A.T.F., Deeg, D.J.H., Smit, J.H., and van Tilburg, W. (1995) Predicting the course of depression in the older population: results from a community-based study in the Netherlands. *Journal of Affective Disorders*, **34**, 41–9.

Fox, J. (2000) *Nonparametric simple regression: smoothing scatterplots.* Sage, Thousand Oaks, CA.

Glynn, R.J. and Buring, J.E. (1996) Ways of measuring rates of recurrent events. *British Medical Journal*, **312** (7027), 364–7.

Matthews, J.N.S., Altman, D.G., Campbell, M.J., and Royston, P. (1990) Analysis of serial measures in medical research, *British Medical Journal*, **300**, 230–5.

Pickering, G.W. (1968) *High blood pressure.* Churchill Livingstone, Edinburgh.

Prince, M., Lewis, G., Bird, A., Blizard, R., and Mann, A. (1996) A longitudinal study of factors predicting change in cognitive test scores over time, in an older hypertensive population. *Psychological Medicine*, **26**, 555–68.

Chapter 16

Critical appraisal

Rachel Churchill

This chapter explains what critical appraisal is, suggests why it is valuable to mental healthcare practitioners and researchers, and briefly describes the general principles involved. Design-specific questions are provided in the form of checklists, alongside guidance on the sorts of strengths and weaknesses that might be identified. Some worked examples using different types of study are provided and further points for discussion are suggested. Developing critical appraisal skills should help readers in structuring and writing their own reports, as well as reinforcing their knowledge about the strengths and limitations of different types of research methodology.

What is critical appraisal?

Critical appraisal helps to establish whether articles are likely to contain reliable and useful information. The questions asked in critical appraisal are designed to identify potential sources of error, and consider what effect these might have had on the findings of a study. The procedures used in critical appraisal assess both the internal and external validity of a study. For internal validity, critical appraisal assesses whether the study has been designed and executed in such a way that we can have some confidence in the results, and their interpretation, with particular reference to the potential effects of bias, confounding, and chance. External validity refers to the applicability of the study findings to specific situations beyond the limited context of the research.

General principles of critical appraisal

Although the questions asked will vary according to the type of study design being evaluated, there are general principles that provide a foundation for the critical appraisal of any study, and these should be clear from particular sections of the report. Being clear about these basic points will facilitate the use of checklists for critical appraisal (presented later in the chapter) and help to decide how useful the article is.

The purpose of the study: *check title/abstract/introduction/background/objectives*

The research question should clearly state why the study is being done. Ideally, this should be tightly focussed, referring specifically to the population of interest, the exposure, intervention, or diagnostic test under study, and the primary and secondary outcomes being assessed. Where appropriate, it should be stated formally as a hypothesis. The introduction or background should present the rationale for undertaking the study.

Study participants and grouping: *check methods section*

A good description of the participants should be given (e.g. age, sex, socio-economic status, ethnic groups, religious beliefs and behaviours, severity of illness). The source from which participants were recruited (e.g. community, primary care, hospital) can affect both the internal validity and applicability of the study. It is also important to establish whether the methods used to recruit participants (e.g. volunteers, referrals) could have introduced bias. The eligibility criteria for entry into the study have implications not only for internal validity (e.g. specific inclusion or exclusion of patients previously exposed to one of the factors under study), but also for applicability (e.g. over-restrictive inclusion/exclusion criteria). The procedures used to ensure that participants are assigned to the appropriate group (e.g. confirming that 'controls' are definitely not 'cases' in a case–control study) and the methods used to allocate participants to groups (e.g. randomization to intervention or control groups in a trial) can have considerable impact on the validity of the comparisons being made in the study and consequently on the validity of the findings.

Data: *check methods section*

The article should demonstrate that appropriate data were collected (e.g. not just 'surrogate end-points' indirectly relating to benefit or harm) and that relevant data were not omitted (e.g. data that might be more relevant to a patient's overall functioning and quality of life). Data on potential confounders should have been collected and taken into account in the analysis. The measures used to collect the data should be referenced and the validity of these (in this particular setting and with these patients) as well as their reliability (particularly when 'soft' outcomes, such as anxiety are being measured) should be demonstrated.

Data collection: *check methods section*

The information in the methods section should indicate the accuracy of the data collection process. It is important to establish who was responsible for providing the data (e.g. patient, informant, GP) and whether there was potential for the introduction of bias (e.g. recall bias, where the disease or exposure status of the informant influences the accuracy of the data). Those responsible for assessing and recording the data could also have introduced bias (e.g. observer bias, where the investigator asked different questions according to the status of the participant). These sorts of information biases can result in inaccurate information being collected on either the exposure, or the disorder, or both. Some data might be less accurate because it has come from existing sources (e.g. routinely collected data) where bias has already been introduced during collection. To limit the scope for bias, the assessors might have been 'blinded' or could have been trained to record the data accurately, and ideally there should have been a check of inter-rater reliability (in case any individual assessors were making systematic or random errors). Efforts should have been made to ensure that comprehensive data are collected at all points of follow-up to diminish the influence of attrition bias (e.g. those not contributing data, such as dropouts, might have been more likely to have got better or worse). It is also worth considering whether follow-up data might have been collected too early or too late to demonstrate any genuine positive or important negative differences.

Statistical analysis: *check methods and results sections*

Since studies involving too few people can lead to Type II errors (false negative), to demonstrate whether a study has adequate power to detect any real differences, a sample size (or 'power') calculation should be presented, along with the figures used in calculating it. Statistical tests are used to determine the role of random error, or chance, in producing an estimate of effect different from the truth. It is important to establish whether the statistical methods used were appropriate and properly executed. The authors should have described what they did in the analyses and why. All statistical analyses make assumptions that may not be justified by the data collected in the study (e.g. that the data is normally distributed, that the data points are independent). Skewed data should have been handled appropriately, the correct statistical methods should have been used to manage multiple measures and any outliers (unusually high or low values) should have been investigated.

Study findings: *check results and discussion sections*

The basic data should be described—if the authors launch straight into impenetrable complex statistical analyses without explanation this might suggest that such analyses were not appropriate to the data. Although confidence intervals (indicating how small or large the true size of the effect might be) are more useful in interpreting the results, many articles only present p-values. If the article states only p-values, the exact p-value should provided and used as the basis for a 'significant' finding, since $p < 0.05$ would produce a significant result by chance alone one in 20 times. This is particularly important if there is evidence of multiple testing, where chance observations might be presented as though they were tests of hypotheses. It is helpful to check whether the stated (or assumed) aims of the study have been fulfilled—where the authors have focused on reporting some unrelated outcome this may be evidence of 'data-dredging'. Examples might be undue emphasis given to the results of subgroup analyses, particularly where these have been conducted *post hoc*. You will need to decide whether the explanation provided by the authors is supported by the data. It is important to look at the role of potential confounders (what they were, how have were measured and presented, whether there are others not considered by the authors), and whether these might be responsible for the findings. Consider also the possibility of 'reverse causality', where the study has identified a causal relationship, but in the opposite direction from that proposed by the investigators.

What are the implications of the study? *check discussion/conclusions*

When critically appraising an article, we are interested in whether the study reports results deemed to be of clinical importance. Keep in mind that a statistically significant result might not be clinically important, whilst a clinically important result might not be statistically significant. Based on your appraisal of the study and your knowledge of the field, you will need to decide whether the study is relevant and has real implications for clinical practice.

Why are critical appraisal skills so important in practice and research?

A large proportion of medical research, however methodologically rigorous, is not sufficiently relevant to answer questions arising in clinical practice. Critically appraising a study often exposes the difficulties of trying to balance the concepts of internal validity and external validity. For example, to enhance internal validity, clinical studies are often performed on a homogeneous study population, excluding clinically complex cases—yet clinically complex cases may well be the type of patients seen in clinical practice and to whom the results of the study might be applied. Day-to-day clinical practice should be directly informed by the findings from good primary and secondary research. Critical appraisal of the best information is an essential component of practicing evidence-based medicine. For the practitioner, critical appraisal facilitates the use of the best evidence in providing clinical care, enabling the appropriate application of the study in developing clinical practice. For the researcher, by taking account of the limitations of previous studies, critical appraisal can contribute to the design, development, and conduct of new high quality and clinically relevant research.

Checklists for use in critical appraisal

The questions below have been adapted from a range of critical appraisal skills resources to provide comprehensive assessments of important aspects of study validity (references to sources and resources are provided at the end of the chapter). Checklists for the appraisal of cohort studies, case–control studies, cross-sectional surveys, qualitative studies, clinical trials, and systematic reviews are provided. Although such questions are often designed to prompt 'yes', 'no', 'don't know' answers, it is helpful to be aware of what specific problems they identify and what influence these might have. The appendix to this chapter demonstrates how these questions might be used in practice. For each design-specific checklist, a study reference has been suggested. Worked examples using the suggested references provide answers to the checklist questions for a cohort study, a clinical trial and a systematic review. Further work and points for discussion are provided for all six types of study design.

Critical appraisal of a cohort study

Cohort studies can be used to examine associations with the onset or course of a disease, or to investigate the consequences of medical interventions (although it should be noted that a controlled trial is the most appropriate for the latter, cohort studies can be used in certain situations). Appraisal questions establish exactly what the aims of the study were, who was studied, where they were recruited, whether they were representative of the source group and on what basis comparisons were made (Box 16.1). Of paramount importance is the accuracy and breadth of the exposure and outcome information and whether all relevant variables have been measured. A common problem with cohort studies is loss to follow-up—this not only affects the power of the study to observe genuine associations, but can also result in imbalances between groups due to differential attrition. It is also important examine the adequacy of the length of follow-up (you might regard it as being to short or too long). Finally, alternative explanations for any observed associations must be considered.

Box 16.1 **Checklist for appraising a cohort study**

A. Internal validity of the study

(1) Did the study address a clearly focused question (including target population, exposure/intervention and outcome)?

(2) Was the sample size justified?

(3) Who has been studied, how were they recruited and were they appropriate?

(4) When, and how accurately was exposure measured and was it recorded independent of outcome?

(5) How accurately was outcome measured and was it recorded independent of exposure?

(6) Was follow-up adequate (do the numbers add up) and is there any indication that the attrition could it have resulted in an imbalance between groups?

B. What were the results?

(7) How large was the effect of the exposure?

(8) How precise was the estimate of the exposure effect (confidence intervals, p-values)?

C. Relevance, applicability, and external validity

(9) Are all important outcomes (to patient, policy-maker and clinician, family/carers and wider community) considered by group?

(10) Are alternative explanations considered?

(11) Does the study help with local decision-making?

Critical appraisal of a case–control study

Case–control studies investigate factors that are associated with certain behaviours or the development of a specific illness. They are not generally an efficient design for evaluating rare exposures (unless the study is very large or the exposure is common amongst those with the outcome of interest) and are also not usually appropriate to calculate directly the incidence of the disease in the exposed and unexposed groups (unless the study is population-based). Furthermore, the temporal relationship between exposure and disease is difficult to establish using a case–control design. Case–control studies involve

collecting data retrospectively, after the development of the outcome of interest, and of all the analytical study designs they are the most prone to bias,
particularly selection and recall bias. It is therefore important to establish how
cases and controls were obtained (e.g. if they were from the same source), and
whether the general characteristics of both groups are similar. The data for
both cases and controls must have been collected using exactly the same methods
to limit the effects of observation and recall bias (if possible, blinding the data
collectors to case–control status). The role of potential confounders must be
considered along with the possibility of reverse causality (where factors that
are actually the result of the outcome are mistaken for, and analysed as, potentially causal explanatory variables—an example might be two alternative
explanations for an apparent association between job loss and depression).
Finally, case–control studies can involve the investigation of many potential
associations and it is worth considering whether statistically significant
findings might be the result of multiple significance testing (Box 16.2).

Critical appraisal of a cross-sectional study

Cross-sectional surveys are descriptive (like correlational studies and case-
reports/series) rather than explanatory studies. They aim to examine outcomes
of interest in relation to variables such as person, place and time. It is important to recognize that cross-sectional surveys measure exposure and outcome
information simultaneously, and it is generally not possible to determine
whether one preceded the other, or whether the presence of the outcome affected
the level of the exposure. While features inherent in their design usually
preclude the ability to test epidemiological hypotheses, descriptive studies can
be useful for examining patterns of disease or behaviour as well as formulating
research questions. The aim of the study and the source of the sample therefore
need to be clear. To avoid selection bias, the population in a cross-sectional
study should be well-defined and representative of the source population
(e.g. using a rigorous process of random sampling so that each individual has
an equal chance of being chosen), and to increase confidence that the effects of
response bias were limited, the authors should have demonstrated a high
response rate. Again, where multiple analyses have been carried out, it is worth
checking that both significant and non-significant findings are presented,
particularly where analyses have been carried out post hoc (Box 16.3).

Critical appraisal of qualitative studies

Whilst quantitative research seeks to use reliable data to draw conclusion
through a process of deduction, qualitative research aims to explore, and gather
information to generate ideas and hypotheses through 'inductive reasoning'.

Box 16.2 **Checklist for appraising a case–control study**

A. Internal validity of the study

(1) Did the study address a clearly focussed question (including target population, exposure and outcome)?

(2) Is the design appropriate to the stated aims?

(3) Was the sample size justified?

(4) How were the cases and controls obtained and were they appropriate?

(5) How valid and reliable was the exposure information and was it recorded independent of outcome?

(6) Was follow-up adequate (do the numbers add up) and is there any indication that the attrition could it have resulted in an imbalance between groups?

B. What were the results?

(7) How large was the effect of the exposure?

(8) How precise was the estimate of the exposure effect (confidence intervals, p-values)?

(9) Is there evidence of data-dredging?

C. Relevance, applicability, and external validity

(10) Are all important outcomes (to patient, policy-maker and clinician, family/carers and wider community) considered by group?

(11) Are alternative explanations considered?

(13) Does the study help with local decision-making?

The validity of the 'data' in a qualitative study is therefore paramount, and is greatly improved if a combination of methods is used (e.g. using both in-depth interviews and focus groups, often referred to as 'triangulation') and if the data is independently analysed by more than one person. Qualitative research often involves an 'iterative approach' (modification of research methods and hypotheses in light of incoming data), a concept strongly discouraged in quantitative methods. Therefore, one of the first things to establish is whether a qualitative approach was appropriate, that is, did the study ask how or why something was taking place (e.g. how people experience illness) and a clear research question will help establish this. Due to the nature

Box 16.3 **Checklist for appraising a cross-sectional study**

A. Internal validity of the study

(1) Did the study address a clearly focussed question?

(2) Is the design appropriate to the stated aims?

(3) Who has been studied, how were they recruited and were they appropriate (could selection bias have arisen)?

(4) How accurate was the information collected?

(5) What was the response rate, is the data complete and do the numbers add up?

B. What were the results?

(6) What were the results?

(7) Was statistical significance assessed and was the precision of the estimate given (confidence intervals, p-values)?

(8) Is there evidence of data-dredging?

C. Relevance, applicability, and external validity

(9) Are all important outcomes (e.g. to patient, policy-maker and clinician, family/carers and wider community) considered?

(10) Are alternative explanations considered?

(11) Can the results be generalized?

of qualitative research, it is difficult to develop a fully comprehensive and universally applicable critical appraisal checklist, although there are some basic principles that are helpful in determining the validity of a study. The method of sampling used (for subjects and setting) must be adequately described to allow consideration of whether the investigators studied a representative range of individuals and settings relevant to their question (e.g. be aware of the use of 'convenience samples'). It is important to recognize that there is no way of avoiding or controlling for observer bias in qualitative research, and it is essential that the researcher has provided a clear statement of their own background and perspective and taken account of this in the analysis, considering how it could have influenced the results. The methods used to collect the data need to be described in detail (e.g. field observation, interview).

Box 16.4 **Checklist for appraising a qualitative study**

A. Internal validity of the study

(1) Was there a clearly formulated question (could have been extended or refined in view of accumulating findings)?

(2) Was a qualitative approach appropriate?

(3) Was the sampling strategy (the subjects and the setting) clearly defined and justified?

(4) Has the researcher critically examined their own perspective, role, potential bias and influence?

(5) What methods did the researcher use for collecting data (e.g. field observation, interview) and are these adequately described?

(6) What methods did the researcher use to analyse the data and what quality control measures were implemented?

B. What were the results?

(7) What were the results and were they credible and important?

C. Relevance, applicability, and external validity

(8) Were the conclusions justified by the results?

(9) Are the findings of the study transferable to other clinical settings?

A systematic approach should have been used to analyse the data (e.g. content analysis) and efforts should have been made to identify and explore data that contradicted the majority findings. Ideally, the data analysis should have been corroborated by more than one investigator. The results reported should justify the conclusions (Box 16.4).

Critical appraisal of a randomized controlled trial

Trials compare the efficacy of treatments, and the study question (preferably stated as a hypothesis) should state explicitly the types of patients, interventions, and particularly the outcomes that are of interest. Information about the source and nature of the patients need to be fully described, not only to help the reader decide the extent to which the study findings can be applied in practice, but also because the choice of patients can influence the size of any observed treatment effect. To ensure a fair comparison is made and prevent systematic differences between groups, patients allocated to the different treatment groups must be similar at baseline. If sufficient numbers are involved, the use of random allocation procedures should ensure that the groups are balanced in terms of factors that might influence outcome, both known and unknown to the investigators. The randomization process should have been carried out in such a way that the groups to which patients are being allocated is concealed from the investigators. Except for the intervention under study, the treatment received by patients in the trial should be identical, and this is made easier if the staff and study personnel are 'blinded' the group assignment (to prevent performance bias). Blinding also prevents observer bias, in which the investigator's knowledge of the treatment assigned to the participant influences the way he or she ascertains the outcome. As in any other analytical study design, it is essential that RCTs have adequate power to detect a difference between treatments. The power calculation should be provided in the methods section. All patients need to be accounted for to establish that systematic differences have not been introduced by systematic differences in dropout or missing information (attrition bias). To protect the balance between groups introduced at randomization, the statistical analysis should have been carried out using an intention to treat approach. It is worth remembering that a single randomized trial rarely provides sufficiently robust evidence to recommend changes to clinical practice or within health policy decision-making (Box 16.5).

Critical appraisal of a systematic review

The review question should be stated in terms of patients, interventions, and outcomes. *A priori* inclusion and exclusion criteria should be explicitly stated to demonstrate how bias was avoided in the selection of studies. An exhaustive and repeatable search strategy likely to have identified all articles relevant to the review question should be presented, to demonstrate that certain types of studies were unlikely to have been systematically omitted (due, e.g. to publication bias, poor indexing on electronic databases, or because they reported 'unfavourable' findings). The strength of the evidence provided by any individual study (and consequently the review itself) will depend upon the research method used, and a reproducible and explicit assessment of the validity (quality) of included studies should have been undertaken by more than one independent assessor, to help establish that the review results were not biased in favour of misleading poor quality studies. Efforts should have been made to obtain missing information and improve the comprehensiveness of the review. One great strength of this method is that in many cases, a meta-analysis can be conducted (the statistical synthesis of the numeric results of several studies examining the same question), substantially

Box 16.5 **Checklist for appraising a clinical trial**

A. Internal validity of the trial

(1) Did the trial address a clearly focussed question (including the population, interventions and outcome)?

(2) Was the source and type of patients properly described and could the choice of subjects have influenced the outcome?

(3) Was the assignment of patients to the intervention and control group randomized and was the randomization list concealed?

(4) Were the groups similar at the start of the trial?

(5) Were participants, staff, study personnel and observers 'blinded' to group assignment (was the trial single, double, or triple blinded and if not, could it have been)?

(6) Aside from the intervention, were the two groups treated equally (were there systematic differences other than those under study in experience of the groups)?

(7) Did the study have adequate power to see an effect if there was one?

(8) What was the attrition rate and were all the patients who entered the trial properly accounted for?

B. What were the results?

(9) Were all patients analysed in the groups to which they were randomized (were they analysed by intention to treat)?

(10) What was the effect of treatment (note which outcomes are used to demonstrate this) and how large was this effect?

(11) How precise was the estimate of the treatment effect (confidence intervals, p-values)?

C. Relevance, applicability, and external validity

(12) Are all important outcomes (to patient, policy-maker and clinician, family/carers and wider community) considered by group, including side effects and other negative outcomes?

(13) Could the intervention be applied in practice (e.g. is sufficient detail about the application of the intervention given and are there economic considerations)?

(14) Does the study help with local decision-making?

Box 16.6 **Checklist for appraising a systematic review**

A. Internal validity of the review

(1) Did the review address a clearly focussed question (including the population, interventions, and outcome)?

(2) Were a priori inclusion and exclusion criteria explicitly stated (including the population, interventions, and outcomes of interest)?

(3) Were appropriate studies included, was a thorough and comprehensive search strategy used and could important studies have been missed (including unpublished and non-English language studies)?

(4) Were data extracted accurately?

(5) Was the validity (or quality) of the included studies assessed properly?

(6) Was missing information sought?

(7) Was clinical and statistical heterogeneity examined and investigated?

(8) Were sensitivity analyses undertaken to explore the possible introduction of bias in the way the review was conducted?

B. What were the results?

(9) What are the overall results in this review (how large was the treatment effect)?

(10) How precise were the results (confidence intervals, p-values)?

C. Relevance, applicability, and external validity

(11) Are all important outcomes (to patient, policy-maker and clinician, family/carers, and wider community) considered by group, including side effects and other negative outcomes?

(12) Does the review help with local decision-making (check that it is up-to-date)?

increasing the power of the review to provide an answer to the question. Heterogeneity between the studies should have been properly examined to establish whether included studies were statistically and clinically comparable. Sensitivity analyses explore whether decisions taken by the reviewers in conducting the review (e.g. which studies to include/exclude and which comparisons should be made) influence the results and conclusions of the review to ensure that the results of the review were not biased by studies that are systematically different (e.g. high versus low quality studies or published versus unpublished studies). The outcomes that are examined should reflect those that are important to patients, policy-maker and clinician, family/carers and wider community and should include side-effects and other negative outcomes. It is also important to ensure that the review is up-to-date before deciding how useful it is in decision-making (reviews published on the Cochrane Library, should be updated regularly to take account of newly published or newly identified data) (Box 16.6).

Conclusions

Critical appraisal skills are essential for interpreting studies and performing research. Each study design is susceptible to its own problems, and this chapter has summarized some of these areas of weakness, so that, for example, when reading a case–control study the immediate consideration should be whether there is recall or selection bias. However the essential characteristic of good research which has been well reported is that the reader is able to understand each stage of the process from setting out the aims of the study to reporting its conclusions.

Appendix: Further study and points for discussion

Worked example of appraising a clinical trial

Appraised article: Hollon, S.D., DeRubeis, R.J., Evans, M., Wiemer, M.J., Garvey, M.J., Grove, W.M., and Tuason, V.B. (1992) Cognitive therapy and pharmacotherapy for depression: singly and in combination. *Archives of General Psychiatry*, **49**, 774–81.

A. Internal validity of the trial

(1) Did the trial address a clearly focused question (including the population, interventions and outcome)?

The aims were not explicitly stated and no hypothesis was given (worth remembering for the Results section). The text indicates the investigators were comparing CT, imipramine and a combination of the two for depression.

(2) Was the source and type of patients properly described and could the choice of subjects have influenced the outcome?

The source and demographics of the patients are clearly described. The levels of severity of depression were high. Previous antidepressant treatment failures (within 3 months) were excluded, potentially biasing sample in favour of antidepressants (although this is not evident from the results, with dropout from imipramine condition at 44% vs. 36% in both other conditions).

Sixty-four percent of patients had had previous psychotherapy, suggesting a positive attitude potentially influencing compliance. There is no mention of the patients' previous success with psychotherapy. Other baseline characteristics of the subjects might also have been influential (see later discussion).

(3) Was the assignment of patients to the intervention and control group randomized and was the randomization list concealed?

Patients were randomly assigned to interventions but the method was not described, casting doubt on procedure. The allocation procedure was not concealed, once more suggesting potential for bias in allocation procedure.

(4) Were the groups similar at the start of the trial?

Groups should have been comparable with regard to age and chronicity of index episode since randomization stratified on these variables. Severity of depression at baseline was taken into account in part of the analysis. However, although the total sample was described thoroughly, no information given about the composition of the different groups in terms of background factors such as psychiatric history, family history, and marital, employment and socio-economic status. Number of patients per group probably insufficient to balance these characteristics using randomization.

(5) Were participants, staff, study personnel and observers 'blinded' to group assignment (was the trial single, double or triple blinded and if not, could it have been)?

No. The nature of the interventions meant neither patient nor clinician could be blinded to allocated treatment. This would have involved a radical change in design (e.g. drug placebo and CT 'placebo' arms, although in fact, the clinical management element of the pharmacotherapy arm may have achieved this by providing an unstructured psychological treatment). However, placebos were probably not appropriate here, since there was no attempt to tease out the 'active' ingredient in different types of therapy or to establish whether any intervention was better than no intervention at all. Evaluators were blind to treatment condition (although the blind was not tested) and same procedures were used to assess outcome in all patients. In addition, evaluations were video-taped and inter-rater reliability checked.

(6) Aside from the intervention, were the two groups treated equally (were there systematic differences other than those under study in experience of the groups)?

No. Direct comparison cannot be made between the two single modality treatments (CT and imipramine). Those not receiving pharmacotherapy did not receive additional time in which pharmacotherapy and clinical management was provided. Clinical management comprised brief supportive counselling and limited advice (it is not clear what this was). These sessions were quite long, lasting between 30 and 50 min and could have had some beneficial (or harmful) effect on those receiving imipramine. Even if this was only an attention placebo, all treatment groups in the trial received it except those allocated CT only.

(7) Did the study have adequate power to see an effect if there was one?

There is no mention of an *a priori* sample size calculation. Sample size would have been particularly important in this trial since it compares three 'active' treatments, and the difference between them might be expected to be small. Furthermore, one of the main attributes of a properly conducted randomization procedure is that it should ensure that groups are evenly distributed according to baseline characteristics (both known and unknown) that might influence outcome. Groups would have been comparable with regard to age and chronicity of index episode (since randomization stratified on these variables), and severity of depression at baseline was taken into account in part of the analysis. However, although the total sample was described thoroughly, no information was given about the composition of the different groups in terms of background factors such as psychiatric history, family history, and marital, employment, and socio-economic status. The number of patients per group was probably insufficient to balance these characteristics using randomization. It is also worth noting that the imipramine groups were combined for the analysis, increasing the possibility of a potential imbalance between groups in the analysis.

(8) What was the attrition rate and were all the patients who entered the trial properly accounted for?

The attrition rate was high at 40% (43/107). Dropout was likely to have occurred on non-random basis. All numbers add up and all patients are accounted for.

B. What are the results?

(9) Were all patients analysed in the groups to which they were randomized (were they analysed by intention to treat)?

The data were analysed both for completers only and by intention to treat, and withdrawals were presented by group.

(10) What was the effect of treatment (note which outcomes are used to demonstrate this) and how large was this effect?

The results are presented using some sort of composite measure of several outcomes and it is not clear how this was calculated or whether such a procedure is valid. The difference between the two single treatment modalities was negligible on measures at all assessment points (effect sizes no greater than 0.10 in either sample). In the ITT analysis, non-significant differences were observed at post-treatment assessment that appeared to favour combination treatment (comb vs. imipramine = 0.44, comb vs. CT = 0.35). The authors concluded there was no evidence that CT was less effective than pharmacotherapy in the treatment of the more severely depressed patients (this suggests a possible sub-group analysis).

(11) How precise was the estimate of the treatment effect (confidence intervals, *p*-values)?

No statistically significant differences were found between groups although no indication is given of the precision of effect sizes (however, adequate raw data and spread scores enable re-analysis). Not properly considered is the lack of power to observe a potentially small effect, or whether the clinical management could have diluted differences between groups. The authors suggest this non-significant finding might still be clinically important.

Relevance, applicability, and external validity

(12) Are all important (to patient, policy-maker and clinician, family/carers and wider community) outcomes considered by group, including side effects and other negative outcomes?

The main outcome is level of depression (assessed using standard measures). Only one global measure of psychosocial functioning is reported and this is not used to calculate an effect size other than as part of a composite measure. Patients may not notice (or care about) a shift of several points on the HRSD, but may value an improvement in overall functioning, ability to work, or improved relationships with family members. Also, acceptability of treatment is not adequately reported. Side effects are only mentioned if they were severe enough to result in withdrawal from the trial (although it is interesting that all 10 patients withdrawing for this reason came from imipramine only group) and no information is given about the specific side-effects experienced by any of the patients. Furthermore, the trial reports three suicide attempts (two successful) and that the medical director withdrew a further two patients (again in the imipramine only group) due to increased suicide risk. Finally, the economic implications of this treatment strategy are not considered.

(13) Could the intervention be applied in practice (e.g. is sufficient detail about the application of the intervention given and are there economic considerations)?

A detailed account of the therapists and treatments was given. CT patients received a maximum number of 20 sessions, each 50 min, over 12 weeks (two sessions per week for first four weeks, one to two for second four, and one for third four). Missed sessions were rescheduled. Therapists had special training according to study protocol and adherence to the protocol was checked.

Imipramine was provided at 75 mg/d increasing to 200–300 mg/d by end of week three. Plasma levels were checked to assess dosing and compliance. Pharmacotherapy management was provided once a week by a psychiatrist who provided information about medication and dosing, and discussed side-effects. Clinical management was also provided to review overall functioning and give brief supportive counselling with limited advice. Psychiatrists received no additional training for undertaking this role. Also, the authors do not report whether additional or adjunctive treatments were available to, or received by patients.

(14) Does the study help with local decision-making?

In many respects this study was unusually well executed and reported. However, the results are not overwhelming, there being only a tendency towards improvement in the combination group and lack of power makes it difficult to know whether the finding is due to random error. Poor differentiation between interventions also casts doubt on validity of the conclusions. Readers will need to decide whether the patients in this trial are similar enough to their own patients (e.g. with respect to diagnosis, age, and socio-economic status, sex, number of previous episodes, duration of current episode, and severity). Readers also need to judge how applicable the treatments evaluated in the trial are to their local setting (e.g. imipramine might to be the drug of choice, same degree of drug supervision might not be available, and the application of the interventions, particularly CT, might be quite different).

Points for discussion

If you were designing a new study with the same objectives, how would you improve on the one reported?

Hint

Consider the study participants, adjunctive treatments, the role and influence of clinical management, the feasibility of the interventions and the appropriateness of the outcomes).

Appraising a cohort study

Weich, S., Churchill, R., Lewis, G., and Mann, A. (1997) Do socio-economic risk factors predict the incidence and maintenance of psychiatric disorder in primary care. *Psychological Medicine*, 27, 73–80.

Points for discussion

(1) Use the above checklist for appraising a cohort study to appraise this article.

(2) Can you think of alternative explanations for the findings?

(3) If you were designing a new study with the same objectives, how would you improve or build upon the one reported?

Hint

Consider the study design, recruitment of subjects and the collection of exposure outcome measures.

Appraising a case–control study

Appraisal article: Cheng, A.T.A., Chen, T.H.H., Chen, C.C., and Jenkins, R. (2000) Psychosocial and psychiatric risk factors for suicide. Case-control psychological autopsy study. *British Journal of Psychiatry*, **177**, 360–5.

Points for discussion

(1) Use the above checklist for appraising a case–control study to appraise this article.

(2) Can you think of alternative explanations for the findings?

(3) Are there other potential exposures you would have liked data on?

Hint

♦ Consider the breadth of the exposure data.

♦ Consider the classification of cases and the suitability of the controls.

Appraising a cross-sectional study

Appraisal article: Cornwall, P.L. and Doubtfire, A. (2001) The use of the Royal College of Psychiatrists' trainee's log book: a cross-sectional survey of trainees and trainers. *Psychiatric Bulletin*, **25**, 234–6.

Points for discussion

(1) Use the above checklist for appraising a cross-sectional study to appraise this article.

(2) Can you think if alternatives reasons for the poor use of log books?

(3) Consider how you might design a study to provide information on promoting the use of the log book by both trainers and trainees.

Hint

♦ Consider whether other study designs might be more appropriate to answer this question (are significant differences in opinion between trainers and trainees likely to be the most important factor?).

◆ Consider what questions you might ask to obtain valid, accurate and reliable information.

Appraising a qualitative study

Appraisal article: Barry, C.A., Bradley, C.P., Britten, N., Stevenson, F., and Barber, N. (2000) Patients' unvoiced agendas in general practice consultations: qualitative study. *British Medical Journal*, **320**, 1246–50.

Points for discussion

(1) Use the above checklist for appraising a qualitative study to appraise this article.

(2) Do you agree with the authors' conclusions?

(3) Can you think of alternative explanations for the observations?

(4) How might you explore these in further research?

Hint

◆ Consider how you might obtain valid, accurate and reliable information.

◆ Consider the perspective of the researchers and how this might influence data-collection and interpretation.

Appraising a systematic review

Appraisal article: Lima, M.S. and Moncrieff, J. (2001) Drugs versus placebo for dysthymia (Cochrane Review). In The Cochrane Library, Issue 4, 2001. Update Software, Oxford.

Points for discussion

(1) Use the above checklist for appraising a systematic review to appraise this article.

(2) The authors of this review suggest the need for future well-designed, executed and reported RCTs specifically addressing the use of a severity threshold and other outcomes including quality of life and longer-term outcomes. Consider how such objectives might be met in further research.

Hint

These are separate issues—it may not necessarily be appropriate to address both objectives in a single study. Remember the need to balance internal and external validity to provide both high-quality, yet relevant information.

References

EBM Working Group Users' Guides to the Medical Literature series:

Barratt, A., Irwig, L., Glasziou, P., *et al.* (1999) Users' guide to medical literature: XVII. How to use guidelines and recommendations about screening. *Journal of the American Medical Association,* **281**, 2029.

Bucher, H.C., Guyatt, G.H., Cook, D.J., Holbrook, A., and McAlister, F.A. (1999) Users' guides to the medical literature: XIX. Applying clinical trial results. A. How to use an article measuring the effect of an intervention on surrogate end points. *Journal of the American Medical Association,* **282** (8), 771–8.

Dans, A.L., Dans, L.F., Guyatt, G.H., and Richardson, S. (1998) Users' guides to the Medical Literature. XIV. How to decide on the applicability of clinical trial results to your patient. Evidence-based Medicine Working Group. *Journal of the American Medical Association,* **279** (7), 545–9.

Drummond, M.F., Richardson, W.S., O'Brien, B.J., Levine, M., and Heyland, D. (1997) Users' guides to the medical literature. XIII. How to use an article on economic analysis of clinical practice A. Are the results of the study valid? Evidence-Based Medicine Working Group. *Journal of the American Medical Association,* **277** (19), 1552–7.

Giacomini, M.K. and Cook, D.J. (2000) Users' guides to the medical literature. XXIII. Qualitative research in health care A. Are the Results of the Study Valid? *Journal of the American Medical Association,* **284** (3), 357–62.

Giacomini, M.K. and Cook, D.J. (2000) Users' guides to the medical literature. XXIII. Qualitative research in health care B. What are the results and how do they help me care for my patients? *Journal of the American Medical Association,* **284** (4), 478–82.

Guyatt, G.H. (1993) Users' guides to the medical literature [editorial]. *Journal of the American Medical Association,* **270** (17), 2096–7.

Guyatt, G., Rennie, D. and the Evidence-Based Medicine Working Group. Why Users' Guides? EBM Working Paper Series #1. Only available on the Internet as: *http://www.cche.net/principles/content_why.asp*

Guyatt, G.H., Sackett, D.L., and Cook, D.J. (1993) Users' guides to the medical literature. II. How to use an article about therapy or prevention A. Are the results of the study valid? *Journal of the American Medical Association,* **270**, 2598–601.

Guyatt, G.H., Sackett, D.L., and Cook, D.J. (1994) Users' guides to the medical literature. II. How to use an article about therapy or prevention B. What were the results and will they help me in caring for my patients? *Journal of the American Medical Association,* **271**, 59–63.

Guyatt, G.H., Sackett, D.L., Sinclair, J.C., *et al.* (1995) Users' guides to the medical literature. IX. A method for grading health care recommendations. *Journal of the American Medical Association,* **274** (22), 1800–4.

Guyatt, G.H., Naylor, C.D., Juniper, E., *et al.* (1997) Users' guides to the medical literature. XII. How to use articles about health-related quality of life. Evidence-Based Medicine Working Group. *Journal of the American Medical Association,* **277** (15), 1232–7.

Guyatt, G.H., Sinclair, J., Cook, D.J., and Glasziou, P. (1999) Users' guides to the medical literature. XVI. How to use a treatment recommendation. *Journal of the American Medical Association,* **281** (19), 1836–43.

Guyatt, G.H., Haynes, R.B., Jaeschke, R.Z., Cook, D.J., Green, L., Naylor, C.D., and Wilson, M.C. (2000) Users' guides to the medical literature. XXV. Evidence-based medicine: Principles for applying the users' guides to patient care. *Journal of the American Medical Association,* **284** (10), 1290–6.

Hayward, R.S.A., Wilson, M.C., Tunis, S.R., Bass, E.B., and Guyatt, G. (1995) Users' guides to the medical literature. VIII. How to use clinical practice guidelines A. Are the recommendations valid? *Journal of the American Medical Association,* **274** (7), 570–4.

Hunt, D.L., Jaeschke, R., and McKibbon, K.A. (2000) Users' guides to the medical literature: XXI. Using electronic health information resources in evidence-based practice. Evidence-Based Medicine Working Group. *Journal of the American Medical Association,* **283** (14), 1875–9.

Jaeschke, R., Guyatt, G., and Sackett, D.L. (1994) Users' guides to the medical literature. III. How to use an article about a diagnostic test A. Are the results of the study valid? *Journal of the American Medical Association,* **271** (5), 389–91.

Jaeschke, R., Gordon, H., Guyatt, G., and Sackett, D.L. (1994) Users' guides to the medical literature. III. How to use an article about a diagnostic test B. What are the results and will they help me in caring for my patients? *Journal of the American Medical Association,* **271**, 703–7.

Laupacis, A., Wells, G., Richardson, S., and Tugwell, P. (1994) Users' guides to the medical literature. V. How to use an article about prognosis. *Journal of the American Medical Association,* **272**, 234–7.

Levine, M., Walter, S., Lee, H., Haines, T., Holbrook, A., and Moyer, V. (1994) Users' guides to the medical literature. IV. How to use an article about harm. *Journal of the American Medical Association,* **271** (20), 1615–19.

McAlister, F.A., Laupacis, A., Wells, G.A., and Sackett, D.L. (1999) Users' guides to the medical literature: XIX. Applying clinical trial results. B. Guidelines for determining whether a drug is exerting (more than) a class effect. *Journal of the American Medical Association,* **282** (14), 1371–7.

McAlister, F.A., Straus, S.E., Guyatt, G.H., and Haynes, R.B. (2000) Users' guides to the medical literature. XX. Integrating research evidence with the care of the individual patient. *Journal of the American Medical Association,* **283** (21), 2829–36.

McGinn, T.G., Guyatt, G.H., Wyer, P.C., Naylor, C.D., Stiell, I.G., and Richardson, W.S. (2000) Users' guides to the medical literature. XXII: How to use articles about clinical decision rules. *Journal of the American Medical Association,* **284** (1), 79–84.

Naylor, C.D. and Guyatt, G.H. (1996) Users' guides to the medical literature. X. How to use an article reporting variations in the outcomes of health services. Evidence-Based Medicine Working Group. *Journal of the American Medical Association,* **275** (7), 554–8.

Naylor, C.D. and Guyatt, G.H. (1996) Users' guides to the medical literature. XI. How to use an article about a clinical utilization review. Evidence-Based Medicine Working group. *Journal of the American Medical Association,* **275** (18), 1435–9.

O'Brien, B.J., Heyland, D., Richardson, W.S., Levine, M., and Drummond, M.F. (1997) Users' guides to the medical literature. XIII. How to use an article on economic analysis of clinical practice B. What are the results and will they help me in caring for my patients? Evidence-Based Medicine Working Group [published erratum appears in *Journal of the American Medical Association,* **278** (13), 1064]. *Journal of the American Medical Association,* **277** (22), 1802–6.

Oxman, A., Sackett, D.L., and Guyatt, G.H. (1993) Users' guides to the medical literature. I. How to get started. *Journal of the American Medical Association,* **270** (17), 2093–5.

Oxman, A.D., Cook, D.J., and Guyatt, G.H. (1994) Users' guides to the medical literature. VI. How to use an overview. Evidence-Based Medicine Working Group. *Journal of the American Medical Association,* **272** (17), 1367–71.

Randolph, A.G., Haynes, R.B., Wyatt, J.C., Cook, D.J., and Guyatt, G.H. (1999) Users' guide to medical literature. XVIII. How to use an article evaluating the clinical impact of a computer-based clinical decision support system. *Journal of the American Medical Association,* **282**, 67–74.

Richardson, W.S. and Detsky, A.S. (1995) Users' guides to the medical literature. VII. How to use a clinical decision analysis A. Are the results of the study valid? *Journal of the American Medical Association,* **273** (16), 1292–5.

Richardson, W.S. and Detsky, A.S. (1995) Users' guides to the medical literature. VII. How to use a clinical decision analysis B. What are the results and will they help me in caring for my patients? *Journal of the American Medical Association,* **273** (20), 1610–13.

Richardson, W.S., Wilson, M.C., Guyatt, G.H., Cook, D.J., and Nishikawa, J. (1999) Users' guides to the medical literature: XV. How to use an article about disease probability for differential diagnosis. *Journal of the American Medical Association,* **281** (13), 1214–9.

Richardson, W.S., Wilson, M.C., Williams, J.W., Moyer, V.A., and Naylor, C.D. (2000) Users' guides to the medical literature. XXIV. How to use an article on the clinical manifestations of disease. *Journal of the American Medical Association,* **284** (7), 869–75.

Wilson, M.C., Hayward, R.S.A., Tunis, S.R., Bass, E.B., and Guyatt, G. (1995) Users' guides to the medical literature. VIII. How to use clinical practice guidelines B. What are the recommendations and will they help you in caring for your patients? *Journal of the American Medical Association,* **274** (20), 1630–2.

Bibliography

Other useful books on critical appraisal and evidence-based medicine

Crombie, I.K. (1997) *The pocket guide to critical appraisal: a handbook for healthcare professionals.* BMJ Publishing Group, London.
An excellent book which covers critical appraisal of the main types of study design and provides information on the sorts of problems to look for. The checklists contained in this book were used as the basis for some of the critical appraisal checklists in this chapter.

Donald, A. and Greenhalgh, T. (1999) *Evidence-based healthcare workbook.* BMJ Publishing Group, London.
Useful because it provides some worked examples of critical appraisals.

Greenhalgh, T. (1998) *How to read a paper: The basics of evidence-based medicine.* BMJ Publishing Group, London.
This book contains a series of BMJ papers on critical appraisal. The individual references for these are listed in the resources section below. Some of these articles were used in compiling the checklists presented in this chapter.

Guyatt, G.H., Rennie, D., Sande, M.A., Gilbert, D.N., and Moellering, R.C. (ed). (2001)
   Users' guide to the medical literature: a manual for evidence-based clinical practice (Book
   with CD-ROM), AMA Press.
This book also brings together a series of JAMA papers on critical appraisal and evidence-based medicine. Again, the individual references for these are listed in the resources section below. Some of these articles contributed to the development of the checklists presented in this chapter.

Sackett, D.L., Richardson, W.S., Rosenberg, W., and Haynes, R.B. (1997) *Evidence-based
   medicine. How to practice and teach EBM.* Churchill Livingston, New York.

Websites resources

The Critical Appraisal Skills Programme Oxford
   Website address *http://www.phru.org.uk/~casp/*
Centre for Evidence-Based Mental Health
   Website address *http://www.psychiatry.ox.ac.uk/cebmh/index.html*
School of Health and Related Research (ScHARR)
   Website address *http://www.shef.ac.uk/~scharr/*
   Includes a guide to psychotherapy and a psychotherapy reference library, and introduction to medical statistics, a guide to finding evidence for EBM and information on free databases of interest to NHS staff.

Section 4

Special topics

Chapter 17

Genetic epidemiology 1: behavioural genetics

Frühling Rijsdijk and Pak Sham

Introduction

Behavioural genetics is the study of the genetic basis of behavioural traits including both psychiatric disorders and 'normal' personality dimensions. Behavioural genetics derives its theoretical basis from population genetics. Soon after the laws of Mendelian inheritance were re-discovered in 1900, the implications of these laws on the genetic properties of populations were worked out. Such properties include segregation ratios, genotypic frequencies in random mating populations, the effect of population structure and systems of mating, the impact of selection, the partitioning of genetic variance, and the genetic correlation between relatives. Some appreciation of population genetics is necessary for a deep understanding of behavioural genetics.

Because of the complexity of behavioural traits, genetic factors cannot be regarded in isolation, or as static. Instead, it is important to consider: (i) the relative contributions of genetic and environmental factors, (ii) the interplay between genetic and environmental factors, and (iii) the changing role of genetic factors in different stages of development from infancy to old age. The major study designs in behavioural genetics will be discussed in this chapter, namely family studies, twin studies, and adoption studies. Behavioural genetics, augmented by molecular genetics has the potential to identify specific genetic variants which influence behaviour. This will be considered in detail in Chapter 14.

Mendelian inheritance

Gregor Mendel first demonstrated the genetic basis of biological inheritance by studies of simple all-or-none traits in the garden pea. These traits were particularly revealing because they were completely determined by the genotype at a single chromosomal locus. Diseases caused by genetic mutation at a single locus are commonly called Mendelian or single-gene disorders.

A dominant disorder is expressed when an individual has one or two copies of the mutant allele, whereas a recessive disorder is expressed only when both alleles at the locus are the mutant variant. Examples of Mendelian disorders of clinical significance in psychiatry are Huntington's disease and fragile X syndrome. Mendelian disorders tend to be relatively rare because they are usually subjected to severe negative selective pressure, due to their increased mortality. Most common disorders and continuous traits of interest in psychiatry have an aetiology involving multiple genetic and environmental factors.

Categorical and dimensional traits

Behavioural genetics is rooted in both psychiatry and psychology. Psychiatrists traditionally adopt a medical model where diseases are defined as categorical entities and diagnoses are either present or absent. Psychologists on the other hand prefer quantitative measures of cognitive ability, personality and other traits. The methodology of behavioural genetics research reflects this duality, although there is a trend to integrate the two approaches, especially for traits such as anxiety and depression where both diagnostic criteria and quantitative measures exist.

Family studies

The aim of family studies is primarily to demonstrate familial aggregation of a disease or trait. If this is confirmed, then the pattern of disease in families can be used to infer its likely mode of inheritance.

Basic design of family studies

The importance of systematic ascertainment in family studies cannot be overemphasized. It is easy to imagine biases that might lead to the over-inclusion of families with several affected individuals ('multiplex' families) into a study. This would obviously lead to a false impression of familial aggregation. In order to prevent such biases, the standard methodology is to adopt a two-stage sampling scheme:

- In stage 1 a random sample of individuals with the disease is obtained. These affected individuals are called index cases or 'probands'.
- In stage 2 the relatives of the probands are assessed for the presence or absence of the disease (as well as other related traits). Relatives found to have the disease are called secondary cases.

An ideal study would include a comparison group, in which the probands are individuals from the same population as the index cases but whom do not have the disease. Where possible, the diagnoses of both probands and relatives should be made according to operational criteria using information obtained from personal interviews with standardised instruments (e.g. the DIGS, Diagnostic Interview for Genetic Studies). However, some relatives may be deceased or for other reasons unavailable for direct interview. In order to avoid bias it is important to obtain information on these individuals from informants (e.g. their parents, siblings or children) using standardised instruments (e.g. FIGS, Family Interview for Genetic Studies), supplemented by medical notes. It is also important that the assessment of relatives should be blind to the affected/unaffected status of the proband.

Measures of familial aggregation

The risk of disease in a relative of a proband is called 'morbid risk' or 'recurrence risk'. For a disease with variable age at onset, there is the problem of 'censoring'—namely that some unaffected individuals of a relatively young age may yet develop the disease in later life. There are two classes of methods for making an 'age-adjustment' in the calculation of morbid risk. The simpler methods, introduced by Weinberg and modified by Stromgren, require making assumptions about the age-at-onset distribution. The more sophisticated methods use some form of survival analysis (lifetable or Kaplan–Meier estimators) and do not require prior assumptions to be made about the age-at-onset distribution. A measure of familial aggregation is the relative risk ratio, which is the ratio of morbid risk among the relatives of cases to the relatives of controls, for a specific class of relatives (e.g. parent, sibling, offspring). Schizophrenia, for example, has relative risk ratios of about 10 for siblings and offspring, and about three for second-degree relatives.

Weinberg and Stromgren methods

These methods are of historical interest and are therefore described briefly here. For both members, the morbid risk (MR) is given by:

$$MR = \frac{\text{Number of affected relatives}}{\text{Number of lifetime–equivalents lived through by relatives}}$$

Weinberg's method defines lower and upper limits for age of onset. A relative contributes 0 lifetime-equivalent if his age is below the lower limit, 0.5

lifetime-equivalent if his age is between the lower and upper limits, and 1 life-time–lifetime equivalent if his age is above the upper limit. Stromgren's method specifies for each age the cumulative risk up to that age as a proportion of the cumulative risk at a grand old age. The contribution of a relative is simply this proportion. Full details of these methods can be found in Slater and Cowie (1971).

Multiple ascertainment

The systematic ascertainment of families through probands can lead to the complication that some families may have two or more probands. In the extreme case, if sampling is exhaustive and all affected individuals in the population are included as probands, then a family will have as many probands as affected members. This situation is known as *complete ascertainment*. At the other extreme, only a small proportion of the affected individuals in the population are included as probands, and almost all ascertained families will have only one proband, a scenario known as *single ascertainment*. In between these two scenarios, the situation is called *multiple incomplete*.

The standard method for estimating morbid risk under multiple ascertainment is attributed to Weinberg and is called the '*proband method*'. In this, each relative is counted in both the numerator and the denominator of the morbid risk estimate as many times as there are probands in the family that could have led to the ascertainment of the relative. As an example, if a sibship has three affected individuals two of whom are probands, then each proband will contribute once to the numerator and the denominator (since each could be regarded as the sibling of one proband). However the non-proband sibling will be counted twice, since this individual is the sibling of two probands.

Inferring mode of inheritance

Simple Mendelian modes of inheritance such as autosomal dominant and recessive have predictable patterns of relative risk ratios. For a rare autosomal dominant disease, the ratios are $\frac{1}{2}$ for parents, siblings and offspring, $\frac{1}{4}$ for second-degree relatives, and so on. For a rare recessive condition, the ratio is $\frac{1}{4}$ for siblings, and other classes of relatives are rarely affected. Most behavioural traits do not show such simple Mendelian ratios. Their mode of inheritance is sometimes called non-Mendelian or complex. The complexity refers to the likely involvement of multiple genes and environmental factors (Box 17.1).

Box 17.1 **Modes of inheritance for complex traits**

- **Simple Mendelian inheritance:** Autosomal/sex-linked; dominant/recessive. Generally confined to rare disorders
- **Single major locus model:** A single gene with a major influence but neither necessary nor sufficient for the disorder
- **Polygenic model:** Multiple genes with small effects
- **Oligogenic model:** Fewer genes involved
- **Mixed model:** Major locus with polygenes

Although the true complexity of behavioural traits is likely to be great, attempts have been made to fit data to idealized models that might represent approximations to reality. The two extreme types are the *single major locus model* and the *polygenic model*. In a single major locus model, the genetic component is due is a single gene that has a major influence on risk but is nevertheless neither necessary nor sufficient for the disease. Technically, the absence of disease among some genetically predisposed individuals is called *incomplete penetrance*, while individuals who are affected despite being genetically non-predisposed are called *phenocopies*. At the other extreme, the *polygenic model* posits a very large number of genes each of small effect. The cumulative effects of multiple genes lead to a continuous distribution, which fits well with quantitative characteristics, but is not directly applicable to categorical traits. The *liability-threshold model* proposes that polygenes exert their influence on an unobserved normally distributed variable (called liability), and that the disease develops if the liability exceeds a certain threshold value. In between these extremes are *oligogenic models*, in which a small number of genes are involved, and *mixed models*, in which a major locus is present among a background of polygenes.

Discrimination between different genetic models depends on assessing the goodness-of-fit of the models to family data. For some disorders such as schizophrenia and bipolar affective disorder, morbid risk data on many classes of relatives from multiple studies have been summarized and tabulated. These figures provide convenient data for model-fitting. When raw pedigree data are available, however, a statistically more powerful approach is *complex segregation analysis*. However the results of such analyses are often inconsistent, with some studies favouring a single major locus model and others favouring a polygenic model. It appears that the analysis of disease phenotypic data alone (without the help of molecular genetic markers) is limited in power to resolve different genetic models. Power is more favourable for quantitative traits: for example, a locus that accounts for a substantial (over 1/3) of the phenotypic variance is likely to be detectable by segregation analysis.

Aetiological heterogeneity

Psychiatry has yet to accomplish a fully medical model since most diagnoses represent syndromes rather than diseases. It is possible that a major diagnostic category such as schizophrenia may in fact represent a number of different diseases. In an attempt to dissect out aetiological heterogeneity, patients with a certain diagnosis are often sub-classified according to clinical and other variables. Features that may help resolve aetiological heterogeneity include age-at-onset, symptomatology (e.g. positive versus negative schizophrenia), and family history (familial–sporadic dichotomy). The validity of these typologies depends on finding additional variables that differ between the subtypes. For example, there is some evidence that early onset in schizophrenia is modestly correlated between relatives and is predictive of higher familial morbid risk.

Comorbidity

A possible scenario with other implications is that different diagnostic categories may in fact have similar genetic or environmental determinants. The frequent co-occurrence of schizophrenic and affective symptoms, and of anxiety and depressive symptoms, suggest common aetiological factors. Family studies of comorbidity help to discriminate common aetiological factors within the family (which are possibly genetic) from others outside the family (random individual environment). For example, generalized anxiety disorder and major depression are frequently comorbid at the level both of individuals and of families.

Adoption studies

A limitation of the family study is its inability to discriminate genetic from shared environmental factors. Familial resemblance or similarity in risk for a particular disorder may be due to shared environmental factors (such as diet and social class) as well as shared genes. If adoption occurred early in life, then shared environmental factors are less likely, and familial resemblance more attributable to shared genes. There are several varieties of adoption studies.

The *adoptees design* compares the adopted-away children of affected and unaffected biological parents. An improved version of this design incorporates the affection status of the adoptive parents. If the affection status of the biological parents is related to morbid risk in the adoptee, after adjusting for the affection status of the adoptive parents, then genetic factors are implicated.

The *adoptees' family design* compares morbid risk in the biological and adoptive families of affected adoptees. An improved version of this design includes the biological and adoptive families of unaffected adoptees. A greater morbid risk among biological than adoptive family members of affected, but not unaffected, adoptees would implicate genetic factors.

Adoption studies are essentially family studies with the added complication of adoption that enables family resemblance to be interpreted as genetic rather than merely familial. Similar issues such as aetiological heterogeneity and comorbidity can therefore be addressed by adoption studies.

Twin studies

The classical twin method is the most popular design used in behavioural genetics. The existence of two types of twin pairs, monozygotic (MZ) and dizygotic (DZ) provides a natural experiment for untangling genetic from environmental factors. MZ twins are developed from the same fertilized ovum and are therefore genetically identical; DZ twins are developed from two separate fertilized ova and share on average 50% of their genes. There are two main types of twin studies: (i) those based on twin pairs ascertained through affected probands, and (ii) those based on population twin registers. The former is appropriate for investigating relatively rare diseases, whereas the latter is better suited for studying common traits and quantitative dimensions.

The inference of a genetic component from proband-ascertained twin pairs is usually based on a difference between MZ and DZ concordance rates. The probandwise concordance rate is defined as

$$\text{Probandwise concordance rate} = \frac{\text{Number of probands whose cotwins are affected}}{\text{Number of probands}}$$

An age adjustment can be incorporated in this calculation, although this is less important than in family studies because the cotwin is of the same age as the proband twin is. Some earlier twin studies used a 'pairwise' definition of concordance rate.

$$\text{Probandwise concordance rate} = \frac{\text{Number of pairs where both twins are affected}}{\text{Total number of twin pairs}}$$

The pairwise concordance rate cannot be interpreted without knowing the intensity of ascertainment and is now obsolete.

Assumptions of the twin method

There are a number of assumptions made in the classical twin study. It is important to be aware of the implications of such assumptions and of the extent to which they are realistic in relation to a trait. The assumptions are that:

* MZ and DZ twin pairs share their environments to the same extent.
* Gene–environment correlations and interactions are minimal for the trait in question.
* Twins are no different from the general population in terms of the trait in question.

When these assumptions are met, the classical twin design is the most powerful tool for detecting genetic and environmental factors on a trait. Procedures for testing these assumptions will be discussed later in this chapter.

The co-twin control method

This method studies differences in MZ twins who are discordant for a particular disorder. The ill and healthy twins are genetically identical, so differences within these pairs can be used to study environmental reasons why individuals may develop a disorder. For schizophrenia it has been found that affected co-twins are more likely to have experienced birth complication.

Quantitative behaviour genetics

Quantitative behaviour genetics investigates the relative contribution of genetic and environmental influences to quantitative individual differences in traits using family, adoption, twin data or a combination of these different designs. Quantitative analysis is becoming increasing important in psychiatry because many diagnoses such as anxiety and depression are likely to represent the extreme of a continuum of symptom severity.

From biometrical genetic theory we are able to write structural equations relating observed traits of family members and twins to their underlying genotypes and environments. We can infer the relative importance of these 'latent' factors by comparing the observed correlations between family members with predicted correlations if different sources of genetic and environmental factors were to play a role.

The sources of genetic and environmental variation considered in behavioural genetics are:

* Additive genetic influences, **A**, represent the sum of the effects of the individual alleles at all loci that influence the trait.
* Non-additive genetic influences which represent interactions between alleles at the same locus (dominance genetic variation, **D**) or on different loci (epistasis).

- Environmental influences shared by family members (common environmental variation, C), for example, socio-economic status, parenting style, diet.
- Unique environmental influences (E), that will result in differences among members of one family, for example accidents, differential parental treatment, and measurement error.

The total phenotypic variance (P) of a trait is the sum of these variance components (P = A + D + C + E). To unravel the sources of variance and estimate their contribution, information from genetically informative participants is essential.

Biometrical genetics and the twin method

How do twins enable the different variance components to be estimated? The answer is that MZ and DZ twins have different degrees of correlation for the genetic components A and D but the same degrees of correlation for the environmental components C and E.

Component	Correlation	
	MZ	DZ
A	1	0.5
D	1	0.25
C	1	1
E	0	0

Therefore,

- differences in traits between MZ twins can only be due to unique environmental influences and, thus, gives us an estimate for E;
- assuming that MZ and DZ twins experience the same degree of similarity in their environments, then any excess of similarity between MZ (compared to DZ) twins can be interpreted as due to the greater proportion of genes shared by MZ twins, and thus, gives us an estimate for A;
- an estimate for C is given by the difference in MZ correlation and the estimated effect of A.

Heritability (h^2) is an index for the relative contribution of genetic effects to the total phenotypic variance. In the classical twin method Falconer's formula was used to estimate heritability based on twin correlations: h^2 is $2(r_{mz} - r_{dz})$, where r is the correlation coefficient. The relative contribution of the shared and non-shared environmental effects are: $c^2 = r_{mz} - h^2$; and $e^2 = 1 - h^2 + c^2$. This approach is not adequate for testing, for example, sex differences and was replaced by a more advanced method in which covariance structure models are fitted by special purpose software in which (multivariate) data from a range of different family groupings can be analysed simultaneously by means of maximum likelihood techniques.

Path analysis and structural equations

The method of path analysis was first developed by Wright (1921). The objective was to provide a method for interpreting observed correlations between a set of variables in terms of an *a priori* model of their causal relations. In terms of twin studies, a model predicts a series of expectations for correlations between twins based on the hypothesis to be tested.

The full twin model (for one variable) is depicted in a path diagram (Fig. 17.1) in which the observed trait for twins 1 and 2 is represented in rectangles and the unobserved (latent) genetic and environmental variables in circles. The single-headed arrows pointing from the latent variables to the observed traits represent causal paths. The path estimates (or regression coefficients) indicated by **a, c, d, e** represent the effects of the latent variables on the trait in question. The square of these estimates represents the variance of the trait accounted for by that specific latent factor.

The curved double headed arrows represent correlations among the latent factors (i.e. for MZ pairs $r = 1$ for **A, D** and **C**; for DZ pairs $r = 0.5$ for **A**, 0.25 for **D** and 1 for **C**). The *additive genetic covariance* between twin1 and twin2 is the product of the paths linking the trait scores via **A** (for MZ: $a^* 1^* a = a^2$; for DZ: $a^* \frac{1}{2} {}^* a = \frac{1}{2} a^2$). The covariance due to **C** and **D** can be derived in similar

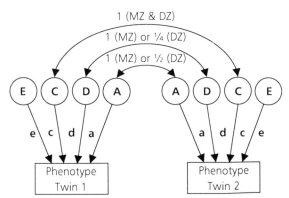

Fig. 17.1 Path diagram for the basic univariate twin model. The additive (**A**) and dominance (**D**) factors are correlated 1 between MZ twins and 0.5 and 0.25 for DZ twins, respectively. Shared family environment (**C**) is correlated 1 for both MZ and DZ twins that are reared together in the same home. Unique environment (**E**) is the source of variance that will result in differences among members of one family and is, thus, uncorrelated between members of MZ and DZ pairs. **a, d, c,** and **e** are the path coefficients for the **A, D, C** and **E** effects, respectively.

way. The total covariance is the sum of these chains via $\mathbf{A}$, $\mathbf{D}$ and $\mathbf{C}$. The expected variances and covariance of the traits within MZ and DZ pairs can then be written in terms of the different variance components:

$$\text{Cov}_{\text{MZ}} = \begin{bmatrix} a^2 + d^2 + c^2 + e^2 & a^2 + d^2 + c^2 \\ a^2 + d^2 + c^2 & a^2 + d^2 + c^2 + e^2 \end{bmatrix}$$

$$\text{Cov}_{\text{DZ}} = \begin{bmatrix} a^2 + d^2 + c^2 + e^2 & \frac{1}{2}a^2 + \frac{1}{4}d^2 + c^2 \\ \frac{1}{2}a^2 + \frac{1}{4}d^2 + c^2 & a^2 + d^2 + c^2 + e^2 \end{bmatrix}$$

Note that, although both $\mathbf{C}$ and $\mathbf{D}$ are included in the diagram and matrices, they are confounded in the classical twin study of MZ and DZ twins reared together and cannot be estimated simultaneously. The twin correlations indicate which of the two components is more likely to be present. When DZ correlations are less than half the MZ correlations, dominance is indicated, because $\mathbf{D}$ correlates perfectly for MZ but only 25% for DZ twin pairs. Common environmental influences, on the other hand, will make the DZ correlations greater than half the MZ correlations. Therefore, DZ correlations of about half the MZ correlations suggest additive genetic influences, but is also consistent with the presence of both $\mathbf{C}$ and $\mathbf{D}$. In other words, data on twins reared together do not contain enough information to tease out the contrasting effects of $\mathbf{C}$ and $\mathbf{D}$. If for example data of adoptive siblings are included (which will give us an independent estimate of $\mathbf{C}$ assuming that observed correlations between adoptive sibs are due to shared family environmental effects) we can estimate the effects of both components. The indices of relative contribution of genetic and environmental effects are normally reported as standardized values: that is if we consider $\mathbf{C}$ rather than $\mathbf{D}$ effects, the *heritability* is given by $a^2/(a^2 + c^2 + e^2)$.

Structural equation model fitting

We have seen that, while path diagrams allow models to be presented in schematic form, they can also be represented as structural equations and covariance matrices and, since all three forms are mathematically complete, it is possible to translate from one to the other (Neale and Cardon 1992). Structural equation modeling (SEM) represents a unified platform for path analytic and variance components models and is the current method that is used to analyze twin data. SEM is a statistical technique that tests hypotheses about relations among observed and latent variables. Many SEM programs are available on the market, but recently a package, Mx, was developed to model genetically sensitive data in a more flexible way (Neale 1999).

SEM programs estimate model parameters by minimizing a goodness-of-fit statistic between observed and predicted covariance matrices. There are different criteria that can be used to test goodness-of-fit, but one of the most common and robust methods is the maximum-likelihood criterion. The log-likelihood function is minimized by iteratively adjusting the values of the unknown parameters. This process, which is called *optimization* or *minimization*, is carried out until parameter estimates are obtained that yield the smallest possible discrepancies between model and data.

The *goodness-of-fit* of the model relative to a perfect fitting (saturated) model can be measured by the likelihood ratio chi-square statistic (χ^2). A non-significant χ^2 value suggests that the model is consistent with the data, whereas a significant χ^2 value suggests that the model poorly fits the data and can be rejected. The degrees of freedom (df) for the χ^2 test are the number of observed statistics (which are typically sample variances and covariances) minus the number of parameters being estimated in the model.

The statistical significance of the difference between two competing models, provided that the models are nested (i.e. the parameters of one model are a subset of the parameters of the other), can be tested by the difference in χ^2 and the difference in df between the two models. In practice this means that we can test whether the components, A, D, C, and E, are significantly greater than zero (i.e. present). For example, it is possible to compare an AE model with an ACE model and in doing so the significance of the shared environmental component is being tested. If the fit of the simpler, nested model (AE) is not significantly worse than that of the full model (ACE), the simpler model is preferred since it provides a more parsimonious explanation of the observed data (Neale and Cardon 1992).

Multivariate genetic analyses

If multiple measures have been assessed in twin pairs, the model-fitting approach easily extends to analyze the genetic–environmental architecture of the covariance between the traits. With multivariate models we can investigate the genetic overlap between different disorders, the continuity of genetic factors at different stages of the illness, and the relationship between genetic factors and mediating or environmental variables (e.g. personality, stressful life events) in the development of illness. For depression and anxiety, two very common and commonly comorbid disorders, it was found that the substantial genetic components for both disorders was due to the same genetic factors. Environmental factors however were different, and therefore important in shaping different outcomes (Kendler *et al.* 1992).

Categorical data for twins

Variance components models can also be applied to categorical twin data by assuming that the ordered categories reflect an imprecise measurement of an underlying *normal distribution of liability*. The liability distribution is further assumed to have one or more *thresholds* (cut-offs) to discriminate between the categories. When the measured trait is dichotomous (i.e. a disorder is either present or not), we can partition our observations into pairs concordant for not having the disorder (a), pairs concordant for the disorder (d) and discordant pairs in which one is affected and one is unaffected (b and c). These frequencies are summarized in a 2×2 contingency table:

Twin2	Twin1	
	0	1
0	00[a]	01[b]
1	10[c]	11[d]

0 = unaffected; 1 = affected

When data on MZ and DZ twin pairs are available, then we can estimate the correlation in liability for each type of twins (known as *tetrachoric correlations*). We can also go further by fitting a model for the liability, that would explain these MZ and DZ correlations. As for continuous traits, a variance decomposition (e.g. into **A, C, E**) can be applied to liability, where correlations in liability are determined by a path model. This leads to an estimate of the heritability of the liability. The often-cited heritability estimates for psychiatric disorders are, strictly speaking, estimates of the *heritability of the liabilities* to the disorders.

Box 17.2 **Methodological issues specific to twin studies**

1. Unequal MZ/DZ environments. MZ twins may be treated differently from DZ. This may exaggerate (or obscure) observed MZ similarity.

2. Associations between gene and environment:

   (a) Assortative mating. Parents may have similar characteristics. DZ similarities (and therefore shared environment effects) may be overestimated.

   (b) Genotype–environment correlation. An individual's genes may affect their environment (active) or their environment may be shaped by their biological relatives (passive).

   (c) Gene–environment interaction. The effect of an individual's genes may be influenced by their environment.

3. Limited generalizability. Twin populations are atypical with respect to obstetric history, and possibly childhood environment.

Checking the assumptions of the twin method (Box 17.2)

Equal environments

The equal environment assumption across zygosities assumes that environmentally caused similarity is roughly the same for both types of twin pairs (MZ or DZ) reared in the same family. This is the most basic assumption of the twin method and has been the subject of great debate over the years. It is generally agreed that MZ and DZ twins do share their environment to the same extent in many respects: they share the womb at the same time, are exposed to the same environmental factors, are raised in the same family and are the same age. However, there is also some evidence that MZ twins are treated more similarly by their parents and have more frequent contact as adults, in comparison to DZ twin pairs (see Plomin *et al.* 2001). The implications are that a more similar treatment of MZ twins will increase their correlations relative to DZ correlations, which can result in an overestimation of the genetic effect and an underestimation of the shared environmental effect. (Note: there are also factors that can have the opposite effect and increase variability between MZ twins. One example, is when MZ twin pairs are forced to attend different classes at school, while DZ twins are allowed to remain in the same class. This could lead to an underestimation of the genetic effect.) This effect can be detected by 'mislabelling'. If parental treatment is more similar for MZ twins, then DZ twins who are mislabeled as MZ twins should be more alike than correctly labeled DZ twins. Conversely, MZ twins mislabeled as DZ should be less alike than correctly labeled MZ twins. Little or no effect of mislabeling has been found. Also, more frequent contact has not been found to result in behavioural similarity in same-sex DZ or MZ twins. Correlations, if present, have been found to be small (Kendler *et al.* 1986). Finally, studies of MZ twins reared apart (e.g. Bouchard and McGue 1990) have found correlations for personality variables which are very similar to those for MZ twins reared together.

Genotype–environment correlation/interaction

Assortative mating   This refers to any non-random pairing of mates on the basis of factors other than biological relatedness. It is included here, since it may be influenced by both genetic and environmental factors and because assortative mating may affect the transmission, magnitude and correlation of both genetic and environmental effects. Apart from assortative mating, social interaction may also cause similarity between mothers and fathers.

The implications of this are that, if people choose partners who are phenotypically like themselves, environmental and genetic correlations between relatives are increased. This means that the correlation between DZ twin pairs, relative to that of MZ twin pairs, is increased and, thus, leads to an *overestimation* of the shared environmental effect. This effect can be detected by investigating the phenotypic correlation between parents for the trait in question. In order to determine whether assortative mating is taking place, it is necessary to trace the change in spouse resemblance over time or analyse the resemblance between the spouses of biologically related individuals (Heath *et al.* 1987).

Genotype–environment correlation   This refers to the genetic control of exposure to the environment. Exposure to environments is not random. Instead, genetic factors influence the probability that individuals will select themselves into certain environments. There are different types of G × E correlation. The most common are the following.

(1) Active G × E correlation: This arises when an individual creates or invokes environments which are a function of his/her genotype. An example in psychiatry is the reported association between genetic liability to major depression and an increased risk for stressful life events (Kendler and Karkowski 1997). The implications are that positive correlations will increase, and negative correlations will decrease estimates of genetic components. There is no way of knowing which genetic effects act directly on the phenotype and which result from the environmental effects that were actually caused by genes unless we have longitudinal trait data and an 'environmental' measure. The first indication is the existence of a genetic overlap between the environmental measures (i.e. life events) and the trait (see multivariate analyses). Kendler and Karkowski (1997) have showed with time survival analysis that 10–15% of the impact of genes on risk for MD is mediated through stressful life events.

(2) Passive G × C correlation: This arises because the environment in which individuals develop is provided by their biological relatives, with whom they are genetically related. An example is the correlated genetic and environmental effects of parents on their children and among siblings themselves. The implications are that positive correlations will tend to increase the estimate for shared family environment effect. This effect is detected by comparing the correlation between a measure of family environment (parental responsivity, encouragement of developmental advance, provision of toys/books, etc.) and offspring traits in non-adoptive and adoptive families. If the correlation is greater in non-adoptive families, it reflects a genetic origin and thus a passive G × C correlation.

Gene–environment interaction   Different genotypes may respond in different ways to the same environment, with some genotypes being more sensitive to changes in environment than others. An example in psychiatry is that the depressogenic effect of stressful life events is substantially greater in those at high compared to low familial risk for major depression (Kendler 1998).

(1) G × E interaction. The implications of a positive interaction will be estimated in E. In practice, it is extremely difficult to detect G × E interactions in humans without explicitly measured environmental indices. However, Jinks and Fulker (1970) have shown that G × E interaction can lead to a relationship between the sum and absolute differences of twin pairs' scores (known as *heteroscedasticity*). This relationship is accompanied by non-normality (skewness) and can often be removed by scale transformation. (*Note*: Sometimes we do not wish to remove this effect, but rather model it as it can give us valuable insight into the aetiology of diseases like the example on major depression given above.)

(2) G × C interaction. The implication of a positive interaction will be estimated in A. As for G × E interaction, it is extremely difficult to detect in humans without explicit environmental measures. G × C interaction may be indicated by a relationship between trait sum and absolute trait difference in DZ but not MZ twins.

Generalizability of twins studies to the general population

Even if the twin method is a valid way of studying the heritability of a trait, it still needs to be shown that twins are representative of the target population from which the researcher has been sampling. There are genuine differences between twins and singletons in terms of pregnancy and the birth process. Twins are on average lighter than singletons, are born on average approximately 3 weeks pre-term, and have more frequent complications, Caesarean sections, and malformations. For many diseases, obstetric, and paediatric complications do not play an important role and so should not necessarily pose a problem. However, for schizophrenia, there is now substantial evidence that there is an excess of obstetric complications among affected participants in comparison to controls. Schizophrenia might therefore be more frequent among twins, and there is now some suggestion that this may be the case.

Practical

Given the following contingency tables summarizing data obtained by complete ascertainment (indicating that all affected individuals are probands):

MZ	0	1	Total	DZ	0	1	Total
0		11	11	0		18	18
1	9	13	22	1	30	9	39
Total	9	24	33	Total	30	27	57

What are the concordance ratios for MZ and DZ pairs? What do these ratios tell us about the genetic basis of this disorder?

Answer

MZ CR 26/(26 + 11 + 9) = 57%
DZ CR 18/(18 + 18 + 30) = 27%

References

Bouchard, T.J. and McGue, M. (1981) Familial studies of intelligence: A review. *Science*, **212**, 1055–9.

Heath, A.C., Eaves, L.J., Nance, W.E., and Corey, L.A. (1987) Social inequality and assortative mating: Cause or consequence? *Behavior Genetics*, **17**, 9–17.

Jinks, J.L. and Fulker, D.W. (1970) Comparison of the biometrical genetical, MAVA, and classical approaches to the analysis of human behavior. *Psychological Bulletin*, **73**, 311–49.

Kendler, K.S. (1998) Major depression and the environment: A psychiatric genetic perspective. Anna-Monika-Prize paper. *Pharmacopsychiatry*, **31**, 5–9.

Kendler, K.S., Heath, A., Martin, N.G., and Eaves, L.J. (1986) Symptoms of anxiety and depression in a volunteer twin population: The etiologic role of genetic and environmental factors. *Archives of General Psychiatry*, **43**, 213–21.

Kendler, K.S., Neale, M.C., Kessler, R.C., Heath, A.C., and Eaves, L.J. (1992) Major depression and generalized anxiety disorder: same genes, (partly) different environments? *Archives of General Psychiatry*, **49**, 716–22.

Kendler, K.S. and Karkowski-Shuman, L. (1997) Stressful life events and genetic liability to major depression: Genetic control of exposure to the environment? *Psychological Medicine*, **27**, 539–47.

Neale, M.C. (1999) *Mx: Statistical modeling*. Box 710 MCV, Richmond, VA 23298: Department of Psychiatry.

Neale, M.C. and Cardon, L.R. (1992) Methodology for Genetic Studies of Twins and Families. Kluwer Academic Publishers, Dordrecht.

Plomin, R., DeFries, J.C., McClearn, G.E., and McGuffin, P. (2001) *Behavioral Genetics*. (4th edition) Worth Publishers, New York.

Slater, E. and Cowie, V. (1971) *The Genetics of mental disorders*. Oxford University Press, Oxford.

Wright, S. (1921) Correlation and causation. *Journal of Agricultural Research*, **20**, 557–85.

Chapter 18

Genetic epidemiology 2: molecular genetics

David Collier and Tao Li

Introduction

The previous chapter has focused on methods for identifying familial clustering of disorders or traits, and on methods for distinguishing between shared genetic and environmental influences. The primary objective for this chapter is to outline techniques for identifying specific genes responsible for an observed phenotype. The theoretical basis of complex and quantitative traits was established many decades ago. However practical methods for the efficient molecular analysis of the human genome have only recently emerged. Alongside these developments, the molecular genetic analysis of human disorders has moved at a rapid pace. Molecular genetics has focused on single gene disorders with great success, whereas for complex psychiatric disorders, few genetic risk factors have been identified. However the tools used by the complex disorder geneticist have evolved rapidly in the last few years and better strategies and statistical methods continue to appear. This chapter outlines some established and novel approaches to the analysis of the genetics of complex human disorders. A basic understanding of genetical statistics will be useful.

Complex genetic disorders

Psychiatric genetics is predominantly concerned with the analysis of complex genetic disorders and traits, which are in general caused by multiple genetic and environmental factors. Each of the genes involved are expected to have a relatively modest effect on risk (i.e. an odds ratio of less than three) and have reduced penetrance, that is, not all those carrying the risk allele will be affected. *Oligogenes* are risk genes with incomplete penetrance but which have a relatively large effect on risk (odds ratios of > 2) whereas *polygenes* have a relatively small effect on risk. It is not reliable to estimate whether the mode of transmission of the oligogenes are recessive or dominant in the classical way, and impossible for

Box 18.1 **Complex genetic disorders**

- Complex disorders are not caused by a single major gene (such as the CF gene in cystic fibrosis) but by multiple genetic and environmental factors acting together.

- The elucidation of a complete aetiological model, including genetic and environmental factors, and their interaction, is the goal of complex disorder research.

- Two types of risk genes are envisaged for complex disorders: oligogenes which have incomplete penetrance but a relatively large effect on risk, and polygenes which have a relatively small effect on risk.

polygenes. This complexity (Box 18.1) raises special problems for genetic analysis, since traditional linkage analysis, which specifies these parameters, cannot be easily used, and alternative methods of genetic analysis have been developed. These methods include *non-parametric linkage* and *allelic association* analysis.

Overview of prinicipal study designs

The key element to any genetic study is its design. Genetic analysis will involve taking blood or other samples from patients to prepare DNA, and the collection of data on clinical and related phenotypes. This work is detailed and labour-intensive, and it is often not practical to return to research participants for more information or samples. Thus, it is imperative that genetic studies are well planned, and this should include realistic power calculations to determine sample size, and careful thought on the type of clinical information to be collected from the research participant. Linkage and genetic allelic association analyses are the two major classes of study design in molecular genetics. These are summarized here and then considered in more detail later in the chapter with respect to the analysis of derived data (Box 18.2).

The objective for *linkage analysis* is to clarify the location of a disorder susceptibility or trait locus in the genome through analysis of the segregation of genetic markers in families. It is usually performed on a genome-wide basis and requires no specific knowledge of aetiology or pathophysiology. Linkage generally requires multiply affected families or affected sibling/relative pairs. Large samples sizes (e.g. more than 400 sibling pair families) may be required to have a good chance of detecting linkage for a complex disorders such as schizophrenia.

The objective for *allelic association analysis* is to investigate the association between specific alleles of polymorphic markers and a particular disorder or

Box 18.2 **Design issues for genetic studies**

- Genetic studies should only be undertaken if the detection of a suscept-ibility gene or locus is feasible; demonstration of heritability is necessary but not sufficient.
- Careful thought should be given to the type of phenotypic information to be collected.
- Systematic genetic linkage and candidate gene allelic association are the two main strategies for genetic analysis.
- Linkage requires no prior knowledge of disorder pathophysiology, unlike candidate gene approaches.
- Power calculations should be performed.

trait. It is usually focuses on candidate genes implicated in disorder pathophysiology, such as the serotonin transporter in depression. It can use a case–control or family-based design. Allelic association has high statistical power to detect genetic effects. However the main disadvantage is the low prior probability of detecting association. If one assumes there are 35,000 genes in the human genome and only a handful are involved in the aetiology of the disorder in question, then the prior probability of correctly picking a 'risk' gene is 1 in many thousands. If large numbers of candidate genes are 'screened', there is a high probability of Type 1 statistical error (false-positive results with 'significant' p-values). It is usually possible to minimize this difficulty by selecting a smaller number of candidate genes based on the pathophysiology of the disorder (such as the insulin gene in diabetes) but this is problematic in psychiatry where little is known about the underlying biological causes. Candidate genes can also be selected from regions of the genome displaying linkage. Systematic analysis of these linked regions is called linkage disequilibrium mapping.

The 'outcome': choice of phenotype in genetic studies

The type and quality of phenotypic information is critical to any genetic study (Box 18.3). First, the disorder or trait measured should have significant heritability, as evidenced by twin or family study. Many different phenotypes can be used, including *axis 1 diagnosis* (e.g. DSMIV schizophrenia), specific *symptoms* (e.g. formal thought disorder in schizophrenia or rapid cycling in bipolar disorder), *pharmacogenetic measures* (i.e. response to or side effects from clinical treatment), or *endophenotypes*, such as the P50 auditory evoked

> ## Box 18.3 **Phenotypes in genetic studies**
>
> - Phenotypes for genetic analysis can include simple diagnosis, specific symptoms or disorder related traits, measures of treatment response, or endophenotypes.
> - Variables can be categorical or quantitative.
> - Both face-to-face or telephone interview, or analysis of written records such as case notes, can be used to measure phenotypes.
> - Longitudinal diagnosis is recommended to increase reliability.

potential or the Continuous Performance Test. These measures may be categorical (e.g. presence or absence of schziophrenia) or quantitative (e.g. the level of positive symptoms or age at onset of disorder).

Phenotypic measures need to be reliable, reproducible and stable, and longitudinal evaluation is often required. DNA does not change, whereas a trait such as the level of depressive symptomatology or positive symptoms of psychosis will vary over time. Consequently measurements at a single time point may be misleading. Even categorical diagnosis may vary—new onset psychosis may resolve into one of many types of psychotic illness, and an initial diagnosis of anorexia nervosa may develop into chronic bulimia nervosa. Consequently careful planning of the method of phenotype assessment is required.

Categorical diagnoses

It is important that the diagnoses are correct for genetic studies, especially for linkage, since misdiagnosis in even a single individual may have a substantial effect on results. Two approaches to diagnosis are used: (i) the examination of patient records such as case notes, and (ii) direct interview of the patient (in person or by telephone). The most rigorous studies will use a combination of both. The use of validated structured interviews to get operational definitions of illness is strongly recommended for aetiological studies, as 'clinical' diagnoses are not reliable enough.

Operational definitions of psychiatric disorders, such as those in the Research Diagnostic Criteria (RDC; Spitzer *et al.* 1978) changed the way psychiatric disorders are defined in research. Operational definitions are included in the two main diagnostic schemes, the Diagnostic and Statistical Manual (DSM) of the American Psychiatric Association and the 10th edition of the International Classification of Diseases (ICD). RDC has been used in many genetic studies but DSM and ICD criteria are currently much more widely used.

A variety of structured interviews for recording the information needed for diagnoses are available. These include the World Health Organisation's Schedules for Clinical Assessment in Neuropsychiatry (SCAN) based on the 10th revision of the Present State Examination (PSE) (Wing *et al.* 1990). There is a SCAN home page on the WHO web site (*http://www.who.int/ evidence/ assessment-instruments/scan/index.htm*), including the text of the recent (June 2001) SCAN program users guide. Also commonly used is the American Psychiatric Association's Structured Clinical Interview for DSM-IV (SCID), formulated as SCID-1 for axis 1 disorders (Spitzer *et al.* 1992), and the Schedule for Affective disorders and Schizophrenia, Lifetime version (SADS-L). These assessment procedures are described by Barnes and Nelson (1993).

An additional option is the use of simple checklists such as OPCRIT (McGuffin *et al.* 1991). These provide information on individual symptoms that can be used to convert between different diagnostic schema such as ICD10, RDC and DSMIV. In OPCRIT, a range of operational definitions has been decomposed into carefully designed constituent items, and a computer program arrives at the diagnosis. The flexibility of a bottom-up polydiagnostic approach can allow refinement of diagnostic categories for genetic evaluation. This is necessary for a beneficial iteration between genetics and psychiatric nosology (McGuffin and Farmer 2001).

Sub-traits and continuous traits

There are also many other disorder-related traits that have a genetic basis, at least in part. Some of these are simple dichotomous measures (e.g. presence or absence of formal thought disorder) whereas others are continuous variables measuring clinical symptoms, neuropsychological or neurophysiological traits. These take into account the level of the trait as well as its presence or absence. Thus each individual gene for a psychiatric disorder may not only contribute to the overall disorder, but also directly to specific traits or symptoms. The use of sub-traits, especially when measured as continuous variables, increases statistical power by providing greater phenotypic information, as well as by reducing complexity through (potentially) a more direct relationship between gene and phenotype.

Many scales for measurement of clinical traits are available (Barnes and Nelson 1993)—these may focus on core symptoms, such as positive and negative symptoms in psychosis, or on related traits such as obsessive compulsive personality disorder in eating disorders. Commonly used scales for the analysis of psychosis include the Positive and Negative Symptom Scale (PANSS), which measures positive, negative and general psychopathology, the Scale for the

Assessment of Positive Symptoms (SAPS) and the Scale for the Assessment of Negative Symptoms (SANS).

Neuropsychological and neurophysiological traits can also be used in genetic studies (Gottesman et al. 2001). For example, the P50 and P300 auditory evoked potentials are neurophysiological measures, and the continuous performance test a neuropsychological measure, all of which are strongly associated with schizophrenia.

Phenotypes in pharmacogenetics

The aim of pharmacogenetics is to identify genetic factors that influence the success of clinical treatment (Arranz et al. 2001). Failure to respond to medication is a common problem in the pharmacotherapy of psychiatry. Two important reasons for treatment failure are lack of efficacy (i.e. failure of a drug to have a clinical effect within the normal therapeutic range), and adverse effects (i.e. toxic or unpleasant side effects). Either of these may result from genetic variation in the receptor pathways at which the drug acts, or in the proteins which break down or activate them. An ideal study would measure response on a prospective basis, that is before and after treatment, although this approach is time consuming and expensive. Retrospective analysis, based on the analysis of case notes, is also possible.

In psychiatry, pharmacogenetics has mainly addressed affective disorders and psychosis. A variety of scales have been used for measuring treatment response in schizophrenia (Barnes and Nelson 1993). The Global Assessment Scale (known as GAS, GAF, or GAFS) is a simplest scale used. The Brief Psychiatric Rating Scale (BPRS), and the PANSS are more detailed and have been used for prospective studies (Masellis et al. 2000). The PANSS measures positive, negative, and general psychopathology. An alternative measure, the Clinical Global Impression scale (CGI) measures the impression of the severity of illness on a seven point scale and is widely used in clinical trials.

Measurement of treatment response in affective disorders is particularly difficult, since the course of these illnesses is variable and unpredictable and many patients have a spontaneous remission (Catalano 1999). The 17-item Hamilton Rating Scale for Depression (HAM-D) is frequently used and is the main assessment tool in more than two-thirds of studies of antidepressant response (Snaith 1977). For bipolar disorder, measurement of both manic and depressive episodes is important. Lithium is the most commonly used and most effective therapy used for bipolar disorder, it has been intensively studied, and there is good evidence that responsiveness to lithium is heritable, since it 'breeds true' in families (Alda 1999). However the criteria for defining response are still controversial. The best strategy is the long-term, prospective assessment of clinical symptoms both before and after lithium treatment, but this requires many years of observation. Retrospective rating is used as an alternative because the time scale of data collection can be much shorter, but response data will be of poorer quality since the methodology relies on the assessment of case notes and patient/clinician recollection. The rate of recurrence of affective episodes during lithium treatment is an important consideration, since it is difficult to gauge response to treatment for a patient whose episodes are infrequent without very long term follow-up.

Ethical issues for genetic studies

As in any other area of research, informed consent must be taken in writing from research volunteers. Genetics differs from other types of research such as epidemiology in that tissue and biological materials (blood and DNA) are taken from the research volunteer and may be stored and used in research for a long period of time. Such samples may consequently be of great value in genetic research that was not envisaged at the time of collection. This raises ethical difficulties, since researchers may wish to undertake research not consented to in the original collection, and it may not be possible to go back to patients for re-consent (Box 18.4). Furthermore the results of genetic research may reveal risk of disorder which has implications both for the research volunteer and their relatives. It is important to note that research is fundamentally different from clinical genetic testing, which includes quality control measures of validated tests together with genetic counselling. These issues are considered in a Medical Research Council policy document, 'Human Tissue and Biological Samples for Use in Research (2001)' which is available as a .pdf file at the MRC web site (*www.mrc.ac.uk/ethics_a.html*).

Box 18.4 **Ethical issues for genetic studies**

- ◆ Written, informed consent is essential.
- ◆ Involvement with commercial companies, and the possibility of collaboration with other investigators in the future, should be declared.
- ◆ The possible use of genetic material for other unforeseeable purposes in the future should be considered and declared if intended.
- ◆ Agreement by participants to non-disclosure of individual results of genetic experiments is advisable.

Collection and preparation of DNA

The main resource for genetic studies, alongside information about the research volunteer, is DNA. This is usually prepared from peripheral blood after venepuncture, but can also be obtained from other tissues such as post-mortem tissue or cheek cell scrapings. Tubes used for taking blood should be anticoagulated with either sodium citrate or potassium EDTA and mixed well. Heparinized tubes should not be used as heparin inhibits the enzymes used to manipulate DNA in genetic analysis. Venous blood is best processed fresh, although it can be stored frozen for a considerable time. DNA is contained in white cells, and these can be prepared by spinning the whole blood in a centrifuge at about 7000 for 25 min or so to obtain the white-cell containing buffy coat layer. The buffy coat can be removed with a pipette and used in a variety of DNA extraction procedures, or frozen for future extraction. The most robust method is phenol–chloroform extraction, but this is labour intensive and the chemical involved are hazardous. White cells can also be preserved by storing the buffy coat in 10% dimethylsuphoxide (DMSO). The buffy coat should be mixed with DMSO and cooled to $-80\,°C$ at a cooling rate of about one degree per minute.

An easier approach is the collection of cheek swab samples. This method involves rubbing cotton buds or brushes on the inside of the cheek, which removes loose cells. The advantages of this method are that it is more acceptable to children or those phobic about venepuncture, and can be used to obtain DNA though the post (Freeman *et al.* 1997).

The 'exposures': obtaining genetic information

The human genome project has made genetic research much easier. The main repository of human DNA sequence and related information are at the National Centre for Biological Information (NCBI), which is accessible on the internet (*www.ncbi.nlm.nih.gov*). This was established in 1988 as a resource for molecular biology information, and contains DNA and protein sequence databases, as well as complete genome assemblies. Expressed Sequence Tags (EST—a reference sequence of known location, that is, a 'genome milepost'), cytoplasmic DNA (cDNA), genomic and protein sequences are available for the majority of human genes and many other organisms are represented. The human genome mapping resource centre in the UK (*www.hgmp.mrc.ac.uk*) and the Sanger Centre (*www.sanger.ac.uk*) also provide a wealth of useful tools and information for genomic analysis and molecular biology. An extensive array of tools is available for the analysis of DNA and protein sequence. For example, programs such as BLAST can be used to search these databases for specific sequences, and programs for the design of primers.

Polymorphisms

Many thousands of human genetic markers are known and can be found through genetic marker databases, such as the SNP consortium Ltd (*http://snp.cshl.org/*). A full list of available databases can be found at the HGMP web site (*www.hgmp.mrc.ac.uk/GenomeWeb/*). *Single nucleotide polymorphism* (SNP) databases have increasing coverage of the human genome, and will eventually obviate the need for screening genes and genetic loci, but at present it is still necessary to search for novel genetic markers, particularly for candidate gene analyses. The most widely used markers in recent decades have been simple sequence repeat or microsatellite markers such as (CA)*n* repeats, which vary in the number of copies of a simple di-, tri-, tetra- or pentanulceotide repeat. They have been used mainly for linkage analysis as they are highly polymorphic and consequently highly informative. Microsatellites are abundant in the human genome and searching for simple repeat motifs using programs such as, Tandem Repeat Finder (Benson 1999) can easily identify novel markers. The longer and more perfect a simple repeat, the more likely it is to be polymorphic. Potential microsatellite repeats can be tested for simply by designing specific polymerase chain reaction (PCR) primers, amplifying the DNA fragment and running out the product on a polyacrylamide gel. Searching for SNPs is a more complex task since these types of polymorphism do not result in changes in DNA fragment length—direct DNA sequencing is required and a pre-screen, such as single stranded-conformation polymorphism analysis or WAVE, is required.

Alleles, genotypes, and haplotypes

Since each person has two chromosomes and these are difficult to distinguish at the molecular level, genotypes are measured, that is, the combination of alleles from both chromosomes. There are three genotypes for any given individual, two homozygotes (*AA* and *aa*) in which the alleles are the same on both chromosomes, and a heterozygote (*Aa*) in which the alleles differ on each chromosome. Allele frequencies in a group of participants are measured simply by counting up the number of *A* and *a* alleles and dividing by the number of chromosomes. For example, if the genotypes for an autosomal biallelic polymorphism are measured in 100 people (who together have 200 chromosomes), and 25 have *AA*, 50 *Aa* and 25 *aa*, then the frequency of *A* and *a* is 0.5. The relationship between alleles and genotypes frequency is expressed as the *Hardy–Weinberg equilibrium*.

Methods of genotyping

Genotyping is the process of scoring which variant is present at a particular polymorphic site, and the method chosen will depend on the type of genetic variant under test. Almost all methods for genotyping require *amplification* of DNA using a *polymerase chain reaction* before or during analysis. Markers which differ in size, such as CA repeats, can be separated simply by gel or capillary electrophoresis, whereas there are dozens of methods for genotyping SNPs.

Statistical analysis: linkage studies

Linkage analysis (Box 18.5) depends on the principle that alleles of two or more genetic loci which are close together on the same chromosome tend to segregate (i.e. be passed on) together. This is because they are physically linked to each other on the same strand of DNA. The closer two loci are together, the lower the chance of their being separated by a recombination event during meiosis, and the stronger the observed linkage. This phenomenon can be applied to the detection of loci for genetic diseases. If a genetic marker is close to a disorder causing gene, alleles of the marker will tend to co-segregate with the disorder, or be shared between affected relatives.

Analytic procedures

Two principal methods are used for linkage analysis: either (i) the pattern of allele transmission in families relative to the pattern of disease transmission, or (ii) the extent of allele sharing between affected family members (Sham 1998). Many programs are available to perform linkage analysis and related activities: a list of these and how to access the software can be found at *http://linkage.rockefeller.edu/soft/*. Some of the most commonly used programs are listed in Table 18.1.

Box 18.5 **Linkage analysis**

- The aim of linkage analysis is to make inferences about the relative positions of two or more loci. In the mapping of a disorder or trait, the inference is about the relative positions of the genetic markers and the causative gene(s).

- Linkage analysis is principally performed in multiply affected families or affected relative pairs.

- Parametric methods based on likelihoods and non-parametric methods based on allele sharing are both used.

- Linkage requires no information on the pathophysiology of disorder, but can only localize susceptibility genes for complex disorders to relatively large areas of the genome.

Table 18.1 Commonly used programs for statistical analysis of genetic data

Program	Function	Author	Location
CLUMP	Monte Carlo method for assessing significance of a case–control association with multi-allelic markers	David Curtis	*http://www.mds.qmw.ac.uk/statgen/dcurtis/software.html*
EH1	Estimating haplotype-frequencies	Xiaoli Xie, Jurg Ott	*ftp://linkage.rockefeller.edu/software/eh* *http://linkage.rockefeller.edu/ott/eh.htm* (user guide)
ERPA	Non-parametric extended relative pair analysis	David Curtis	*http://www.mds.qmw.ac.uk/statgen/dcurtis/software.html*
ESPA	Extended sib pair analysis	Lodewijk Sandkuijl	*sandkuyl@rullf2.leidenuniv.nl*
ETDT	TDT test on markers with more than two alleles using a logistic regression analysis	PC Sham, Dave Curtis	*http://www.mds.qmw.ac.uk/statgen/dcurtis/software.html*
GENEHUNTER	Multipoint analysis of pedigree data including: non-parametric linkage analysis, LOD-score computation, information-content mapping, haplotype reconstruction	Leonid Kruglyak, Mark Daly, Mary Pat Reeve-Daly, Eric Lander	*http://www.fhcrc.org/labs/kruglyak/Downloads/index.html*
QTDT	Performs linkage disequilibrium (TDT) and association analysis for quantitative traits	Goncalo Abecasis	*http://www.well.ox.ac.uk/asthma/QTDT*
TDT/S-TDT	Transmission disequilibrium test and sib transmission disequilibrium test—provides separate results for TDT, S-TDT, and the combined (overall) test, as appropriate	Richard Speilman	*http://spielman01.med.upenn.edu/TDT.htm*
TRANSMIT	TRANSMIT tests for association between genetic marker and disorder by examining the transmission of markers from parents to affected offspring. It can deal with transmission of multi-locus haplotypes	David Clayton	*http://www.mrc-bsu.cam.ac.uk/pub/methodology/genetics/*

Linkage analysis is based on levels of statistical significance. The most widely used approach is based on likelihood ratios, and compares the odds of segregation between the marker and the disorder being the result of chance, or the result of linkage. This is commonly expressed as a logarithm, so that statistical scores from various families, which may have different pedigree structures, can simply be added together to provide a summary statistic. This test is expressed as the *logarithm of odds* (LOD). The level of statistical significance conventionally required to support linkage for major loci (e.g. those for Mendelian disorders) is a LOD score of ≥ 3. A LOD of 3 is roughly equivalent to a *p*-value of 0.0001 (and a LOD score of 2 to a *p*-value of 0.001). A LOD of 3 is necessary but not sufficient to draw a reliable conclusion, although, with rare exceptions, linkage at a correctly computed LOD score of ≥ 3 is true (Morton 1998).

The situation differs a little for complex disorders, where major genetic loci are not expected. LOD scores of 3 may provide adequate evidence for linkage for a complex disorder if assumptions are valid and the sample size large, whereas a LOD score of 2 can be regarded as suggestive and a LOD score of 4 unnecessarily conservative (Morton 1998). Others have argued that a slightly higher LOD score of 3.3 is necessary for a complex disorder (Lander and Kruglyak 1995).

The LOD score method is usually parametric, and it is necessary to specify the disorder gene frequency and three penetrances (one for each marker genotype) which define whether the putative disorder gene is dominant or recessive. This is clearly not a good representation of the causal system for complex disorders, and mis-specification of parameters can have a substantial effect on the resulting LOD score. Consequently, non-parametric *allele sharing methods*, such as affected sibling pair methods, were suggested by Penrose in 1935. Alternatively, the robustness of the likelihood method, combined with the use of flexible parameters, has been used for complex disorders.

Power to detect linkage

Statistical power is a key issue in designing a linkage study, that is, the information content of the families under study. It is desirable to assess the power of the sample *a priori*: (i) to assess the magnitude of genetic effects that the sample might detect, (ii) to see if effort can be saved through not genotyping individuals who will not contribute to linkage information, and (iii) to reveal areas where more makers might be genotyped (Sham 1998). Commonly assessed factors include the number of fully informative gametes, the expected LOD scores, Fisher's information and entropy-based information content mapping (as used by GENEHUNTER). Power calculation programs for quantitative linkage can be found at the Institute of Psychiatry statistical genetics website *http://statgen.iop.kcl.ac.uk/gpc/*.

Linkage analysis with large families

Traditionally, large families with multiply affected members have been used for linkage analysis (Fig. 18.1(A)), and this approach is exemplified by successful linkage analysis in Mendelian disorders such as Huntington's disease. However linkage in large families was designed for Mendelian disorders, caused by single genes with predictable patterns of inheritance. Because the pattern of inheritance for complex disorders cannot be specified, parametric LOD scores methods are less appropriate, as mis-specification of parameters has a major effect on the resulting LOD score. Therefore most investigators prefer to use non-parametric methods which mainly apply to the analysis of small family units. However it is worth noting that the most important linkage results in psychiatric genetics have been obtained using large families. This may be because large, multiply affected families have higher genetic loading but also because small family designs have less statistical power than larger families.

Sibling pair analysis

Sibling pair analysis was first proposed almost 70 years ago and relies on the relationship between the pairs of sibling for (i) disorder status and (ii) the genetic markers under test (Sham 1998). If a marker is linked to the disorder, then sibling pairs who are both affected or unaffected will be more alike than siblings discordant for the disorder. This method has been refined to the *affected sibling method* (ASP), which considers only pairs of affected siblings

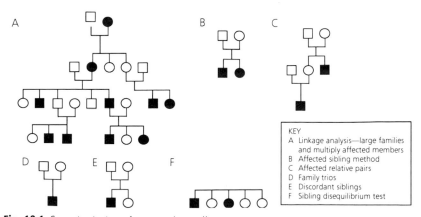

Fig. 18.1 Sample designs for genetic studies.

and uses *identity by descent* (IBD) rather than *identity by state* (IBS) (Fig. 18.1(B)). IBS is measured when a sibling pair is simply alike for two marker alleles; identity by descent occurs when the two alleles are shown to come from the same chromosome in the previous generation (i.e. they are replicates of each other). The ASP method is very popular and gives greater power than looking at sibling pairs with one or none affected. Many programs are available for this type of analysis, such as ESPA. The significance of ASP linkage is often expressed as a *p*-value.

Affected relative pair analysis

For some disorders with low *sibling relative risk* (λs: the risk of a disorder in a sibling relative to the general population), such as anorexia nervosa, affected sibling pairs are rare. Instead, affected relative pairs can be used (Fig. 18.1(C)). Different statistical methods to ASO methods are required, however. One approach is the affected pedigree member (APM) method, which uses an IBS method (Weeks and Lange 1992). Alternative methods of affected relative pair analysis use IBD information, and can implemented by the programs ERPA (Curtis and Sham 1994) which calculates the prior and posterior IBD probabilities of alleles IBD for the relative pair, or in the NPL procedure of GENEHUNTER (Kruglyak *et al.* 1996), a more conservative test.

Statistical analysis: association studies

If a particular allele of a polymorphism is associated with a disorder, then it should be more common in the disorder population than in the control population, that is, associated with the disorder. Association analysis can be used to examine specific candidate genes, or to attempt to map the location of disorder genes from within a region showing linkage. Genome-wide association studies have also been proposed (Box 18.6).

Formally, allelic association is the occurrence of specific combinations of alleles along the same chromosome more often than expected, that is, specific alleles of genetic markers are physically (and hence genetically) associated with each other (Sham 1998). This is also termed *linkage disequilibrium* (LD). When a new mutation arises on a chromosome, it does so on a background of the alleles of existing polymorphisms. Because of linkage, short chromosomal segments tend to be inherited from parent to offspring. These chromosomal segments may be preserved over many generations, resulting in some combinations of alleles (i.e. *haplotypes*) being common in the population. In general LD acts across short distances (<1 million base-pairs or megabases), compared to linkage which can be detected across 10s of megabases.

Box 18.6 Genetic association studies

- Association analysis aims to detect association between specific alleles of genetic polymorphisms and disorders or traits.

- Association analysis can be used to examine candidate genes, to map the location of disorder genes from within linked regions. Genome-wide association studies have also been proposed.

- Case–control methods are popular but prone to selection bias.

- Family based methods which avoid stratification have become increasingly popular.

- Haplotypes can also be used for association analysis and may detect associations missed by the analysis of single polymorphisms.

An observed association between an allele of a polymorphism and a disorder occurs may arise for various reasons:

(a) The allele is a causative factor for the disorder.

(b) The allele is in linkage disequilibrium with the true causative allele. Since LD acts across short distances, the disorder causing polymorphism must be nearby.

(c) The polymorphism is part of a haplotype associated with the disorder (which is caused by this allele and other surrounding alleles with which it is in LD).

The extent of LD between markers can be measured using the D *statistic*, and its normalized derivative D'. D' indicates the level of LD from 0 to 1, where 1 is complete disequilibrium and 0 is no disequilibrium, that is, random association between the markers.

Case–control genetic studies

The aim of a genetic case–control study is to detect association between alleles, genotypes or haplotypes of a gene (or genetic locus) and the disorder in question. Two groups of participants are recruited: affected cases and unaffected controls. If a particular allele of a polymorphism is associated with a disorder, then it should be more common in the disorder population than in the control population. The excess frequency can be tested by a simple χ^2 test, although for polymorphisms with multiple makers, Monte Carlo methods such as CLUMP should be used. A particular problem with case–control analysis is population stratification, where the case and control populations are not well matched. Populations from different geographic regions or ethnic groups have different allele frequencies at many polymorphisms—thus false association (selection bias) may occur if the populations are ethnically stratified. Careful matching of cases and controls is required to avoid this, and there are methods to test for and correct for stratification (Pritchard and Rosenberg 1999). An alternative is to use family-based controls.

Family-based tests of association and linkage

Family based tests attempt to overcome the problem of hidden population stratification by comparing cases with their relatives rather than with unrelated controls, thus ensuring matching for genetic background . In addition it is possible to find association with family-based tests when linkage is too weak to be detectable. The relatives may be siblings or other relatives, but the use of parents is the most popular. All of these methods use a basic sampling unit of the parents as 'controls' and a single affected offspring as the case (often termed family trios) (Fig. 18.1(D)), but can be adapted to take into account families with more than one case. One potential bias in these family-based methods might arise through the selection of less severely affected cases. It is important that the diagnosis of the parents providing control alleles is not important for the test. A full description of these methods is provided by Sham (1998).

The haplotype relative risk and haplotype-based relative risk

Most methods of genetic analysis have confusing names, and haplotype relative risk (HRR), a genotype-wise method and haplotype-based relative risk (HHRR), an allele-wise method are no exceptions. The HRR method (see Sham 1998) uses the genotype of the offspring as the 'case' genotype and the two remaining non-transmitted alleles of the parents as the 'control' genotype. These are considered as two independent samples, which are treated as unmatched cases and controls. HRR thus provides an unbiased estimate of the population relative risk for the putative risk genotype. HHRR is a commonly used variation of the HHRR that uses alleles rather than genotypes (see Sham 1998). The HHRR statistic is a powerful test of linkage disequilibrium when the recombination fraction theta (θ) is near to zero. Both of these methods can simply be performed by counting up the transmitted versus non-transmitted alleles and performing a χ^2 test.

The transmission disequilibrium test

The transmission disequilibrium test (TDT; Sham 1998) also examines the transmission of alleles from parents to affected offspring but unlike the HRR and HHRR, is a matched pair test. It uses the McNemar test for matched pairs, which only considers heterozygous parents (i.e. those where the transmitted and non-transmitted alleles are different). Evidence for the preferential transmission of one allele over the other is assessed. It was originally known as the transmission distortion test, but was renamed since it is sensitive to linkage disequilibrium (as well as linkage) in sets of unrelated family trios. However in a large single pedigree it only measures linkage. The TDT has been extended to include genetic markers that have more than two alleles, and the computer program used to implement this test is called the Extended Transmission Disequilibrium Test (ETDT). TDT analysis using quantitative traits is also possible (Abecasis *et al.* 2000).

The sibling disequilibirum test

In late onset disorders, it is usually not possible to get DNA from the parents. Consequently, tests which use siblings as controls have been developed, and these use the family design shown in Fig. 18.1(F). These include the sibling association test (SAT) and the sibling disequilibrium test (SDT; Horvath and Laird 1998). This latter test has been usefully combined into a single test by Curtis *et al.* (Table 18.1) which can use data from SDT and TDT approaches. The use of discordant siblings is particularly helpful for the analysis of gene-environment interaction (Fig. 18.1(E)).

Analysis of haplotypes

There are good arguments to suppose that genetic associations with disorder may be easier to detect with the analysis of haplotypes. The use of haplotypes will allow efficient genotyping of only the most informative polymorphisms in order to test the hypothesis that common genetic variants cause common disorders. In addition, if susceptibility is encoded by a series of rare variants from within the same gene, haplotype analysis may improve statistical power by combining their information. If disorder susceptibility is dependent on *cis* interaction with other loci (i.e. concerning the 3D structure of the encoded protein rather than simply its amino acid sequence), then disorder association may not be detected unless haplotypes are examined. Finally, the analysis of haplotypes across ethnically different populations may be valuable in pinpointing the actual disorder-causing DNA variants. A number of programs are able to analyse the transmission of haplotypes, including TRANSMIT (Table 18.1).

Power to detect association

Power in case-control studies and haplotype relative risk methods is much simpler to calculate than in linkage samples (Box 18.7). For unmatched

Box 18.7 **Summary**

General principles

- Most psychiatric disorders are complex disorders, thought to be caused by interaction between genes of moderate effect, and environmental factors.
- Psychiatric genetics aims to find variation in the genome that alters the risk of developing psychiatric illness.
- This concept can be extended to include genetic variation that affects disorder onset, symptomatology, severity and outcome, clinical response to treatments, as well as behavioural, neurophysiological and neuropsychological traits related to psychiatric disorders.

Specific design issues

- Careful choice of phenotypes, such as diagnostic instruments.
- Careful consideration of ethical issues.
- The use of linkage analysis.
- The use of case–control association and family-based association analysis.
- The necessity for power calculations.

case–control studies, programs such as the STACALC program, part of Epi2000, can be used (*www.cdc.gov/epiinfo/*). This can estimate the samples size required to detect a particular odds ratio for exposure to a risk genotype. For family-based methods, approaches using simulation can be used, but statistical large sample theory can also be used to give precise analytical power (Knapp 1999). Power calculation programs for case–control and TDT analysis can be found at the Institute of Psychiatry statistical genetics web site *http://statgen.iop.kcl.ac.uk/gpc/*.

Practicals

Allelic and genotypic association

ApoE is a lipoprotein containing a polymorphism with three alleles, e2, e3, and e4. The e4 allele is a risk factor for the development of Alzheimer's disease. The following table shows the genotype frequencies of the polymorphism in cases and controls from two populations: Group A and Group B.

Ethnicity	Diagnosis	e2/e2	e2/e3	e3/e3	e2/e4	e3/e4	e4/e4
Group A	Dementia	20	65	245	10	140	20
	Control	10	60	230	5	170	5
Group B	Dementia	10	45	275	20	130	20
	Control	10	65	315	5	95	5

Questions

1. Calculate the allele frequencies for e2, e3, e2+e3 and e4 from the genotype frequencies and express them as fractions. Allele frequences will always sum to 1, so round up or down.

2. Calculate the allele-wise odds ratio for the e4 allele vs the other alleles combined in each ethnic group, using the epi-info program statcalc (*http://www.cdc.gov/epiinfo/*).

3. Calculate the odds ratio in each group of carrying at least one e4 allele on developing AD using the same program.

4. Calculate the odds ratio for developing AD if you have two copies of the e4 allele compared to all other alleles combined in each group.

Answers

1. Allele frequencies

Ethnicity	Diagnosis	e2	e3	e2 + e3	e4
Group A	Dementia	115 (0.12)	695 (0.69)	810 (0.81)	190 (0.19)
	Control	110 (0.11)	700 (0.70)	810 (0.81)	190 (0.19)
Group B	Dementia	85 (0.08)	725 (0.73)	810 (0.81)	190 (0.19)
	Control	90 (0.09)	790 (0.79)	880 (0.88)	120 (0.12)

2. Allele-wise risk e4 allele vs. others combined

   A: Odds ratio 1.00 (95% CI 0.8–1.3, p-value = 1)

   B: Odds ratio 1.72 (1.3–2.2, $p = < 0.0001$)

3. Risk from carrying one or more e4 alleles

   A: Controls 180 e4 carriers vs. 320 non-carriers; cases 170 vs. 330

   Odds ratio 0.92 (0.7–1.2, $p = 0.51$)

   B: Controls 105 e4 carriers vs. 395 non-carriers; cases 170 vs. 330

   Odds ratio 1.94 (1.44–2.6, $p < 0.00001$)

4. Risk from carrying two copies of e4 compared to all other alleles

   Odds ratio 4.13 (1.5–12.6, $p = 0.002$) in both groups

Power calculation

Questions

1. You are designing an unmatched case control allelic association study. Using the 'sample size and power, unmatched case–control' routine in statcalc, determine how many cases you would need to detect a risk allele with 95% confidence and 80% power if the exposure in the control group was 20% and the exposure in the case group was 30%.

2. You have 200 cases with disorder X and 200 controls without the disorder collected for an unmatched case–control study of genetic risk factors. Determine the smallest percentage exposure in the ill group and the corresponding odds ratio you can detect with 95% confidence and 80% power if 20% of the controls have the risk allele (exposure).

Answers

1. 313 cases and 313 controls

2. Percentage exposure 33%. Detectable odds ratio 1.95

References

Abecasis, G.R., Cardon, L.R., and Cookson, W.O. (2000) A general test of association for quantitative traits in nuclear families. *American Journal of Human Genetics* **66**(1), 279–92.

Alda, M. (1999) Pharmacogenetics of lithium response in bipolar disorder. *Journal of Psychiatry and Neuroscience* **24**(2), 154–8.

Arranz, M.J., Munro, J., Osborne, S., Collier, D., and Kerwin, R.W. (2001) Applications of pharmacogenetics in psychiatry: personalisation of treatment. *Expert Opinion on Pharmacotherapy* **2**(4), 537–42.

Barnes, T.R.E. and Nelson, H.E. (1993) *The Assessment of Psychoses.*

Benson, G. (1999) Tandem Repeat Finder, a program to analyse DNA sequences. *Nucleic Acids Research* **27**(2), 573–80.

Catalano, M. (1999) The challenges of psychopharmacogenetics. *American Journal of Human Genetics* **65**(3), 606–10.

Curtis, D. and Sham, P.C. (1994) Using risk calculation to implement an extended relative pair analysis. *Annals Human Genetics* **58**, 151–62.

Freeman, B., Powell, J., Ball, D., Hill, L., Craig, I., and Plomin, R. (1997) DNA by mail: an inexpensive and noninvasive method for collecting DNA samples from widely dispersed populations. *Behaviour Genetics* **27**(3), 251–7.

Gottesman, I.I. and Erlenmeyer-Kimling, L. (2001) Family and twin strategies as a head start in defining prodromes and endophenotypes for hypothetical early-interventions in schizophrenia. *Schizophrenia Research* **51**(1), 93–102.

Horvath, S. and Laird, N.M. (1998) A discordant-sibship test for disequilibrium and linkage: no need for parental data. *American Journal of Human Genetics* **63**(6), 1886–97.

Knapp, M. (1999) A note on power approximations for the transmission/disequilibrium test. *American Journal of Human Genetics* 64(4), 1177–85.

Kruglyak, L., Daly, M.J., Reeve-Daly, M.P., and Lander, E.S. (1996) Parametric and nonparametric linkage analysis: a unified multipoint approach. *American Journal of Human Genetics* 58, 1347–63.

Lander, E. and Kruglyak, L. (1995) Genetic dissection of complex traits: guidelines for interpreting and reporting linkage results. *Nature Genetics* 11(3), 241–7.

Masellis, M., Basile, V.S., Ozdemir, V., Meltzer, H.Y., Macciardi, F.M., and Kennedy, J.L. (2000) Pharmacogenetics of antipsychotic treatment: lessons learned from clozapine. *Biological Psychiatry* 47(3), 252–66.

McGuffin, P., Farmer, A., and Harvey, I. (1991) A polydiagnostic application of operational criteria in studies of psychotic illness. Development and reliability of the OPCRIT system. *Archives of General Psychiatry* 48(8), 764–70.

McGuffin, P. and Farmer, A. (2001) Polydiagnostic approaches to measuring and classifying psychopathology. *American Journal of Medical Genetics* 105(1), 39–41.

Morton, N.E. (1998) Significance levels in complex inheritance. *American Journal of Human Genetics* 62(3), 690–7.

Pritchard, J.K. and Rosenberg, N.A. (1999) Use of unlinked genetic markers to detect population stratification in association studies. *American Journal of Human Genetics* 65(1), 220–8.

Sham, P.C. (1998) *Statistics in human genetics*. Arnold, London.

Snaith, R.P. (1977) Hamilton rating scale for depression. *British Journal of Psychiatry* 131, 431–2.

Spitzer, R.L., Williams, J.B., Gibbon, M., and First, M.B. (1992) The Structured Clinical Interview for DSM-III-R (SCID). I: History, rationale, and description. *Archives of General Psychiatry* 49(8), 624–9.

Weeks, D.E. and Lange, K. (1992) A multilocus extension of the affected-pedigree-member method of linkage analysis. *American Journal of Human Genetics* 50, 859–68.

Wing, J.K., Babor, T., Brugha, T., Burke, J., Cooper, J.E., Giel, R., *et al.* (1990) SCAN. Schedules for Clinical Assessment in Neuropsychiatry. *Archives of General Psychiatry* 47(6), 589–93.

Chapter 19

Health economics for psychiatric epidemiology

Daniel Chisholm and Paul McCrone

Introduction

This chapter examines the interface between psychiatric epidemiology and health economics, particularly in relation to mental health service evaluation. We discuss the issues inherent in conducting an economic evaluation and conclude with a summary of the applications of economic analyses.

The relationship of health economics and psychiatric epidemiology

The application of economics to mental health is a relatively recent addition to ways of thinking about psychiatric disorders. Economic evaluation provides insight into the adverse risks and consequences of psychiatric morbidity, fairer ways of allocating available resources and improved modes of service delivery, thus representing a necessary and valuable component of modern mental health policy-making. Psychiatric epidemiology represents a common starting point for many economic analyses of mental health care, which may use socio-economic risk factors for psychiatric morbidity, underlying incidence, prevalence and other data for modelling cost-effectiveness, or collaborative study design for clinical and economic evaluations. While the ultimate objectives of the two disciplines may differ, both are essentially pitched at understanding the consequences of disorder and its treatment at the level of the population at-risk. As such, the two disciplines can be viewed as offering complementary perspectives to mental health policy, planning, and evaluation.

Estimating the burden of psychiatric disorders

Epidemiological perspective: burden of disease studies

Nowhere is the link between health economics and epidemiology more apparent than in the estimation of national and global disease burden. The Global

Burden of Disease study, conducted by the World Health Organization and the World Bank, set out to provide estimates of incidence, prevalence, duration, and case-fatality for 107 conditions and their 483 disabling consequences, which could be used to generate summary measure of population health to inform resource allocation decisions (Murray and Lopez 1996). The main summary measure used was the disability adjusted life year (DALY), consisting of years of life lost (YLL) by premature death and years of life lived with disability (YLD). The disability component of this summary health measure (YLD) was weighted according to the severity of the disorder's sequelae. Disability caused by major depression was found to be equivalent to blindness or paraplegia, whereas active psychosis was estimated as somewhere between paraplegia and quadriplegia in severity of disability. Following this incorporation of disability into disease burden estimates, mental disorders ranked as high as cardiovascular and respiratory diseases, and exceeded all malignancies combined or HIV (Murray and Lopez 1996). This study posed new challenges to mental health policy by highlighting unmet and growing needs in both developed and developing countries (Patel 2000).

The results of the Global Burden of Disease study have been extremely influential and have been widely used as a justification for greater investment in psychiatry and related fields as a result of the high burden attributed to neuropsychiatric disorders (see Table 19.1). However, there are limitations to the approach used and its data sources. For example, some of the basic parameters for psychiatric epidemiology, such as incidence, duration and treatment effect, do not exist for many developing countries. In common with other disease categories, good-quality data on disability due to mental disorders were lacking at the time of the study. In addition, the appropriate inclusion of co-morbidity was limited, which given the high rates of co-morbidity of mental disorders and physical disorders, is problematic. Finally, DALYs have also been criticised about the placement of values on states of health and the scales along which these values are measured.

Economic perspective: cost of illness studies

Disease burden has also been gauged from an economic perspective for many years by 'cost of illness' studies, which attempt to attach monetary values to a variety of societal costs associated with a particular disorder, often expressed as an annual estimate aggregated across all involved agencies (see Table 19.2). Such studies aim to influence policy-making and resource allocation by demonstrating the relative economic burden associated with a particular

Table 19.1 DALY ('000) by WHO region and neuropsychiatric cause for the year 2000

Region[1]	World	Africa	The Americas	Eastern Mediterranean	Europe	South-East Asia	Western Pacific
Population (millions)	6045	640	827	482	874	1536	1687
Neuropsychiatric conditions	181,951	15,481	33,659	14,323	31,132	46,964	40393
1. Unipolar major depression	64,963	4060	11,487	4691	9256	19,955	15,516
2. Bipolar disorder	13,645	1595	1702	1164	1537	3693	3956
3. Schizophrenia	15,690	1559	1934	1409	1592	4594	4601
4. Epilepsy	7090	1120	1302	532	837	1904	1395
5. Alcohol dependence, harmful use	18,506	1229	6335	322	5254	2219	3147
6. Dementia	12,503	581	2234	629	4558	2310	2191
7. Parkinson disease	1496	67	280	79	425	285	360
8. Multiple sclerosis	1478	90	225	106	300	382	375
9. Drug dependence, harmful use	5833	1128	1713	605	1170	632	586
10. Post-traumatic stress disorder	3230	299	407	258	461	884	922
11. Obsessive–compulsive disorders	4761	798	837	510	807	993	815
12. Panic disorder	6591	722	838	571	801	1840	1818
13. Sleep disorders	3361	284	615	184	620	953	705
14. Migraine	7539	419	1366	537	1237	2021	1960
15. Other neuropsychiatric disorders	15,265	4081	3342	555	8136	2653	2166
All Causes	1,485,780	355,028	143,491	134,175	155,868	428,530	268,688
Neuropsych as % all causes	12.2%	4.4%	23.5%	10.7%	20.0%	11.0%	15.0%

[1]For list of countries by region, go to *http://www.who.int/whr/2001/main/en/memberstates.htm.*

Source: Annex Table 3, WHO (2001).

Table 19.2 The economic burden of depression and schizophrenia: cost of illness studies

Authors	Country	Year	Type (I/P)[a]	Direct costs	Indirect costs	Total costs	Ratio Dir:Indir	Comment
Depression								
West (1992)	UK	1990	P	£333 million	—	—	—	NHS costs only; crude method of calculation
Kind and Sorensen (1993)	UK	1991	P	£417 million	£2.97 billion	£3.39 billion	12:88	ICD-9 codes 296, 311 only; underestimation
Jonsson and Bebbington (1994)	UK	1990	P	£222 million	—	—	—	Major depression only
Stoudemire (1986)	USA	1980	P	$2.1 billion	$14.2 billion	$16.3 billion	14:86	
Greenberg et al. (1993)	USA	1990	P	$12.4 billion	$31.3 billion	$43.7 billion	28:72	Updated/extended version of Stoudemire et al.
Rice and Miller (1995)	USA	1990	P	$19.8 billion	$10.5 billion	$30.4 billion	35:65	ICD-9 codes 296, 298.0, and 311
Schizophrenia								
Andrews et al. (1985, 1991)	NSW, Australia	1975	I	$24.6 million	$114 million	$139 million	18:82	NSW data converted into $US; estimates sensitve to scenario analyses (Andrews 1991)
Goeree et al. (1999)	Canada	1996	P	C$1.1 billion	C$1.2 billion	C$2.35 billion	48:52	Comprehensive; Friction cost method used
Evers and Ament (1996)	Holland	1989	P	G 778 million	G 66 million	G 844 million	92:8	Mortality costs not included
Davies and Drummond (1994)	UK	1991	I	£397 million	£1.7 billion	£2.1 billion	19:81	Non-NHS agency costs excluded
Knapp (1997)	UK	1993	P	£1.4 billion	£1.2 billion	£2.6 billion	54:46	Not complete (mortality); aggregation not clear
Guest and Cookson (1999)	UK	1997	I	£88 million[b]	£84 million[b]	£172 million[b]	51:49	Comprehensive; discrete event model of first 5 years
Gunderson and Mosher (1975)	USA	1975	P	$2–4 billion	$9–11 billion	$11–19 billion	33:66	
Rice and Miller (1995)	USA	1990	P	$15.9 billion	$17.1 billion	$32.5 billion	48:52	Includes mortality and non-health agency costs
Wyatt et al. (1995)	USA	1991	P	$19 billion	$46 billion	$65 billion	29:71	Similar methods / data to Rice and Miller (1995) but future earnings not discounted

[a]Type of study: I = Incidence-based study; P = Prevalence-based study; [b]Mean annual cost, discounted at 6%.

disorder, in its simplest form by multiplying case prevalence by cost per case. Since no measures of outcome enter into these analyses, cost of illness studies are not true economic evaluations as the latter involves the *comparison of costs to outcomes attained*. However, cost of illness studies can serve as a benchmark against which to compare the costs of future interventions.

Psychiatric disorders impose a range of costs on individuals, households, employers, and society as a whole. A proportion of these costs are self-evident, including the varied contributions made by service users, employers, and tax-payers/insurers towards the costs of treatment and care, and the productivity losses resulting from impaired work performance or inability to work. However there are other significant costs that are not so readily quantifiable, including informal care inputs by family members and friends, treatment side-effects, and mortality. Most recent cost of illness studies attempt to account for these costs, with lost productivity being the biggest item in most studies as others are more problematic to estimate. Where a comprehensive estimate of overall economic burden for depression has been attempted, total estimated costs (1990 price levels) amount to £3.4 billion in the UK, and between $30 and 40 billion in the US (Kind and Sorensen 1993; Rice *et al.* 1995). A common feature of these studies is that the lost productivity costs exceed the direct costs of care and treatment, sometimes by as much as six or seven times.

Cost of illness studies in mental health have focused mainly on schizophrenia, depression, and dementia in a handful of countries and thus have limited relevance to the economic burden associated with a broader range of psychiatric disorders in the global population. Some researchers are concerned that the *human capital approach* to costing lost productivity, based on the assumption that when an individual is absent from work there is a corresponding reduction in national productivity, leads to over-estimation since lost work may be 'made-up' when the individual returns, or replacement workers can be employed temporarily. An alternative approach, the *friction-cost* method, takes these counterbalancing influences into account. For example, Goeree *et al.* (1999) in Canada, estimated that the cost of lost productivity resulting from schizophrenia related mortality was $1.53 million, as opposed to $105 million if the human-capital approach had been used.

Due to these methodological complexities with cost of illness studies, DALYs currently constitute the more internally consistent and globally applicable metric for assessment of the burden of disease. However, it is important to emphasise that cost of illness and burden of disease estimates alone provide insufficient information for allocating resources or setting priorities.

A disorder can place a considerable burden on a population but if appropriate interventions were absent or extremely expensive in relation to the outputs achieved, large-scale investment would be misplaced on economic grounds alone. Scarce resources could be more efficiently channelled to other burdensome conditions for which cost-effective responses were available. For example, dementia represents a large and growing cause of disability and premature mortality, but the proportion of current burden avertable through health care intervention remains low but costly. However, efficiency concerns represent only one set of criteria for health care decision-making, which will also be informed by ethical and other social considerations.

Applying health economics to mental health

Much of the need for a health economics perspective arises out of the *scarcity of resources* relative to needs, which translates into a requirement to make choices about how to allocate resources. At the most aggregated level, a government could decide to increase its budgetary allocation to mental health care. While this would have many positive impacts, it would be unlikely to completely eliminate unmet mental health need in the population, because the extra investment in mental health care would be likely to increase the detection of mental health problems. Moreover, the decision to allocate a greater volume of resources to mental health care in a constrained, publicly funded system impacts on the resources available for other health or welfare programmes. At the level of mental health purchasers, resource scarcity prompts the need to gather evidence with which to evaluate the clinical and cost-effectiveness of new and current therapies.

Macro-analyses: assessment of mental health systems

Core functions of a health system include the generation and allocation of resources, the provision of services, and overall stewardship of these various components (WHO 2000). Economic analysis of these key functions as they relate to mental health care include:

+ the availability of mental health care personnel, psychotropic medications, and basic infrastructures;
+ the relative merits of different methods for financing healthcare;
+ the respective roles of public, private, voluntary, and informal providers and their interaction;
+ the impact of clinical practice guidelines, strategic frameworks, and national mental health policies.

Many of these issues remain poorly researched at an international level, with current evidence almost entirely coming from the US and the UK (Frank and McGuire 2000; Chisholm and Stewart 1998).

The importance of a systems approach to mental health policy and planning is apparent from the following illustration. Cheap, effective drugs exist for key neuropsychiatric conditions, including tricyclic anti-depressants, conventional neuroleptics, and anti-convulsants, which are affordable even to resource-poor countries. The prescription of these drugs to those in need is determined by the extent to which they have been distributed and the ability of health care providers to detect and treat the underlying condition. Access to and use of such medication may be hampered by the private cost of seeking and receiving health care, particularly if it is 'out-of pocket'. User fees, provider incentives, and clinical practice are in turn influenced by the availability of national legis-lation, regulation, and treatment guidelines. Comprehensive mental health service models that have attempted to link these separate functions have been developed in a number of high-, middle-, and lower-income countries includ-ing Guinea Bissau, Iran, Tanzania, and the UK.

A health economics perspective can aid the distribution of healthcare resources within economies. A substantial literature has arisen exploring the factors that influence the demand for health care, which could lead to effective mechanisms for predicting resource use at the individual level. However, in mental health services research to date, such predictive tools function poorly since analyses have focused primarily on diagnosis, which is only capable of predicting approximately 10% of the observed variation in resource use (McCrone 1995). In many countries mental illness tends to accumulate in areas of high social deprivation and economists are involved in the generation of allocation formulae that incorporate ecological characteristics.

Micro-analyses: economic evaluations of mental health care interventions

Economic evaluation provides a set of principles and analytical techniques used to assess the relative costs and consequences of different interventions or treatment strategies. Despite the need for cost-effectiveness evidence, there remains a paucity of mental health economic evaluations from both developed and developing countries (Evers *et al.* 1997; Shah and Jenkins 1999). The majority have been concerned with specific treatment modalities for psy-choses and affective disorders, in particular the cost-effectiveness of different psychotropic drugs and, more recently, various psychotherapeutic approaches (Box 19.1).

Box 19.1 **Cost-effectiveness trials of mental health care interventions**

Although the volume of completed studies remains modest, particularly in middle- and low-income countries, there is increasing economic evidence to support the argument that interventions for schizophrenia, depression and other mental disorders are not only available and effective but also affordable and cost-effective.

Schizophrenia care

Controlled cost-outcome trials of family therapy for schizophrenia carried out in the UK, USA, and China have each identified greater reductions in relapse rates, hospital re-admission and family burden for study subjects in receipt of the family intervention as compared to standard care. In the China study, for example, researchers developed a family-based intervention appropriate to the Chinese context and showed that, in comparison to patients receiving standard care, such an approach reduced the need for inpatient hospital care, improved employment and saved an estimated US $149 per family (Xiong *et al.* 1994).

Depression and anxiety in primary care

A recent study conducted in India and Pakistan piloted methods for, and showed the feasibility of, applying economic analysis to community mental health programmes in low-income countries (Chisholm *et al.* 2000). These methods have subsequently been incorporated into a randomised controlled trial of the efficacy and cost-effectiveness of anti-depressant and psychological treatment for common mental disorders in general health care settings in Goa, India. Anti-depressants were found to be significantly superior to placebo on symptom and disability levels at 2 months and were also significantly more cost-effective both at 2 months and one year follow-up. Psychological treatment, on the other hand, was not appreciably superior to placebo (Patel *et al.* 2003).

A series of prospective trials undertaken in Seattle and elsewhere in the US have shown that important gains in clinical outcomes and functioning can be achieved for a modest investment via the pursuit of disease management and quality improvement programs for depression in primary care settings (Rosenbaum and Hylan 1999; Simon *et al.* 2001).

Cost-effectiveness trials of mental health care interventions *(continued)*

Suicide prevention

An educational programme to prevent depression and suicide introduced on the island of Gotland in Sweden resulted in a significant reduction in the suicide rate and produced considerable economic savings to society (a cost-benefit ratio of 1 : 30 in direct costs of care, and 1 : 350 in terms of productivity gains and mortality reductions), although initial improvements faded gradually over the longer follow-up study period (Rutz *et al.* 1992).

Alcohol misuse

A controlled trial of brief physician advice to problem drinkers in primary care carried out in the USA produced a cost-benefit ratio of 1 : 5.6, with savings made up of reduced use of hospital services and avoided crime and motor accidents in broadly equal measure (Fleming *et al.* 2000).

Pharmacotherapy

Most economic studies have focused on the cost-effectiveness of newer classes of anti-depressant and anti-psychotic medications over their older counterparts. Synthesis of the available evidence indicates that these newer psychotropic drugs may have less adverse side-effects but are not significantly more efficacious, and that the higher acquisition costs of the newer drugs are offset by a reduced need for other care and treatment (Knapp *et al.* 1999; Rosenbaum and Hylan 1999). The inconclusive evidence arising out of experimental and simulated studies to date suggests that the choice of drug, particularly in localities where evidence has not been accrued, remains a question of preference and affordability. What is less in question is the superior efficacy of pharmacotherapy over no treatment or placebo in reducing psychotic or depressive symptoms, associated disabilities, and service costs in the acute phase of illness, and if appropriately managed, over the longer-term as well.

Psychological interventions

Encouraging evidence is emerging in relation to the cost-effectiveness of psychotherapeutic approaches to the management of psychosis and a range of mood and stress-related disorders, with or without pharmacotherapy (Miller and Magruder 1999). A consistent research finding is that psychological interventions lead to improved satisfaction and treatment concordance, which contributes significantly to reduced rates of relapse, hospitalization, and unemployment. For example, controlled cost-outcome trials of family therapy for schizophrenia carried out in the UK, USA, and China each identified appreciably greater reductions in relapse rates, hospital re-admission and family burden for study subjects in receipt of the family intervention (Knapp *et al.* 1999). As with the newer psychotropic medications, the prevailing, if not fully substantiated view is that the additional costs of psychological treatments are countered by decreased levels of other health service contact (Miller and Magruder 1999; Rosenbaum and Hylan 1999). A controlled trial of brief physician advice to problem drinkers in primary care, for example, produced a cost-benefit ratio of 1 : 5.6, with savings made up of reduced use of hospital services and avoided crime and motor accidents in broadly equal measure (Fleming *et al.* 2000). Perhaps the greatest challenge here is the introduction of effective psychological interventions into routine practice. There is typically a lack of staff trained in family therapy and cognitive behavioural therapy and this means that many patients may receive sub-optimal treatment.

Care management approaches

Key challenges in the effective management of common mental disorders include their recurrent nature and the high rate of treatment discontinuation, suggesting the need for a proactive, chronic disorder management model. A series of studies undertaken in the US have shown that important gains in clinical outcomes can be achieved for a modest investment via disease management and quality improvement programmes for depression in primary care settings (Rosenbaum and Hylan 1999; Simon *et al.* 2001). For more persistent and severe disorders including schizophrenia, various permutations of an assertive or intensive community treatment model have been tested as an alternative to hospital-based care. Research suggests a positive if slowly declining impact on the clinical outcomes and satisfaction of patients, as well as on the costs and processes of care (Knapp *et al.* 1999). A similar finding emerged from the evaluation of an educational programme to prevent depression and suicide in Sweden. The programme resulted in considerable economic savings to society; a cost–benefit ratio of 1 : 30 in direct costs of care, and 1 : 350 in terms of productivity gains and mortality reductions using a human capital approach; but initial improvements gradually faded over the follow-up study period (Rutz *et al.* 1992).

Conducting an economic evaluation

The merit of an economic study in terms of its coverage and generalizability is determined to a significant extent by three parameters. As in clinical evaluation,

Table 19.3 Study design parameters

Parameter 1 Type of clinical data (What ratings are based on)	Parameter 2 Costing scope/perspective (What costs are included)	Parameter 3 Type of economic evaluation (How costs & outcomes combined)
Non-empirical (e.g. claims database)	Single care agency (e.g. health service only)	Cost-minimization analysis (CMA) (outcomes are the same)
Observational (e.g. cross-sectional study)	All formal care agencies (e.g. voluntary sector included)	Cost-effectiveness analysis (CEA) and cost-consequences analysis (e.g. cost per change in depression score)
Quasi-experimental (e.g. retrospective study)	Formal & informal care agencies (e.g. lost employment included)	Cost-utility analysis (CUA) (e.g. quality adjusted life year)
Experimental (e.g. RCT)	All societal costs (e.g. user/carer distress included)	Cost-benefit analysis (CBA) (all costs and outcomes monetized)

an important consideration for the review, assessment, and interpretation of economic evidence is the study design. For economic studies, the type of economic evaluation, and the scope or perspective of the study are equally important (Table 19.3).

Study design

Since economic analyses often take place alongside clinical evaluations or trials, the design of the study needs to be agreed with other evaluators. The ideal design is a randomized controlled trial which is the 'gold standard' of clinical and economic evaluation, since changes in outcome measures are attributable to the intervention, as opposed to other possible explanatory factors or 'confounding' variables. Where it is not practicable to carry out an experimental study, observational studies may have better external validity by preserving the context in which care is provided, but shift the focus of the analysis towards identifying associations between the intervention and changes in costs or outcomes (Black 1996).

Alongside the sample size needed to show a statistically significant clinical difference, investigators are increasingly required to demonstrate that there is sufficient power to show that a real cost-effectiveness difference has been observed. What constitutes a worthwhile difference in cost or cost-effectiveness will depend on several factors such as the perspective of the study and the burden of the disorder under investigation. The sensitivity of power calculations to the variance of the parameter(s) under investigation means that the numbers needed to show a statistically significant cost difference may be very large, and may exceed the number necessary to show a clinical difference (Sturm *et al.* 1999). Gray *et al.* (1997), for example, showed that at 80% power, their case management study ($n = 30$) was sufficient to detect between-group differences of approximately 30% for total costs, but to detect a 20% difference in health care costs alone over 700 subjects per arm would have been required. Concern that studies may be underpowered to detect differences in costs suggests two possible solutions. Sample sizes could be increased to generate enough power to detect both clinical and cost differences, although there are ethical considerations in increasing the number of people recruited to a trial simply to test for economic differences. Alternatively we can accept a lower level of confidence when analysing cost data, as we may be more ready to accept a greater probability of an incorrect cost finding than an incorrect clinical finding.

Mode of economic evaluation

Cost-minimization analysis is the simplest economic evaluation and establishes the least costly method of achieving given outcomes. However it is only appropriate if all outcomes are known or found to be identical, which is unlikely given the multi-dimensional nature of mental health outcome studies.

A much more common type of economic evaluation in the field of mental health care is cost-effectiveness analysis, which assesses the outcome of an intervention in addition to costs, expressed in terms of cost per reduction in symptom level, or cost per life saved. Where there is more than a single measure of outcome being investigated, as is often the case in psychiatry, it is more correctly called a cost-consequences analysis. This kind of economic evaluation is the first choice in most contexts, and has the advantage of presenting an array of outcome findings to decision-makers (Box 19.2).

Box 19.2 **Types of economic analyses**

Types of economic analysis:

- Cost-minimization analysis—the least costly method of achieving the same known outcome.
- Cost-effectiveness analysis—cost per unit of (principal) outcome.
- Cost-consequences analysis—cost per unit of (several) outcomes.
- Cost-utility analysis—cost per unit of 'utility' (summary measure allowing comparison across different fields of healthcare).
- Cost-benefit analysis—converts outcomes into monetary units to establish if monetarized benefits exceed costs.

Cost-utility analysis has considerable appeal for decision-makers since it generates a combined index of the mortality and quality of life effects of an intervention, upon which priorities can then be based. This would allow, for example, cost-utility findings for an intervention for schizophrenia to be compared to an intervention for asthma or cancer. However, there are technical difficulties in using this approach, and where it has been used in psychiatry, it has not performed very well to date (Chisholm *et al.* 1997).

Cost-benefit analysis includes all costs and outcomes valued in monetary units, thereby allowing assessment of whether a particular course of action is worthwhile, based on a simple decision rule that benefits must exceed costs. The difficulty of this approach is quantifying all outcomes in monetary terms, and consequently is rarely found in mental health care evaluation. Nevertheless, methodologies are now being developed which aim to obtain direct valuations of health outcomes by patients or the general public, such as 'willingness-to-pay' techniques, where an individual states the amount they would be prepared to pay to achieve a given health state (Healey and Chisholm 1999). These modes of economic evaluation allow us to determine the relative efficiency of different interventions. However, comparing the efficiency of different services can produce problematic results. The Oregon prioritization exercise in the United States, for example, resulted in tooth-capping receiving a higher ranking than appendectomies (Hadorn 1991). The general public will often want to prioritize interventions that preserve life, although they could be relatively inefficient. This 'rule of rescue' needs to be considered alongside evidence from economic evaluations.

Costing scope and perspective

The clinical and social burden imposed on individuals, families, and communities by mental health problems contains an economic dimension. This covers not only the costs associated with health and social care support of users, in the past referred to as 'direct' costs, but the knock-on effects or 'indirect' costs of mental disorder, such as the impact on someone's ability to work. Inconsistent definition of what constitutes 'direct' as opposed to 'indirect' costs has led to a move away from the use of these terms, to be replaced by the more useful distinction between health care (and other formal sector) costs and patient/family costs.

A key decision to make at the design stage of an economic study relates to the scope or perspective of the evaluation or the viewpoint from which the analysis is being taken. The scope might be that of a particular agency or government department, the formal sector as a whole, or a societal perspective that assesses the impact of the intervention on all involved agencies. The choice of viewpoint influences what costs and outcomes are measured, and is determined by the extent that the intervention under study exerts a differential impact on these various agencies/sectors. Since comprehensive mental health care requires multi-disciplinary inputs, the adoption of a single agency perspective is not appropriate for most evaluations and the most suitable perspective will seek to identify the costs falling to the multiplicity of care agencies involved, plus any costs incurred by users or carers.

Measurement of resource utilization

Individual profiles of service use can be constructed using a retrospective service receipt instrument, a prospectively kept diary of any contacts made or the examination of patient records, particularly if these records are computerized. Sole reliance on patient records is difficult due to the multiplicity of databases on which an individual's service contact(s) may appear and the potential for under-reporting. However, they can act as useful validation of data obtained through interview. Despite concerns expressed over the accuracy of data provided by patients, the evidence suggests that inaccuracies are limited (Calsyn *et al.* 1993).

The disparate needs of different client groups are reflected in patterns of service use. The service demands of people with common mental disorders may be quite modest, focusing on primary health care-based counselling or psychological therapy. In contrast, the needs of users with more severe mental disorder, such as schizophrenia, are likely to encompass a wide range of services, such as psychiatric inpatient and outpatient hospital services, social care, housing or residential care, structured day care support and activities and sheltered employment. The extensive range of services that people with mental health problems may use means that most evaluations should adopt a wide coverage, emphasizing the usefulness of an instrument that is similarly broad based.

Calculation of unit costs

For each item of resource utilization, a unit cost estimate is required, such as a cost per inpatient day, day care attendance or professional contact. Theoretically, the appropriate level of cost analysis is 'over the long-run' and 'at the margin', since it is the *incremental change* in resources implied by an intervention that is of interest. The difficulty associated with deriving costs in this way often results in a reliance on average revenue costs, adjusted to include capital and overhead elements. Economic theory suggests that in the long-run these average costs may be approximately equal to long-run marginal costs (Knapp 1993). In some countries and for certain services, unit cost data of this kind have been calculated, otherwise they need to be computed from sources like national/local government statistics, health authority figures and specific facility accounts. In practical terms, the main categories of cost that need to be quantified are:

+ wages of professional staff;
+ facility operating costs where the service is provided such as cleaning and catering;
+ overhead costs such as personnel and finance;
+ capital costs of the buildings and equipment where the service is provide.

The aggregation of these components amounts to the total cost of a service and this total is divided by the appropriate unit of service provision, such as number of patient contacts, to give the unit costs.

Measurement of outcomes

Intermediate outcomes, also known as process indicators, should not normally be the focus of the analysis, since positive changes in attendance or detection rates, for example, may not necessarily result in improved patient welfare or mental health. Final outcomes are concerned with detecting changes in the physical, psychological or social well-being of individuals, and commonly revolve around the measurement of symptoms, functioning and disability, quality of life, and service satisfaction. A further, population-level of outcome assessment are the composite indices of health such as the quality adjusted life-year (QALY) or DALY, which weight time spent in a certain state of health by the severity of the health state. With the further development and refinement of cost-utility methods, such measures of outcome will be more routinely included as a corollary to more condition- or domain-specific measures.

Comparative analysis of costs and outcomes

Economic evaluation compares the costs and outcomes of a mental health care intervention in an explicit framework, enabling decision-makers to assess whether the intervention offers a good use of resources. An analysis of costs or outcomes alone does not provide such information. In analytical terms, there are a number of possible scenarios:

+ If one intervention is both less costly and more beneficial than a comparison intervention, one can immediately conclude that this intervention is preferable.
+ If the costs and outcomes are equivalent, then either is acceptable. If costs alone are equivalent, then the more effective intervention is preferable, and if clinical outcomes are equivalent, then the cheaper intervention is preferable.

Box 19.3 **The incremental cost-effectiveness ratio**

$$\text{Incremental cost-effectiveness ratio} = \frac{\text{Difference in costs between treatments}}{\text{Difference in outcomes between treatments}}$$

And is used to assess whether additional costs are a good investment when one treatment is both more effective and more costly

- ◆ When the evidence shows that one intervention is more costly and more effective, we need to assess whether the additional costs are worth the greater effectiveness. This can be established by calculating an incremental cost-effectiveness ratio (see Box 19.3). A negative cost-effective ratio has little meaning since it implies that one intervention is dominant over, or dominated by the other in terms of cost or outcome.

The usefulness of economic analysis depends on the validity of the evidence about the study population, which is never perfect. A key stage of an economic evaluation is a *sensitivity analysis*, which involves the introduction of alternative values to key study parameters to assess the robustness of the conclusions.

The uptake of services is highly variable, so that pooled individual service use and cost data tends to be highly positively skewed, reflecting the heavy use of services by a small number of individuals. As parametric statistical approaches may not be appropriate, non-parametric approaches or data transformation may be required. The median is commonly used as the key measure of central tendency, or data is transformed onto a log or other scale. While use of the median may be useful for showing the 'typical' cost of a study subject, it is based on ranked data rather than actual values, ignores the influence of outliers and does not capture the total or (arithmetic) mean cost of treatment and care (Barber and Thompson 1998). Likewise, while log-transformation of costs data may resolve the problem of skewness, tests of differences between groups are on the geometric rather than the arithmetic mean. An alternative approach is the non-parametric 'bootstrap', which makes no distributional assumptions, yet is able to generate standard errors and confidence intervals for the parameter of interest (Mooney and Duval 1993).

Conclusion: the uses and limitations of economic analyses

The results of well-conducted economic evaluations can inform decision-making processes at many levels, from users and care-givers to government and society. However, it is important to mention some limitations of the approach. Conclusions based on a small-sample randomized trial can often only be tentative, while the failure to measure the wider non-health, non-service costs associated with two or more alternative treatments may produce misleading results. There are also a number of ongoing methodological debates such as the alternative techniques available for measuring health state preferences which are essential for both cost-utility and cost-benefit analyses. Given the low priority and stigma that is commonly associated with mental health care, a further desirable feature of studies yet to be achieved is that cost-effectiveness data should be comparable to interventions for physical conditions, in order to provide a firmer basis for new investment of resources. Even without these limitations, economic evaluation should not be viewed as a panacea for making difficult allocative and policy decisions. It is one additional tool that can facilitate explicit, evidence-based decision-making.

Practical

You are requested by local government to prepare a protocol for the economic evaluation of a day hospital programme for acute psychiatric illness as an alternative to inpatient treatment. Construct a 2-page summary protocol answering the following questions:

1. What are the specific aims and hypotheses of your planned economic evaluation? What is your chosen study design?

2. What is your chosen scope, duration and perspective for the evaluation? How might your choice of time scale and viewpoint affect the end results?

3. What are the main categories of cost that you would include in the evaluation? Are there any economic costs that you are not including, and if so, why?

4. What are the key measures of outcome that need to be considered, and by which mode of evaluation will you link these outcomes to cost data?

5. How would you propose to deal with the potential uncertainty surrounding key findings?

Once the exercise has been completed, the following study provides an illustration of how the questions raised were dealt with by a team of researchers in actual clinical practice:

Creed, F., Mbaya, P., Lancashire, S., Tomenson, B., Williams, B., and Holme, S. (1997) Cost-effectiveness of day and inpatient psychiatric treatment: results of a randomised controlled trial. *British Medical Journal*, **314**, 1381–5.

References

Andrews, G. (1991) The cost of schizophrenia revisited. *Schizophrenia Bulletin*, 17, 389–94.

Andrews, G., Hall, W., Goldstein, G., *et al.* (1985) The economic costs of schizophrenia; implications for public policy. *Archives of General Psychiatry*, 42, 537–43.

Barber, J. and Thompson, S. (1998) Analysis and interpretation of cost data in randomised controlled trials: review of published studies. *British Medical Journal*, 317, 1195–200.

Black, N. (1996) Why we need observational studies to evaluate the effectiveness of health care. *British Medical Journal*, 312, 1215–18.

Calsyn, R.J., Allen, G., Morse, G.A., Smith, R., and Tempelhoff, B. (1993) Can you trust self-report data provided by homeless mentally ill individuals. *Evaluation Review*, 17, 353–66.

Chisholm, D. and Stewart, A. (1998) Economics and ethics in mental health care: traditions and trade-offs. *Journal of Mental Health Policy and Economics*, 1, 55–62.

Chisholm, D., Healey, A., and Knapp, M.R.J. (1997) QALYs and mental health care. *Social Psychiatry and Psychiatric Epidemiology*, 32, 68–75.

Chisholm, D., Sekar, K., Kishore Kumar, K., Saeed, K., James, S., Mubbashar, M., Srinivasa Murthy, R. (2000) Integration of mental health care into primary care: a demonstration cost-outcome study in India and Pakistan. *British Journal of Psychiatry*, 176, 581–8.

Davies, L. and Drummond, M. (1994) Economics and schizophrenia: the real cost. *British Journal of Psychiatry*, 165 (Suppl. 25), 18–21.

Evers, S.M. and Ament, A.J. (1995) Costs of schizophrenia in the Netherlands. *Schizophrenia Bulletin*, 21, 141–53.

Evers, S.M., Van Wilk, A., and Ament, A.J. (1997) Economic evaluation of mental health care interventions: a review. *Health Economics*, 6, 161–77.

Fleming, M.F., Mundt, M.P., French, M.T., Manwell, L.B., Stauffacher, E.A., and Barry, K.L. (2000) Benefit-cost analysis of brief physician advice with problem drinkers in primary care settings. *Medical Care*, 38, 7–18.

Frank, R.G. and McGuire, T. (2000) Economics and mental health. In *Handbook of health economics* (ed. A. Culyer and J. Newhouse). Elsevier Science, Amsterdam.

Goeree, R., O'Brien, B., Blackhouse, G., *et al.* (1999) The valuation of productivity costs due to premature mortality: a comparison of the human-capital and friction-cost method for schizophrenia. *Canadian Journal of Psychiatry*, 44, 464–72.

Gray, A., Marshall, M., Lockwood, A., and Morris, J. (1997) Problems in conducting economic evaluations alongside clinical trials. *British Journal of Psychiatry*, 170, 47–52.

Greenberg, P.E. *et al.* (1993) The economic burden of depression in 1990. *Journal of Clinical Psychiatry*, 54, 405–18.

Guest, J.F. and Cookson, R.F. (1999) Cost of schizophrenia to U.K. society: an incidence-based cost of illness model for the first five years following diagnosis. *PharmacoEconomics*, 15, 597–610.

Gunderson, J.G. and Mosher, L.R. (1975) The cost of schizophrenia. *American Journal of Psychiatry*, 132, 901–6.

Hadorn, D.C. (1991) Setting health care priorities in Oregon: cost-effectiveness meets the rule of rescue. *Journal of the American Medical Association*, 265, 2218–25.

Healey, A. and Chisholm, D. (1999) Willingness to pay as a measure of the benefits of mental health care. *Journal of Mental Health Policy and Economics*, 2, 55–8.

Jonsson, B. and Bebbington, P. (1994) What price depression? The cost of depression and the cost-effectiveness of pharmacological treatment. *British Journal of Psychiatry*, **164**, 665–73.

Knapp, M.R.J. (1993) Background theory. In *Costing community care: theory and practice* (ed. A. Netten and J. Beecham). Ashgate, Aldershot.

Knapp, M.R.J., Almond, S., and Percudani, M. (1999) Costs of schizophrenia. In *Evidence and experience in psychiatry, Vol. 1* (ed. M. Maj and N. Sartorius). John Wiley and Sons, London.

McCrone, P. (1995) Predicting mental health service use: Diagnosis-based systems and alternatives. *Journal of Mental Health*, **1**, 31–40.

Miller, N. and Magruder, K. (ed.) (1999) *Cost-effectiveness of psychotherapy*. Oxford University Press, New York.

Mooney, C. and Duval, R. (1993) *Bootstrapping: a nonparametric approach to statistical inference*. Sage Publications, London.

Murray, C.J.L. and Lopez, A.D. (1996) *The Global Burden of Diseases: A Comprehensive Assessment of Mortality and Disability from Diseases, Injuries and Risk Factors in 1990 and Projected to 2020*. Harvard School of Public Health, WHO and World Bank; Boston.

Patel, V. (2000) The need for treatment evidence for common mental disorders in developing countries. *Psychological Medicine*, **30**, 743–6.

Patel, V., Chisholm, D., Rabe-Hesketh, S., Dias-Saxena, F., Andrew, G., and Mann, A. (2003) Efficacy and cost-effectiveness of drug and psychological treatments for common mental disorders in general health care in Goa, India: a randomised, controlled trial. *Lancet*, **361**, 33–9.

Rice, D., Kelman, S., and Miller, N. (1995) *The Economic Costs of Alcohol and Drug Abuse and Mental Illness, 1985*. Publication No. (ADM) 90-1694. Alcohol, Drug and Mental Health Administration, Rockville, USA.

Rosenbaum, J.F. and Hylan, T. (1999) Costs of depressive disorders: a review. In *Evidence and Experience in Psychiatry (Volume 2)*, (ed. M. Maj, N. Sartorius) John Wiley and Sons, London.

Rutz, W., Carlsson, P., von Knorring, L., *et al.* (1992) Cost-benefit analysis of an educational program for general practitioners given by the Swedish Committee for Prevention and Treatment of Depression. *Acta Psychiatrica Scandinavica*, **85**, 457–64.

Shah, A. and Jenkins, R. (1999) Mental health economic studies from developing countries reviewed in the context of those from developed countries. *Acta Psychiatrica Scandinavica*, **100**, 1–18.

Simon, G.E., Katon, W., VonKorff, M., *et al.* (2001) Cost-effectiveness of a collaborative care program for primary care patients with persistent depression. *American Journal of Psychiatry*, **158**, 1638–44.

Stoudemire, A. (1986) The economic burden of depression. *General Hospital Psychiatry*, **8**, 387–94.

Sturm, R., Unutzer, J., and Katon, W. (1999) Effectiveness research for study design: sample size and statistical power. *General Hospital Psychiatry*, **21**, 274–83.

West, R. (1992) *Depression*. Office of Health Economics, London.

WHO (2000) *The World Health Report 2000; Health Systems: Making a Difference*. WHO, Geneva.

WHO (2001) *The World Health Report 2001; New understanding: new hope*. WHO, Geneva.

Wyatt, R.J., Henter, I., Leary, M.C., and Taylor, E. (1995) An economic evaluation of schizophrenia—1991. *Social Psychiatry and Psychiatric Epidemiology*, **30**, 196–205.

Xiong, W., Phillips, M., Xiong, H., *et al.* (1994) Family-based intervention for schizophrenic patients in China: a randomised controlled trial. *British Journal of Psychiatry*, **165**, 239–47.

Chapter 20

Qualitative research

Joanna Murray

Background

Qualitative research is an increasingly popular method of enquiry in biomedical, clinical and behavioural research. Once regarded as the preserve of social scientists and psychologists, qualitative methods have entered the mainstream of epidemiology and clinical research, as evidenced by the publication of a series of papers in the *British Medical Journal* (Britten 1995; Mays and Pope 1995; Pope and Mays 1995; Pope *et al.* 2000). The qualitative methods to be described in this chapter offer a scientific approach to understanding and explaining the experiences, beliefs, and behaviour of defined groups of people. The contrasting features and the complementary roles of qualitative and quantitative methods of enquiry will be described.

While the majority of chapters in the present volume are concerned with research methods designed to answer questions such as 'how many?' or 'how frequently?', qualitative methods enable us to explore the 'why?', 'what?', and 'how?' of human behaviour. Since the aim is to understand the meaning of the phenomena under study from the perspective of the individuals concerned, the direction of enquiry is guided more by respondent than researcher. This approach is particularly appropriate to complex phenomena such as the range of beliefs that underlie illness behaviour and the aspects of health care that matter to different service users. Qualitative enquiry would focus on identifying beliefs and describing the circumstances that surround particular behaviours, while quantitative research would focus on measurable characteristics of the sample and the frequency and outcome of their behaviour.

An example of the contribution of the two methodological approaches is the study of variations in treatment of depression in older people. Epidemiological studies in the community and in primary care settings have found that the prevalence of depression in older adults far exceeds the prevalence of the disorder among those consulting their general practitioners. To identify the factors associated with this disparity, qualitative researchers would set out to explore the reasons why older people with depression do and do not present their symptoms to the GP. The aim would be to describe the range of beliefs about depression among attenders and non-attenders. The quantitative approach would involve establishing the strength of associations between personal characteristics, external factors, and behaviour of older people with depression. It is clear from this example that both approaches are complementary in identifying the nature of the disparity.

Qualitative research is based on the premise that each individual's experience is unique and the beliefs that underlie illness behaviour can only be measured once identified and described from a variety of individual perspectives. When information of this type is combined with data on prevalence and variable risk, more appropriate services and outcome measures can be developed.

Qualitative methodologies

The three most commonly used methods of data collection are in-depth interviews, focus groups, and observation. There are no rigid criteria for the application of the three methods; each has particular strengths to bring to certain situations.

In-depth interviews allow for a detailed exploration of an individual's beliefs, attitudes and feelings. Although the researcher is guided by a set of topics for exploration during the interview, their role is to enable each respondent to focus upon the areas that are important to them. To return to the example of depression in older people, the researcher would set out to explore the respondent's understanding of depression, the symptoms, causes, treatments, and their own experiences.

The personal interview is preferable to focus groups for exploring sensitive topics, such as sexual attitudes and behaviour, terminal illness and bereavement, or indeed any topic for which disclosure in the context of a group discussion is likely to cause embarrassment.

Focus groups are in-depth discussions in which groups of between 8 and 12 people who share a particular set of characteristics or experiences are brought together, under the guidance of a facilitator, to discuss a topic of importance to them. As in the individual in-depth interview, the facilitator uses a set of guidelines to steer the group discussion to ensure that the essential topics are covered. The content of the discussion emerges from the dynamics and interaction of each particular group. The discussion usually opens with general issues, for instance well-being in old age, and moves towards the specific area, the experience of depression among older people. The facilitator may ask more probing questions towards the end or may seek to clarify the variety of opinions expressed within the group.

The composition of the group depends upon the research topic. Participants may be selected on the basis of a shared health problem or because they have experience of a particular treatment; they may belong to an age group for whom the subject of enquiry has special relevance. To ease the flow of discussion, it is recommended that participants share similar socio-demographic characteristics; the atmosphere should be relaxed and the setting as natural as possible. The discussion should be tape-recorded and a second researcher, who is familiar with the objectives of the study, should be present to take notes on non-verbal interactions. The note taker should also be involved in annotating the transcriptions of the taped discussion to extend the data for analysis.

The focus group can be a particularly rich source of information on how different groups perceive their status or shared experiences; the method is also suited to generating ideas for service development. Group discussions are used to generate hypotheses, to test the relevance of topics as a preliminary step in a quantitative study and to clarify the use of terms and descriptors. When a study involves cross-cultural comparisons, focus groups enable the researcher to explore cultural differences in concepts and language.

Observational research is carried out in the natural setting with the researcher becoming a temporary member or an active participant in that setting. The objective is to understand the social functioning of the place from the perspectives of the people within it. As in the two methods described, the research process is one of inductive theory building from the bottom up rather than hypothesis testing. Fieldwork of this type is particularly suited to study the range of interactions in an institutional setting and may combine a number of types of data collection. Apart from the procedure for recording on checklists and diaries the actions of the various participants, the observer may record conversations and interviews for later transcription and content analysis since it is important to understand the participants' perceptions of what is going on. This can be most clearly demonstrated in the context of day care or residential institutions, in which the staff and clients' perspective on events and interactions are likely to be different. Focus groups and interviews can be used to clarify the meaning of observed behaviours and the significance to the individuals concerned. In situations where some participants are less able to speak for themselves, because of cognitive impairment for instance, participant observation can be a particularly useful method of inclusion.

The research process

General principles

As in all studies, a thorough literature review should be carried out to help the investigator to formulate the research question and to select a population best suited to answering it. A qualitative study may be designed to meet a number of objectives:

- Exploration of concepts: Finding out what particular concepts mean to different people (e.g. what does 'stress' mean to people in different demographic groups and how does it affect their illness behaviour?).

- Hypothesis or theory development: There may be a lack of relevant data from which to develop a hypothesis or no existing theoretical model to underpin the design of a quantitative study. A qualitative study forms the exploratory stage.

- Development of research tools: potential respondents' understanding of key concepts, use of colloquial descriptions and sociocultural variations need to be explored so that research instruments ask the right questions in a comprehensible way.

- Explanation: to clarify the findings of a quantitative survey (e.g. why are spouses caring for an older person with dementia less willing to accept support services than other carers? Why do some subjects drop out of a treatment trial at a differential rate? Why are potential service users from minority ethnic groups underrepresented?).

Although a representative sample is not required for qualitative research, it is of obvious importance that the sample be drawn from the target population. When a study is concerned with a broad range of subjects (e.g. people living in the catchment area of a hospital), efforts should be made to include individuals from the different gender, age, ethnic, and socio-economic groups within that population so that the spectrum of individual experiences and attitudes is explored. In contrast, the target population may be narrowly defined, for example, people attending a specialist clinic or parents of children with a particular disorder; the aim should be to include as broad a range of informants as possible. The number of interviews should be determined by the likely range of responses; the range of views and experiences may emerge after a small number of interviews but it is necessary to continue to interview further subjects until you are confident that the range has been fully explored.

As personal data will often be sought, the interviewer must establish good rapport before beginning the interview. An explanation of the importance of the research and the respondent's unique contribution should be stressed. The researcher should be aware that their own characteristics may influence the course of the interview; the respondent may wish to present themselves in a particular light and to avoid intrusion into certain areas of their life. Empathic listening, respectful and tactful probes should be used. Challenging questions are *not* appropriate and it is important to make clear that they, not you, are the experts on these topics.

An example

The design and method of the following study will be used to illustrate the research process:

Murray, J. and Livingston, G. (1998) A qualitative study of adjustment to caring for an older spouse with psychiatric illness. *Ageing and Society*, **18**, 659–71.

This study was designed to increase understanding of the adaptation of older people to living with a spouse who has a mental illness. There were a number of starting points for the study:

- A community prevalence survey in North London had found that spouses of older people with mental illness were significantly more likely to suffer from depression than those who were caring for a spouse with a physical illness (Livingston *et al.* 1996).

- A review of the literature indicated that spouses of older people with mental illness were at higher risk of depression than other carers and that, in spite of undertaking more intensive levels of care, they tended to seek and accept help at a later stage than other family carers.

- A randomized controlled trial of the efficacy of multi-disciplinary support to the spouses of those suffering from a mental illness was underway (Murray *et al.* 1997).

- The two studies raised questions about adjustment to caring for a spouse in later life: what makes some partners adjust to the role without negative consequences for their mental health while others in similar circumstances become depressed?

The aim of the qualitative study, therefore, was to identify aspects of the past and present relationship that might affect adjustment to caring for a spouse with a mental illness. There was also a practical purpose to the study: a better understanding of experiential data could help in the development of more acceptable and effective services for this vulnerable group.

The first stage of the research process is the formulation of the interview guide. In the present example, the literature on marriage in later life and caregiving suggested the concepts to be explored. The first concept concerned the common expectation that at times of illness or frailty, the spouse will provide support and try to keep their partner at home (Tower and Kasl 1996). Second, positive perceptions of the marital history, including companionship, affection, reciprocal support, and mutual decision-making, lead to better morale in old age. The interview guide was designed to explore respondents' accounts of their marriages from the early days to the present, encouraging them to describe good and bad aspects and to identify changes in the relationship over time. They were asked about their ways of coping with caring for their spouse.

The sample consisted of couples identified in the community survey (Livingston *et al.* 1996) in which at least one partner was suffering from a mental illness. Twenty interviews were conducted, sufficient to explore the range of experience and attitudes in a relatively homogenous sample. As in quantitative studies, it is essential to point out sample limitations: respondents lived in the same area of North London and shared socio-economic, ethnic, and educational characteristics, thereby limiting the extent to which the findings can be generalized. Had we selected a target population with greater diversity, a larger sample would have been required to explore the range of experiences.

To allow the carer the opportunity for disclosure, a second interviewer carried out an assessment of the mental health of the spouse in a separate room. The interviews were recorded on audio-tape then transcribed in full. Transcription is a lengthy and costly part of the process; each hour of recorded interview takes about 7 hours to transcribe. Notes were also made of any comments made by respondents when the machine was not running and observations of the respondent's behaviour. Interactions between the couple before or after the interview were noted.

Analysing the data

The objective of the lengthy process of content analysis is to identify themes in the area under scrutiny. Themes are generalized statements by respondents about beliefs, attitudes, values and sentiments; they are likely to be culturally bound and help in understanding behaviour. The topics used in the interview guide to elicit respondents' views may be used as the starting point for the analysis. Frequently the analytic process begins during data collection; an iterative process is then underway, in which data already analysed allows the researcher to refine questions for subsequent interviews and pursue lines of enquiry in more depth.

The analytic process begins with reading through transcripts of completed interviews and field notes several times to identify recurrent statements or powerfully expressed feelings. These are then labelled, described and categorized to signify the most important experiences for each individual. Similar themes may emerge from other transcripts and these can be grouped to indicate the frequency of a recurrent theme. Expressions of divergent or opposing views and experiences will be labelled and categorized until a range of experiences is identified. The procedure is applicable to the analysis of data from individual interviews, focus groups, and participant observation. The benefit of thematic analysis is that it directly represents individual points of view. The data can be presented in two modes: preserving the richness of the data by descriptive and interpretative accounts, and summarizing the data into categories which can then be used to represent the strength of a particular theme within a target group.

In the study of spouses' adjustment to care-giving, the topics in the interview guide provided an initial framework through which to explore the content of the interviews. After both authors had independently marked and labelled key passages in the transcripts, the following concepts were identified from respondents' descriptions of their marriages:

 (i) a history of intimacy (confiding, feelings of companionship, affection);

 (ii) a history of reciprocity (mutual support, shared decision making);

(iii) continuity in the relationship;

(iv) coping style (understanding of the spouse's condition and of acceptance of support from others).

The analyses showed that positive appraisals of the pre-morbid relationship, in terms of intimacy and reciprocity, were associated with higher morale and a strong sense of commitment to their partners. Perceived continuity in the relationship, in spite of considerable deterioration in their partners' mental health, was similarly linked to good morale. However, those who were unable to accept the changes in their partner were inclined to blame them for the deterioration and expressed the wish to give up caring for them. Hypotheses concerning the acceptability of support strategies for couples were developed on the basis of these findings.

Data analysis software

Computer software packages, such as ATLAS, ETHNOGRAPH, and QSR— *in vivo*, can assist in the indexing and retrieval of data once expressed attitudes and behaviours have been categorized, although they do not remove the need for close study of the transcripts. A series of key words can be assigned to particular ideas or attitudes and large quantities of text can then be scanned for these key words or phrases. Since it is obvious that a variety of styles of speech and colloquial usage may be found in a single sample, the researcher needs to perform the early stages of labelling sections of the text and categorizing expressions of similar sentiments. Software packages can reduce the volume of material for the later stage of identifying themes, and can retrieve illustrative examples from the labelled passages in the stored transcripts.

Information on training courses in the use of software packages may be obtained from the computer assisted qualitative data analysis software (CAQ-DAS) Centre at the University of Surrey, Guildford, UK.

Reporting the findings

Since the purpose of qualitative research is to explore the phenomenon of interest from the respondent's perspective, it is essential that the findings be placed in the context in which the study took place. This means a full description of the setting, the target population from which the sample was drawn, respondents' characteristics and a detailed account of the procedure. From this account, it should be possible for the reader to judge the reliability of the results. Although the sample was not designed to be strictly representative and the results may not be generalized to a wider population, providing full contextual details should indicate the likelihood of a similar outcome if the study were to be replicated under the same conditions. It is important to report negative evidence emerging from the analysis and to consider alternative explanations before final conclusions are reached. In this way the researcher can avoid the challenge that initial preconceptions may have dictated the outcome. Confirmation of the findings may be obtained from other sources, such as comparisons of aspects of the data with quantitative studies or from similar conclusions reached by other researchers in comparable settings.

References

Britten, N. (1995) Qualitative interviews in medical research. *British Medical Journal,* **311,** 251–3.

Livingston, G., Katona, C., and Manela, M. (1996) Depression and other psychiatric morbidity in carers of elderly people living at home. *British Medical Journal,* **312,** 153–6.

Mays, N. and Pope, C. (1995) Rigour and qualitative research. *British Medical Journal,* **311,** 109–12.

Pope, C. and Mays, N. (1995) Reaching the parts other methods cannot reach: an introduction to qualitative methods in health and health services research. *British Medical Journal,* **311,** 42–5.

Pope, C., Ziebland, S., and Mays, N. (2000) Analysing qualitative data. *British Medical Journal,* **320,** 114–16

Tower, R.B. and Kasl, S.V. (1996) Gender, marital closeness and depressive symptoms in elderly couples. *Journal of Gerontology,* **51**B, 115–29.

Further reading

Denzin, N.K. and Lincoln, Y.S. (1994) *Handbook of qualitative research.* Sage, Thousand Oaks, CA.

Huston, K., Parry-Jones, W., Livinston, M., Hogan, A., and Wood, S. (1998) Qualitative research. *British Journal of Psychiatry,* **172,** 197–9.

Miles, M.B. and Huberman, A.M. (1994) *Qualitative data analysis: an expanded sourcebook.* Saga, Thousand Oaks, CA.

Chapter 21

Psychiatric epidemiology— looking to the future

The Editors

The daunting objective for this chapter is to summarize issues which face the emerging specialty of psychiatric epidemiology, and to suggest broad directions for future research. Some of these have already been highlighted and we are grateful to contributing authors for providing their opinions as to the 'state of play', both in their own contributions and in communications solicited with respect to this chapter. Although the editorial team take responsibility for what is written here, we hope that it can be taken to reflect a wider body of opinion in this field. The issues raised are not intended to be exhaustive, although we hope that any specific omissions can be reasonably included within one or other of the broad themes identified.

Psychiatric epidemiology is a relatively young research specialty. This creates both problems and opportunities. A problem is that it has 'grown up' heavily influenced by prevailing paradigms from other older fields—principally general epidemiology (regarding methodologies) and other areas of psychiatric research (regarding systems of classification and diagnosis). These are not automatically appropriate or helpful and may instead be a source for difficulties encountered in research. An advantage however for a young specialty is that it can perhaps more easily discard the trappings of tradition as it seeks to make its way in the world. Current issues will be considered under three broad headings. First, the need for new methodologies will be considered. Next, interfaces will be summarized both between psychiatric epidemiology and other specialties/agencies and within the specialty itself. Finally possible new directions for psychiatric epidemiology will be considered.

The need for new methodologies

Psychiatric epidemiology has inherited its study designs (ecological studies, case–control studies, cohort studies, randomized controlled trials) largely wholesale from general epidemiology. It is also probably fair to say that most epidemiological psychiatrists have received what formal research training they have from generic institutions or courses. Psychiatric epidemiology remains a small specialty with limited resources to strike out on its own. Statisticians with a specific interest in psychiatric research are relatively few in number and new techniques for data analysis are therefore predominantly developed in other fields. Shortfalls in existing methodologies can be divided into those shared with general epidemiology and those which are more specific to psychiatric research.

Generic problems

Uncertainty regarding future directions for epidemiology has attracted a considerable degree of attention and soul-searching. An important shift of focus from infectious diseases to chronic diseases (such as cardiovascular disease and cancer) occurred in the first half of the twentieth century. While epidemiological research has contributed important information on the aetiology of many of these conditions, there has been a feeling expressed in some quarters that it is now flagging—or at least becoming more difficult (Pearce 1996). In particular it is likely that most 'easy' risk factors (i.e. those with reasonable variance within a given population and with large effects on risk for the outcome in question) have already been identified. Those which remain to be discovered may well be numerous but with more minor effects on the outcome of interest and more complex interactions. Conventional epidemiological techniques may not be adequate for identifying these effects and there is therefore a need for novel approaches both in study design and statistical analysis. Psychiatric epidemiology shares these challenges. Some important considerations are described below.

(1) *Identifying multiple 'small effect' exposures.* The most obvious example of this difficulty is in genetic epidemiology. Conventional techniques for investigating risk factors are adequate if specific exposures can be hypothesized. However they have no usefulness when faced with a polygenic disease and the entire human genome to choose candidate genes from. In the context of multiple analyses, how are small effects on risk (let alone those with complex interactions) to be distinguished from 'significant' associations arising from Type 1 error? And to what extent should scarce research resources be targetted towards replication studies for every reported association? Some approaches to these problems are discussed in Chapter 18 although it is fair to say that progress in identifying undisputed genetic factors has been negligable to date for most common chronic disorders.

(2) *Modelling multiple levels of exposures.* Simple risk factor–outcome relationships are becoming less useful for modelling the aetiology of chronic diseases. For example, physical illness particularly if chronic or disabling

increases the risk of subsequent depression. However the risk for most physical illnesses is determined by factors operating much earlier in life or even *in utero*. Socioeconomic environment in childhood is an important determinant of risk for depression. This effect may be partially mediated by worse physical health. Childhood socioeconomic environment may also *modify* the risk of depression associated with physical illness. This effect modification may in turn depend on other events occurring during the life-course. Psychiatry may be 'ahead' of other medical specialties in this respect since, at least in clinical practice, there has been a tradition of considering multiple aetiological levels for individual outcomes and a 'life-course approach' through the diagnostic formulation. However there is a growing need for techniques to model and test these complexities.

(3) *Identifying population-level risk factors.* While it is recognised that risk factors operate at a population-level for some disorders (e.g. distance from the equator for multiple sclerosis, herd immunity for infectious diseases), there has been a tendency for epidemiology to focus on those exposures which vary *within* populations. A risk factor will be less likely to be identified if there is insufficient variability within the studied sample. For example, if everyone smoked, lung cancer would appear to be a genetic disease (Rose 1985). Developing methods to investigate population-level risk factors is as important in psychiatric research as for other specialties. Examples might include the role of the social milieu in the aetiology and/or course of schizophrenia, the role of national culture in risk of suicide, or the role of a 'western' lifestyle in the aetiology of Alzheimer's disease.

(4) *Evaluating complex interventions.* Service research in all areas of healthcare is faced with the need to evaluate new models of care and interventions. On the one hand evaluation and proof of effectiveness are required by funding agencies and policy makers. On the other, the classical randomized controlled trial is frequently inadequate for this task: (i) service-level interventions are complex and it is generally not feasible to evaluate each aspect individually; (ii) opportunities may be limited for random allocation of the intervention; (iii) numbers of intervention groups (and hence statistical power to detect differences) are limited by the nature of the intervention (which is applied at a group - rather than individual-level). New methods of evaluation are therefore required which are both valid and accessible to policy-makers— either through the development of the classic RCT or using non-randomized approaches.

Problems specific to psychiatric epidemiology

The generic problems discussed above relate predominantly to the investigation of 'exposures', whether in the context of observational or intervention studies. From an epidemiological perspective, an important difference between psychiatry and other medical specialties is in the nature of its 'outcomes'. Some of these issues have been discussed with respect to causation in Chapter 13. For most areas of health research, 'disorders' or 'outcomes' (such as death, the occurrence of a particular type of cancer, or myocardial infarction) are relatively easy to define. Even where these involve more arbitrary criteria (e.g. for hypertension), there is generally an underlying physiological parameter (e.g. blood pressure) which can be measured and quantified. Psychiatry's disadvantage to date has been a lack of these quantifiable parameters (although 'disadvantage' is an entirely subjective description of the state of affairs which could equally be considered as 'fascinating' or 'challenging'). These issues lead to important difficulties in differentiating clinical and non-clinical states.

(1) *Clinical states.* 'Diagnoses' in psychiatry involve the presence of a 'syndrome', that is, the co-occurrence of particular symptoms, none of which are generally *sufficient* and only some of which are *necessary* for the diagnosis. Furthermore this syndrome must generally occur at a sufficient level of severity. Severity may in turn be quantified on the basis of the number of symptoms (e.g. of depressive symptoms), the extent to which they are disabling, or the nature of the symptoms themselves (e.g. the timing of sleep disturbance).

(2) *Non-clinical states.* Most if not all psychiatric diagnoses cannot be distinguished absolutely from 'normality'. Major depression, 'minor' depression, dysthymia, and euthymia, for example, exist as a spectrum with essentially arbitrary distinctions imposed between each category. Where this situation exists in other fields, an underlying parameter can generally be identified to define the borderline state: such as borderline raised blood pressure, impaired glucose tolerance, insulin resistance, and early cell dysplasia. Borderline states are important in psychiatry but frequently difficult to 'measure'. A progressive condition such as Alzheimer's disease is recognized to have a long prodromal phase where pathological changes are occurring which may or may not ultimately result in a dementia syndrome and which, to date, cannot be directly quantified *in vivo*. Conditions such as depression and schizophrenia also have long prodromal phases which are not amenable to quantification. Furthermore, the first 'clinical' episode is usually followed by a complex fluctuation between varying states of health or ill-health. For depression, where earlier episodes may be poorly recalled, the disorder may be identified while already in a state of fluctuation.

The transition from health to ill-health defines the onset of a condition. This has dubious validity in psychiatry where boundaries are less distinct. However these issues are fundamental for a large part of 'mainstream' epidemiological research. Terms such as 'incidence', 'risk ratio' and 'rate ratio' become meaningless without a clear idea of onset. The assumed advantages of prospective over cross-sectional study designs must also be re-appraised. For example, apparent risk factors for a transition from a non-depressed to a depressed state may include factors associated with an earlier depressed state which was not accurately recalled. Apparently causal factors prospectively associated with decline in cognitive function or 'incident' dementia may be those which are associated with previous unmeasured neurodegeneration. Factors associated with 'first onset psychosis' may themselves be secondary to the prodromal syndrome. As discussed in Chapter 13, concepts of induction and latency are also meaningless in psychiatry where disease onset is defined by the manifestation of the clinical syndrome.

The differentiation between states of health and ill-health also depend on how a 'disease' is defined. Uncertainty surrounding 'diagnoses' in psychiatry has important implications for epidemiological investigation. Where a diagnosis is formulated from an observed clustering of symptoms, risk factors for the condition will include: (i) those which influence the likelihood of individual symptoms occurring, (ii) those which influence the co-occurrence of these symptoms, and (iii) those which influence the impact of co-occurring symptoms on an individual's quality of life (since criteria for most diagnoses require a sufficient degree of syndrome severity). These considerations apply both for research into risk factors for a condition and for research into the effects of that condition. The consequences of a diagnosis (e.g. on quality of life) relate to the effects of symptoms both individually and in combination. Through a circular argument, they are also influenced by the syndrome having to cause functional impairment to fulfill diagnostic criteria. For example, dementia is defined on the basis of apparently declining function in more than one cognitive domain. Diagnostic criteria also require that this has had occurred to a sufficient degree to cause difficulty in social and/or occupational functioning. Dementia may therefore be more likely if a process affecting one domain of cognitive function (e.g. early Alzheimer's disease affecting memory function) is accompanied by processes affecting others (e.g. white matter disease affecting executive function). It will also be determined by factors modifying effects on general function, for example, a given stage of cognitive impairment may be less likely to attract a diagnosis of dementia in people who are more healthy in other respects, or in cultures where less is expected of older people.

Diagnoses and health states are particularly fluid entities in psychiatry. Study designs fundamental to general epidemiology involve important assumptions in this respect. Case–control studies assume that cases (e.g. people with a depressive disorder) can be clearly differentiated from controls (people without depression). Cohort studies assume that 'unaffected' people can be identified and that the 'onset' of the disorder can be ascertained during the follow-up period. Intervention studies (e.g. randomized controlled trials) assume that 'recovery' can be ascertained and compared between exposure groups. These traditional research designs have been of enormous value in all areas of epidemiological research. However a long tradition does not imply indefinite usefulness. An important consideration for psychiatric epidemiology is the extent to which it should move away from the 'mainstream' and develop methodologies which are more suited to its own questions.

Epidemiological interfaces

As a discipline, the traditional role of epidemiology has tended to be one of servant rather than master. That is, research directions are generally driven by others' agendas whether these are public health issues, questions of clinical practice, or efforts to elucidate the biological basis of disease. Epidemiology is the tool by which others' questions are answered. This sets it apart from some other research disciplines where scientific enquiry for its own sake is more easily justifiable. The nature of epidemiology is determined by its research questions: that is, by these imposed agendas. As agendas change, the nature of epidemiology will change. This does not imply an entirely passive process— *epidemiologists* have an important role in setting agendas. However factors influencing them (i.e. the questions which they wish to answer) will generally arise from outside the discipline, for example, their own experiences of clinical practice, of public health issues or of collaborations with researchers in other fields. These areas of interface have shaped epidemiology and will continue to do so. The most important are summarized below.

With biological science

The interface with biological science has been a key feature in the changing 'face' of epidemiology. Epidemiology emerged as a discipline strongly linked with public health at a time when biomedical research was in its infancy. Indeed, epidemiological findings have provided an important impetus for biological research. Transmissible agents were hypothesised as causes of infectious diseases long before pathogenic organisms were isolated. Links between dietary deficiencies and ill-health were identified before vitamins were characterized. Associations between smoking and lung cancer were established before carcinogenic processes were understood. However, as the focus of research has moved from population- to individual-level risk factors, it can be argued that biomedical considerations (understanding mechanisms of disease causation) have increasingly determined the directions of epidemiological research. The influence of biological science takes various forms:

(1) *New hypotheses.* Findings from biological science may lead to epidemiological hypotheses, for example, suggestions from neuropathological research of inflammatory processes in Alzheimer's disease leading to observational and intervention studies of anti-inflammatory drug use as a preventative factor. Epidemiological research may of course still give rise to biological hypotheses although it would be fair to say that the direction of information flow is more frequently in the opposite direction.

(2) *New measurements.* A limitation in Psychiatric Epidemiology discussed earlier is the lack of directly measurable physiological parameters related to disease states. Rapid advances in biomedical research will continue to give rise to new measurements which can be applied in an epidemiological context and may ultimately address this limitation. These might concern new measures of exposure status (such as physiological measures of 'stress'), new outcomes (e.g. through the search for disease biomarkers), and measures of 'intermediate' disease states (e.g. through neuroimaging). Advances in technology have meant that measurements which were once confined to case series in tertiary centres (such as genetic assays and neuroimaging procedures) can be applied to large epidemiological samples.

(3) *New disease models.* The traditional epidemiological model of disease causation treated the individual or population as a 'black box' between exposure and outcome. Increasing ability to measure subclinical disease states has led to more sophisticated models of causation. Epidemiological investigation of aetiology has therefore begun to draw closer to biological investigation of pathogenesis. Rapidly advancing biomedical technology and the mapping of the human genome mean that complex gene–gene and gene–environment interactions can now be taken into consideration. The extent to which existing epidemiological research designs and statistical procedures are able to deal with these complexities has been discussed earlier. The shape of epidemiology in the future however is likely to be strongly influenced by further developments in these fields.

With social science

The role of social science in influencing epidemiological research is potentially similar to that of biological science. Findings from social sciences may lead to epidemiological hypotheses. This process is, for example, prominent in cross-cultural research where 'emic' disease models derived from anthropological research are applied in an epidemiological context. Important contributions to epidemiological research have included new methods for quantifying social networks and illness beliefs. From these and other developments, new models of disease causation may arise, for example, concerning the role of childhood social environment in the aetiology of later affective disorders, or the social basis for ethnic group differences in risk of schizophrenia.

A number of articles have highlighted the lack of attention paid to social factors in disease causation, both in general and psychiatric research (Pearce 1996; Susser and Susser 1996; Thomas *et al.* 1996). As discussed earlier, there has been a prominent shift in focus within epidemiology from population- to individual-level risk factors. A danger in this process is that it may fail to identify important risk factors which do not vary sufficiently within a population. Also, a focus on processes occurring between the risk factor and the disease, ignores those giving rise to the risk factor: a whole level of causation which may be more important when it comes to prevention. The social context of disease states may therefore escape identification purely for methodological reasons. In psychiatric epidemiology the situation is compounded by the fact that concepts of disease aetiology (a strong influence on research funding, and hence research directions) have shifted markedly from social to biological models. As part of the debate over future directions for epidemiological research (both generally and within psychiatry), it may be argued that the shift towards the biological interface has been at the expense of links with social science. However are biological science and social science truly at opposite ends of a spectrum? And is epidemiology really defined by a 'tug-of-war' relationship between the two? The future of the specialty will not only be determined by its individual interfaces but by the extent to which it can draw together apparently diverse research disciplines in explaining the distribution and determinants of disease states.

With those who use research

Further back along the process of 'causation' (and therefore potentially more fundamental in shaping the face of epidemiology) are the agencies which pose the questions for scientists to answer. It is at this point where the tension is perhaps most acute between an individual- or population-level focus. Epidemiology has its origins as a population-level science. Research was driven by public health considerations—the need to describe and explain the distribution of disease states within and between populations in order that population-level interventions might be developed and evaluated. Information at a population-level is required by public health and also by policy makers whose decisions will be evaluated in their impact on populations. A clinician, on the other hand, is predominantly interested in individual-level factors, for example, the likelihood of a disease occurring in an at-risk individual or the potential benefits of a drug treatment. Pharmaceutical research also therefore has this focus, since clinicians end up using the treatment under evaluation. Biological research into disease causation follows suit since it is generally directed towards opportunities for pharmacological intervention, however distant a prospect. The nature of epidemiological research depends on these interfaces. However, the level of investigation may not always be so clearly determined as suggested above. Public health workers and policy makers need to take into account individual-level factors in order to evaluate the acceptability and therefore practicability of a given intervention. Clinicians may practice at the level of an individual but are also intimately involved with population-level interventions (such as vaccination programmes, or measures taken to improve the identification of depression). Furthermore their activities are increasingly quantified at a service (i.e. population) level. Pharmaceutical interventions also increasingly are not only evaluated in terms of individual-level efficacy, but also in terms of their cost and effectiveness across populations. Biomedical research may not only identify targets for the treatment of a disorder once it has developed, but also for preventative interventions with important public health relevance (e.g. potentially, the use of anti-inflammatory agents or oestrogen replacement to prevent dementia).

Epidemiology as a discipline may be defined in terms of the questions posed for it to answer. However its nature also depends on the extent to which it is passive in this process. This in turn depends on the extent to which epidemiologists are involved at a given interface, which is by necessity a two-way process. With respect to clinical practice, epidemiologists have a role in *informing* decision-making based on existing evidence, but also in *being informed* of the most pressing clinical questions for further research. The same considerations apply to policy-making bodies, but the clinical interface has traditionally been strongest since most health-related epidemiological research is led by clinicians. This is possibly particularly the case in psychiatry and may go some way towards explaining why influences of epidemiology on policy have historically been weak. The wholesale closure of long-stay psychiatric institutions illustrates the danger of neglecting this interface (a politically driven process with massive public health implications but with little or no attempt at epidemiological evaluation either before or during its implementation). Psychiatric morbidity accounts for a large proportion of any nation's health and social care costs. However 'mental health policy' has tended to focus on preventing rare *consequences* of psychiatric disorders, such as violence and suicide, rather than the disorders themselves. The future of psychiatric epidemiology will be strongly determined by the extent to which it improves its interface with policy making bodies. Other interfaces are important in this respect, in particular that with health economics as discussed at greater length in Chapter 19. It is, for example, increasingly expected that an intervention is described not only in its effects on a condition but with respect to its costs—placed in the context of the costs incurred by the condition in question.

...including the 'general public'

Perhaps more than any other, this interface requires a radical change in the way in which epidemiological research is carried out. Traditionally, communication between researchers and the public has been through intermediate agencies—principally clinicians and politicians. Directions for research have therefore been determined, and results disseminated, by people who felt they knew 'what was best' for the public. This situation has changed and will undoubtedly continue to change with increasing 'lay' involvement in research. This already includes powerful and vocal 'patient' or 'service user' groups (who are in general substantially more proficient at influencing policy than academics), as well as increasing lay representation on research funding bodies and research ethics committees, and an increasing public demand for (and access to) research evidence, particularly via the internet but also through the media (who form a distinct area of interface in their own right). A fundamental change for epidemiology has therefore been that research agendas are driven not only by governments and public health agencies but also directly by the 'public' themselves. Similarly the implications of research findings not only have to be interpreted for other academics, for policy making bodies and for clinicians but also, predominantly through national media, for the public. Two characteristics of epidemiological research present substantial challenges in this respect.

Challenge 1. Findings from single studies are rarely conclusive and 'truth' in epidemiology is attained through the gradual accumulation of evidence. However the traditional process for research publication involves the separate reporting of individual studies. Research journal editors are keen to gain lay publicity to increase the readership (and advertising revenue) of their periodicals. Results from single studies (including findings which are exploratory and not hypothesis-driven) may therefore receive exaggerated attention. Contradictory findings from other studies, or 'failures to replicate' despite being a frequent occurrence in epidemiology, add to the confusion. The end result is that a public health measure based on reasonable evidence will be poorly received because of a general belief that researchers will have changed their minds after a few years. The danger is also a gradual erosion of belief in an 'evidence base' and an increasingly eccentric application of research findings based purely on their attractiveness, novelty, and 'spin'.

Challenge 2. This concerns the individual significance of group-level findings. A difficulty faced by epidemiology is that an association between an exposure and outcome across a population is difficult to translate to the level of the individual because this involves a clear concept of probability and risk. A possible association between beef consumption and variant Creutzfeld–Jacob disease may, for example, be given equal or greater salience to that between dietary fat and myocardial infarction. Schizophrenia as a cause of violence often appears to be viewed as a more pressing concern than alcohol consumption. Poor risk assessment is of course by no means confined to politicians or the lay public (*viz.* rates of smoking by health professionals).

The meaningful interpretation of epidemiological findings will become increasingly important if attention shifts towards smaller and more complex genetic and environmental influences. At present the majority of the explanation is left to a few professionals who have links with the media and an apparently rare ability among academics to communicate with people outside their field. Given that publicity and 'fashion' have always influenced research funding (and therefore the direction of a field of research), and given that public involvement in research is unlikely to diminish, the ability to consolidate and interpret research findings will form an increasingly important aspect of epidemiology in the future.

...and the legal system

An excellent example of one of the challenges facing epidemiology in its relationship with lay bodies was described in a recent Lancet editorial (2002). A UK High Court judge was asked to rule on an action brought by seven women against three pharmaceutical companies, alleging that third-generation combined oral contraceptive pills had caused venous thromboembolism. The case illustrated two points. One was the stark divergence between what is legal and what is scientific proof. The legal standard is that the proposed cause–effect relationship should be 'more probable than not', that is, a relative risk of 2.0 or greater. There appears to be no clear guidance about what to do about sampling variability (e.g. is it the point estimate or the lowest 95% interval which has to be above 2?) and no clear reason why a relative risk of 2.01 should be distinguished from one of 1.99. Six published studies were considered. The judge put his weight behind one industry funded study showing a relative risk below 1.0 and the plaintiffs lost their case. The second 'message' was the clear impatience of the judge with disagreeing experts. It represents a salutory lesson for epidemiologists that rigorous scientific debate and musing is poorly tolerated by those who rely on research for answers. The proceedings appear to make a frank mockery of Bradford Hill's 'verdict of causation'. A verdict was required from the scientific community. This was not forthcoming, leaving nothing but a distinctly un-scientific alternative.

Within epidemiology

The future shape of psychiatric epidemiology will be determined not only by its interfaces with other agencies and scientific disciplines, but also by important inter-relationships within the specialty itself. An important feature will be the extent to which diverse influences can be integrated. For example, to what extent can biological pathways (e.g. neuroendocrine changes) explain an association between factors arising from the social environment (e.g. adverse life events) and risk of psychiatric morbidity? The development of individual interfaces is likely to involve increasing specialization which has implications for the coherence of the discipline. In the first part of this chapter, it has been suggested that psychiatric epidemiology may benefit by taking its own direction as a sub-specialty and by cutting links to an extent with generalism in the main specialty. The next question is whether generalists can continue to exist even within psychiatric epidemiology if they are to keep up with emerging neuroimaging technology and rapid genetic advances, while maintaining links with social science, public health specialists, policy makers, and health economists.

Within medicine

The tradition of western medicine has been to compartmentalise diseases (and those who treat them) according to the organ or physiological system predominantly affected. While this may (or may not) have benefits at a service level, it has important implications for epidemiology since clinicians and clinical concerns strongly influence research directions. Themes for epidemiological research are determined by both the experience and inexperience of its researchers. Psychiatric epidemiology has been affected particularly in this respect since relatively few physicians have had substantial psychiatric experience, and the general medical experience of psychiatrists is also limited. There has also been a prevailing Cartesian paradigm in medicine of mind and body as separate. The interface between psychiatry and general medicine is an important future consideration since it is, for these reasons, poorly conceptualised, despite ample evidence for highly interdependent processes:

(a) Somatic disease is important in the aetiology of psychiatric morbidity (e.g. general physical health and risk for depression, cerebrovascular disease, and dementia).

(b) Somatic symptoms are a common presentation of psychiatric morbidity.

(c) Somatic disease may have a psychiatric presentation.

(d) Psychological factors are important in the aetiology, course and prognosis of somatic disease (e.g. depression and cardiovascular disease).

(e) Psychological factors influence other aetiological factors for somatic disease (e.g. smoking, diet, and alcohol consumption).

(f) Somatic and psychiatric disorders may share common aetiological factors both genetic (e.g. APOE genotype in Alzheimer's and cardiovascular diseases) and environmental (e.g. socio-economic status).

(g) Somatic and psychiatric disorders may share common outcomes (e.g. effects on disablement, quality of life, mortality).

Given the complex nature of these processes, the term 'comorbidity' to describe the co-occurrence of disorders is highly over-simplistic since it implies parallel and independent processes. Future directions in psychiatric epidemiology will depend on its relationship with other areas of epidemiological investigation. Disentangling the complex inter-relationship between somatic and psychological health demands inter-disciplinary research:

(a) to inform the design of the study—with respect to expertise in the background literature but also, in particular, with respect to differing perspectives on the research question;

(b) to develop appropriate measurements for each 'axis' of morbidity;

(c) to consider the clinical implications of results for both specialties;

(d) of necessity where the disorder treated by one specialty occurs principally in the service context of another (e.g. puerperal psychiatric disorders).

The neglect of this interface may have important public health implications. Psychiatric morbidity is recognized to be commonly associated with somatic disease, influences its presentation and prognosis and yet is poorly identified and treated in primary and secondary care settings with potentially substantial financial consequences for health services. The problem is not confined to health service issues but also extends into epidemiological research. Cerebrovascular disease has been assumed to be an important cause of dementia for approximately three decades but has received little research attention until recently. This may partly arise through ageism and therapeutic nihilism, potent factors in determining research directions, but it may also have arisen because 'vascular dementia' falls between traditional medical specialties.

Within psychiatry

Compartmentalization of course also occurs within psychiatry and, again because of the influence of clinicians, is important in determining the nature of epidemiological research. The most prominent interface for most service settings is that between childhood and adulthood. Life-course influences on disease aetiology are likely to be as prominent a theme for psychiatric as for

general epidemiology. The childhood environment is recognised to be important in the aetiology of later psychiatric disease. Psychiatric disorders in childhood may or may not lead to morbidity later in life. The developing
personality has important influences both on the risk of later morbidity and
on the way it is expressed. The childhood–adulthood interface however not
only involves a complex transition of symptoms, but also of the way in which
syndromes are conceptualised (e.g. from conduct disorder to antisocial personality disorder), the types of disorder seen (e.g. hyperkinesis, schizophrenia), the
treatment indicated (e.g. family therapy for anorexia nervosa in adolescence,
against individual cognitive behavioural therapy in adults) and the nature of
the service context. Other areas of compartmentalization also affect the nature
of research which is carried out. Situations where older people are treated by
different research teams, or where people with dementia are treated outside
psychiatry, may lead to similar interfaces. Many research studies impose an
upper age cut-off of 65 with little justification (since dementia incidence does
not start to increase till 5–10 years later), except that it is the age of retirement
in some countries and the age of secondary care service transition in others.
Studies of schizophrenia in later life (whether of early or late onset) are far
outweighed in number by those in early adulthood. A challenge for psychiatric
epidemiology is to move across boundaries between age-groups and individual clinical contexts. This will be particularly important as clinical practice
continues to move towards greater sub-specialization.

New horizons

Substantial challenges for psychiatric epidemiology therefore include the need
to develop methodologies which are adequate for its research questions, and
the need to develop interfaces with agencies posing these questions. The
future nature of psychiatric epidemiology will be shaped to a large part by
these issues. It will also naturally be influenced by entirely new external
developments. While these are to a large extent unforeseeable, the past and
present provide some clues as to the likely future.

New research environments

A lot has changed since the days when an epidemiologist could carry out a
survey, expecting at least 90% response rates with sufficient persuasion and an
assumption by participants that whatever information was gathered was their
duty to provide because it would be used by the research team for the greater
good. Survey response rates have declined gradually but consistently over at least
two to three decades, at least in developed countries. Consent procedures have

moved from being implied by participation to complex considerations concerning the amount of information which can reasonably be transferred and the extent to which consent can ever truly be fully 'informed'. Feedback of survey information is an important consideration now that a large amount is derived from blood tests and other procedures, yielding findings which may or may not have clinical implications (and the dividing line is frequently unclear). There are also important conflicts between allowing participants access to information held on them, sanctioned by principles of data protection, but denying the same access to insurance companies. Bioethics is an influential context in which research is carried out and is likely to grow in importance. From being principally concerned with the issue of informed consent, ethical considerations have gathered a steadily increasing sphere of influence, now involving the nature of the research question itself (e.g. should research be carried out into genetic factors underlying human behaviour?). While there are important bodies now set up to consider these issues (see Chapter 4), the framework is currently inadequate with many complex decisions left to the variable opinions of local committees.

New populations

Like many other research disciplines psychiatric epidemiology has, to date, principally addressed the concerns of the richest nations. As well as unfairly ignoring the majority of people suffering from mental illness throughout the world, this has led to an impoverishment in epidemiological models of aetiology and intervention. Even within developed nations, community studies have tended to have a relatively restricted focus. For example, studies of socioeconomic influences on mental health have tended to focus on urban deprivation, ignoring poverty in rural settings. Diagnostic systems and interventional research are also still strongly influenced by secondary rather than primary care experience. The issue of within- and between-population risk factor variability has been discussed earlier, and it is likely that substantial progress will be made in understanding the aetiology of many disorders through research initiated outside somewhat stereotyped 'Western' environments. As discussed in Chapter 3 cross-cultural research also generates important challenges, as yet largely unfaced, to traditionally held views of disease definition. A crucial issue with geographic expansion in epidemiological research will be the extent to which it addresses the needs of developing nations and builds local research expertise rather than serving the interests of developed nation investigators and funding bodies.

New exposures

Psychiatric epidemiology is a young specialty in a rapidly changing environment. A major test of its worth will lie in its ability to keep pace with these changes and influence the way in which they are evaluated. Many new 'exposures' have been alluded to under previous headings. The mapping of the human genome has generated a virtually limitless number of influences to be evaluated, although with little in the way of adequate methodology to do this. Advances in proteomics and their application in population based research will fuel expectations further. Life-course epidemiology may lead not only to new exposures but also to new ways of modelling the causal influences of existing ones. The expansion of epidemiological research towards a more global focus, as discussed in the previous section, will undoubtedly lead to new concepts of disease causation as well as to an expansion in the variety of health services and systems requiring evaluation. Research into 'upstream' factors, particularly those operating at a population-level will also be influenced substantially if psychiatric epidemiology broadens its focus. This process might include expanded research into mental health influences of social milieu, culture, housing and architecture, income distribution, political systems, or even (with the growing influence of media and mass communication) national and international events. There is also a pressing need to evaluate factors of particular relevance to many developing nations such as military conflict and internal migration. A final important 'exposure' for psychiatric epidemiology which has received relatively little investigation to date is *time*. Temporal trends in disease frequency are of vital importance for policy makers and can also provide valuable information with respect to disease aetiology. The relative youth of psychiatric epidemiology has meant that disease trends have been difficult to measure and that time periods have been limited. Improved disease classification systems and replicable survey procedures potentially increase the opportunities for research in this area.

New outcomes

Of all future directions for psychiatric epidemiology, new outcomes are perhaps the hardest to predict. One important feature of epidemiology in the future may be an increasingly blurred distinction between 'exposure' and 'outcome'. Biomedical research is likely to lead increasingly towards 'intermediate' disease states which can be treated either way around. White matter lesions on magnetic resonance imaging (MRI) are a good example of this, both being investigated as risk factors (for dementia) and as outcomes (e.g. with respect to hypertension or diabetes). MRI is also a good example of biotechnology which is being increasingly used in an epidemiological context. Structural imaging has been of less interest in other areas of psychiatry. However it is not inconceivable that some forms of functional neuroimaging will begin to be used in epidemiological studies of affective and psychotic disorders in earlier life, with similarly ambiguous exposure/outcome status. Another reasonable bet for the future will be that outcome definitions will have changed. Diagnostic concepts have changed throughout the history of psychiatry and there is no reason why they will not continue to do so. A trend in functional neuroimaging research has been to investigate symptoms rather than syndromes. The same process may take hold in epidemiology with studies increasingly investigating, for example, the aetiology of auditary hallucinations rather than schizophrenia. 'Outcomes' will also be detemined by the agency initiating the research question, for example, the growing need by policy makers for health economic analyses, costing the impact of a given disorder or intervention. Least predictably of all, outcomes in psychiatric research may vary according to changes in social, cultural, and political environments. The existence of apparently 'culture-specific' manifestations of psychological morbidity is proof of this. The 'youth' of psychiatric epidemiology creates difficulties in estimating to what extent disorders such as anorexia nervosa or chronic fatigue syndrome are 'new' rather than previously unrecognised. If anorexia nervosa has arisen as a disorder because of cultural changes in attitudes to body image, it is likely that other unforseen 'diagnoses' will arise in the future. As in many areas, the place of psychiatric epidemiology in future research will depend on the extent to which it remains unblinkered by its past.

References

Lancet editorial (2002) Epidemiology on trial. *Lancet*, **360**, 421.

Pearce, N. (1996) Traditional epidemiology, Modern Epidemiology and Public Health. *American Journal of Public Health*, **86**, 678–83.

Rose, G. (1985) Sick individuals and sick populations. *International Journal of Epidemiology*, **14**, 32–8.

Susser, M. and Susser, E. (1996) Choosing a future for epidemiology. II. From black box to Chinese boxes and eco-epidemiology. *American Journal of Public Health*, **86**, 674–7.

Thomas, P., Romme, M., and Hamelijnck, J. (1996) Psychiatry and the politics of the underclass. *British Journal of Psychiatry*, **169**, 401–4.

Index